Tàijíquán 太极拳

by Li Deyin

Singing Dragon
London and Philadelphia

First published in the United Kingdom and the United States of America in 2008 by
Singing Dragon
An imprint of Jessica Kingsley Publishers
116 Pentonville Road
London N1 9JB, UK

Jessica Kingsley *Publishers* Inc.
400 Market Street
Suite 400
Philadelphia
PA 19106, USA

www.jkp.com

First published in the People's Republic of China in 2004 by Foreign Languages Press
24 Baiwanzhuang Road, Beijing 100037, China, flp.com.cn

British Library Cataloguing in Publication Data
A CIP catalogue record for this book is available from the British Library

ISBN: 978 1 84819 004 7

Text by Li Deyin
Translated by Yu Ling, Zhang Shaoning, Wang Qin, Ouyang Weiping, Yan Jing

Edited by Sara Grimes

Demonstrated by
Li Yulin — 81-Step Taijiquan
Li Tianji — 24-Step Taijiquan
Li Deyin — 42-Step Taijiquan
Li Defang — 42-Step Taiji Sword
Faye Yip — 32-Step Taiji Sword

All photographs courtesy of Li Deyin.

Cover designed by Cai Rong. The background photograph shows part of a 10,000-person Taijiquan demonstration in Tian'anmen Square in 1998. The Chinese calligraphy "Taijiquan" on the cover is that of Deng Xiaoping from his inscription "Taijiquan is wonderful," written by the late Chinese leader in 1978.

Disclaimer
This book is for reference and informational purposes only and is in no way intended as medical counseling or medical advice. The information contained herein should not be used to treat, diagnose or prevent any disease or medical condition without the advice of a competent medical professional. The activities, physical or otherwise, described herein for informational purposes, may be too strenuous or dangerous for some people and the reader should consult a physician before engaging in them. The author and Singing Dragon shall have neither liability nor responsibility to any person or entity with respect to any loss, damage, or injury caused or alleged to be caused directly or indirectly by the information contained in this book.

Printed and bound in Great Britain by
Athenaeum Press, Gateshead, Tyne and Wear

This book commemorates our family's devoted journey
of over 100 years to the Martial Arts

And is dedicated to

My grandfather, Li Yulin (1885-1965)
Northeast China Pioneer of Taijiquan

And

My uncle, Li Tianji (1914-1996)
One of China's Top 10 National Martial Arts Masters

CONTENTS

FOREWORD

Taijiquan is a traditional Chinese martial art and a Chinese national treasure. It integrates the physical external and the meditative internal. It is one of the few sports that improves balance, coordination, flexibility, muscle strength, and cardiovascular health. It is gentle enough to be accessible to the elderly and infirm, yet demanding enough to pose a significant challenge to the most professional young athlete. Taijiquan is beneficial to people of all ages and all lifestyles.

But prior to 1988, there was no standard for Taijiquan. It was passed on master-to-student, changing and evolving with time and generation. Everybody practiced Taiji differently.

In international competition, this created a dilemma. How were judges to score Taiji routines that could be as different as pineapples and bananas? A standard was needed.

The 42-Step Taijiquan was created to be that standard. It is a combination-routine of the best of four traditional Taiji styles — the "silk reeling power" of the Chen, the graceful strength of the Yang, the exquisite subtleties of the Wu, and the flexible agility of the Sun — plus eight-hand and five-foot techniques from Push Hands. It was choreographed with harmony and beauty in mind, and a high degree of technical difficulty in practice; competitors must display a broad range of knowledge and skills in order to perform 42-Step well. It is a symphony of motion.

In 1990, China hosted the 11th Asian Games. It was then that they announced 42-Step Taijiquan Competition Routine as the first ever universally standardized Taiji competition routine. This began a new chapter in the history of Chinese martial arts, and the primary author is a man I am lucky enough to call my *shifu* (master): Professor Li Deyin.

Li Deyin is the third generation of famous masters from the Li family. His grandfather Li Yulin, who earned the honorary title "Pioneer of Taijiquan" in Northeastern China, served as president of the Shanghai Shangde Wushu Institute, head coach of the Shandong Wushu Institute, and publisher of the Harbin Taijiquan Press. Professor Li Deyin's father Li Tianchi became a doctor who integrated wushu (martial arts), medical science, and *tui na* (massage). Professor Li's uncle Li Tianji studied wushu with his father, Li Yulin, as well as his father's masters, Sun Lutang and Li Jinglin. Li Tianji graduated from the Shandong Wushu Institute, became a college professor, the head of the Harbin Wushu Federation, and the first head coach of the China Wushu Team. In 1956 Li Tianji created the first standardized Taijiquan forms in Chinese history: the Simplified 24-Step Taijiquan and Simplified 32-Form Taiji Sword. Both forms opened the door of Taiji to novices and nonathletes, and both are now extremely popular all over the world. For this, Li Tianji — honored as one of the "Top 10 Wushu Masters of China" (Zhongguo Shi Da Wushu Mingshi) — also is known as the "Father of Contemporary Taijiquan."

Born in 1938 in Hebei Province, Li Deyin was raised in a culture of wushu and began training when he was eight years old with his grandfather, Li Yulin, under intense training for 12 years that left Li Deyin accustomed to perfection in wushu. As an adult, wushu took him to all different regions and masters in China. He traveled to Shaolin Temple and Mount Wudang to study from advanced abbots; he sought out Master Li Jingwu to learn Chen style Taijiquan, Master Xu Zhiyi to learn Wu style, Master Sun Jianyun to learn Sun style, and Master Hao Jiajun to learn Yang style and Push Hands.

When Li Deyin entered Renmin University in Beijing, his original idea of becoming an economist was eclipsed by his interest in sports, especially Taiji although not much collegiate-level competition was available at the time. Immediately after Li Deyin graduated, Renmin University hired him as one of their youngest professors ever. Thanks to his continued efforts, Taijiquan has become an accredited course at all Chinese universities, and 24-Step Taijiquan has become a required class for physical education majors. Taijiquan has become one of the most popular Chinese university sports.

There is a difference between Taiji for competition and Taiji for health, notes Li Deyin. The former should be strictly accurate according to accepted choreography and held to rigorous standards of strength, flexibility, fluidity, and stability. The latter can be practiced in any style or sub-style of Taiji, performed at any level of physical prowess, and should be given only encouragement. The purpose of competitive Taiji is perfection; otherwise, Taiji is for health and enjoyment.

To make Taijiquan more enjoyable and accessible, Li Deyin had music composed for 24-Step Taijiquan and 32-Form Taiji Sword. He also has rewritten many Taiji books and, at the invitation of video and television producers, made a significant number of instructional videos and television programs. Numerous articles have been written about Li Deyin's contributions and achievements in China and many other countries, especially Japan.

People seek out Li Deyin's materials. His style is simple and profound, accessible to the average person and indispensable to the professional athlete. His instructions are guaranteed to be excellent: he has broken down every stance, form, and transition into clear, distinct movements. He gives precise directions, applicable explanations, and perfect visual examples. His teaching is honest, direct, and very efficient. He addresses real problems encountered in practice and performance, both stylistically and specifically. The way he performs and teaches Taiji is guaranteed to be correct in the eyes of all judges. More importantly, he is one of few who are able to express the passion and strength beneath Taiji's soft veneer.

During my training with Professor Li, he explained the difference between a good and an outstanding Taiji performance. A good Taiji performance demonstrates a high level of flexibility, balance, and fluidity — it should be very elegant. In addition to that elegance, an outstanding Taiji performance will express the internal strengths of *jing*, *qi*, and *shen* (strength, vitality, and spirit). "Taiji without *jing*, *qi*, and *shen* is like reciting a beautiful poem without rhythm or emotion," he told me. "It is beautiful, but still lacking in something important, and elusive."

For the sake of unity and competition, it is good to have standards and requirements. Li Deyin and a wushu committee created, edited and standardized all Taijiquan competition routines, including the 88-form, Yang, Chen, Wu, and Sun styles and Wu Dang Taiji Sword. Among all contemporary and traditional Taiji routines, competition routines are widely considered the best because they include the most important elements of their respective styles with a minimum of repetition.

By 1976, the rapid growth of popular and competitive Taiji demanded a comprehensive routine that would embody all the different styles. The 48-Step Taijiquan was Li Deyin's first attempt at a comprehensive Taiji routine. Working with a committee of Taiji masters, he created this form as a combination of the four major styles plus elements of Push Hands. Though 48-Step Taijiquan did not become the international standard for competitive Taijiquan, it is a beautiful form that has become very popular throughout the world.

In 1989, a committee of great Taiji masters, foremost among whom was Professor Li Deyin, choreographed 42-Step Taijiquan Competition Routine. This routine is stronger, more beautiful, and shorter than 48-Step, which makes it altogether much more appropriate for international competition. The next year, the International Wushu Federation announced 42-Step Taijiquan Competition Routine as the first ever universally standardized Taijiquan competition routine, and the official Taiji competition routine of the 11th Asian Games. Today, 42-Step Taijiquan is still considered the most complete standard by which a Taiji competitor can be judged, as well as one of the most beautiful Taiji forms in existence.

As vice president of the Chinese Wushu Association, Li Deyin holds responsibility for many important events. Li Deyin has established over 200 Taijiquan learning centers in Beijing. In the past 20 years, he has trained thousands of volunteer Taijiquan coordinators and teachers. With the support of his many friends and peers, Li Deyin has organized Taijiquan tournaments all over China. He coordinated a magnificent 10,000-person performance of 24-Step Taijiquan in Tian'anmen Square. For the opening ceremony of 11th Asian Games, Li Deyin organized and led 1,500 Chinese and Japanese practitioners in a performance of 24-Step Taijiquan, the first time that people of these two nations performed together in such a large venue.

Professor Li Deyin has earned numerous titles and awards, among them "International Wushu Judge" and "China's Best Judge." At the 11th Asian Games, Professor Li Deyin was the chief judge. He has trained many judges in classes set up by the International Wushu Federation, and given numerous lectures all over the world explaining the rules, requirements, and standards of Taijiquan competition.

In 1975, Li Deyin collaborated with other Taiji instructors and opened the first international recreational Taiji center in China when classes were established in Beijing for foreign residents who were studying or who worked in China. In just two years, over 600 people from 50 countries participated in Taiji classes, including Barbara Bush whose husband George Bush (40th President of the United States) served from 1974 to 1976 as the top diplomat to the People's Republic of China as head of the U.S. Liaison Office.

But since not everybody can go to China to study Taiji, Li Deyin has traveled nearly everywhere to teach Taiji, including Taiwan, Hong Kong, Macao, Japan, England, the United States, Sweden, and Switzerland.

When the door of China was opened to the world in 1981, Li Deyin, representing the city of Beijing, made his first trip to Japan to teach Taijiquan. Since then, Li Deyin has made special teaching trips to Japan every year for the last 20 years. Over 100,000 Japanese have studied with Li Deyin. Every Taiji practitioner in Japan knows his name. In 1982, on his tour of Beijing, the Japanese Prime Minister Suzuki Yoshiyuki made a special appointment with Li Deyin for a Taijiquan lesson in his hotel room, squeezed into his busy schedule.

Li Deyin first taught in England in 1989, and now his daughter, Faye Yip (Li Hui), has become the fourth generation of her family to teach Taijiquan as the founder of the Deyin Taijiquan Institute in England.

Many of Li Deyin's students have become great Taiji instructors and judges. World renowned Chinese athletes Gao Jiamin, Chen Sitan, Su Zifang, Huo Dongli, Wang Erping, Kong Xiangdong, Fan Xueping, Su Renfeng, and Zhou Yunjian all call Li Deyin their *shifu*. In England, British athlete Simon Watson has won the Taiji grand championship in England and in Europe. Japanese athlete Morita Hisako began as a housewife interested in Taijiquan; under the tutelage of Professor Li Deyin, she won the Japan and Asian Wushu Competition championship.

In my home city of San Diego in the United States live two grateful students of Li Deyin: Cao Fengshan, a Beijing Collegiate gold-medalist, and myself. I have won numerous championships and medals in the USA and in China. The USA Wushu Kungfu Federation awarded me the title "Internal (Taiji) Athlete of the Year" for the year 2000. I attribute my successes to my masters, especially Professor Li Deyin. He teaches wholeheartedly and tirelessly, with amazingly sharp eyes and clear judgment. He truly is the best Taiji coach in the world.

——Siu-Fong Evans

Based on article published by Kung Fu Magazine.com

CHAPTER I
TAIJIQUAN IN CHINA TODAY

A Popular Tradition

People from other countries who visit China are often impressed — both touched and puzzled — by the Chinese enthusiasm for early morning exercise, especially Taijiquan that has been one of the most popular forms of morning exercises in China for ages.

Chinese have been "getting up at the crack of dawn to practice with the sword," as the old saying goes, since ancient times. The story behind the saying can be traced to Zu Di, a Jin Dynasty (265-420) general who from childhood dreamed of doing great things for his country on the battlefield. This ambition inspired him as a youth to get up early on hearing the crow of a rooster and wake up his friends to go practice unarmed combat and sword techniques every morning. Later when the State of Jin was forced to retreat down to the south of the Yangtze River after being invaded by a foreign state, General Zu Di led the Jin army across the Yangtze to recover a large area of lost territory. Stories about Zu Di's exploits have inspired Chinese youth over the generations to dedicate themselves to hard study and training in the service of their country. The stories also helped establish a tradition of practicing the martial arts early in the morning to keep fit.

In Beijing parks in the downtown area like Tiantan Park, Zhongshan Park, and Dongdan Park, people can be seen everywhere doing morning exercises of various kinds. But the most eye-catching are those people wholly concentrated in practicing Taijiquan. Their slow steps and gentle movements seem to carry them to a world above the mortal life, seeing and hearing nothing around them. Only when the exercises are over do they return to the busy life of this world. Many ride bicycles or get on a bus to get back to their work.

The first regular bus to Fragrant Hills, a scenic region in the western suburbs of Beijing about 15 miles from the downtown area, is always crowded with people going to the mountains to do morning exercises. So popular is this activity that the bus company had to add extra buses and open a special line to the Fragrant Hills. Once I went there, too, invited by a friend. Half way up the mountain, I was out of breath but my Taiji friend said that they had yet to start their morning exercises. They practice Taijiquan here everyday for half an hour before going back down the mountain.

On my campus of Renmin University in northwest Beijing, many teachers and students make it a point to take time in the morning to do three things before going to class: Morning exercises, morning reading and breakfast. As an old Chinese proverb goes:

"The plan of the year starts in spring; the plan of the day begins in the morning."

My colleague Wu Qiantao, a professor at the Philosophy Department at Renmin University, offers an example of the many who make it a point to arrange their morning fully in good order. In addition to teaching, his responsibilities include supervising students writing doctoral dissertations and directing the work of the university's information office. Since he has to receive many visitors during the day, he often works until midnight. But still, he never changes his habit of getting up at six every morning to practice Taijiquan, taking a shower at seven, and having breakfast before going to work at eight. It is hard to see how his slow movements in Taijiquan connect with his busy work schedule, yet he says: "No matter how busy I am, I do 30 minutes of Taijiquan in the morning. Otherwise, I don't have the energy and spirit for the whole day."

A Taiji friend who practices in a park early in the morning once told me in a good-natured way:

"People who come fall into three types: The first to arrive like us treasure life and crave good health. After we leave, the second batch includes tourists who come to appreciate the scenery and flowers. They enjoy life and have good health. The third batch that comes in the evening is pairs of lovers. They create life but neglect their health."

Beyond being an important recreational and sports activity, Taijiquan permeates Chinese culture. For instance, in China a friend might ask about someone: "Is he a hot-headed, outspoken person or does he have a Taijiquan temper?" Which means — Is he quick to anger or does he have an even disposition? Also, you might hear: "Don't play Taijiquan with me. Please come straight to the point." This means that the speaker wants you to speak directly and frankly, not in a roundabout way. So to thoroughly understand the life of the Chinese people, one has to understand Taijiquan.

Taijiquan Coaching Centers in Beijing

How many people today are practicing Taijiquan in China? It is hard to tell because of all the ways available: Martial arts schools, individual instruction, public classes organized by the community and the Martial Arts Association, leisure staff activities organized by the trade unions in businesses and factories, organized professional activities in schools, hospitals, and clubs — as well as in all the small self-organized groups and with individuals who practice on their own. At the same time, this very number and variety of ways indicates how popular Taijiquan is today and how easy it is for anyone to learn and practice it in China.

For example, in Beijing some 200 Taijiquan coaching centers have been established by the sports and recreation departments at the district level under the city government as well as the Beijing Martial Arts Association in the parks, neighborhoods and squares where people gather to practice Taijiquan in the morning. While helping to popularize Taijiquan as a sport, these Taijiquan centers have played a significant role in helping people keep fit and enriching the cultural life of the community.

The head of each center is a respected person from the community elected by its members while the instructors are volunteers certified by the Beijing Martial Arts Association, which holds regular technical training and examinations for instructors who are awarded state-authorized certificates as community sports instructors. These public Taijiquan coaching centers offer regular classes and activities year round to the general public at little or no cost. People participating are mostly local residents, including both white- and blue-collar workers. They can join and leave as they like. With no requirement as to a basic skill level, people can choose whatever activities and levels they like among the programs offered by the center. The Haidian District in Beijing where I live has some 51 Taijiquan coaching centers with 3,200 registered members and 356 instructors. In one recent year alone, the centers held 606 short training classes, from which 14,900 trainees graduated.

One of the most successful coaching centers in Beijing is the Beijing Zhongguancun Taijiquan Coaching Center located in the Zhongguancun area of Beijing's Haidian District, an area known for its high concentration of cultural and educational institutions such as Peking University, Tsinghua University, Renmin University and the Chinese Academy of Sciences. Also known as the Martial Arts Association of the Chinese Academy of Science, Zhongguancun Taijiquan Coaching Center has grown to include some 700 members and 50 instructors since its founding in 1975 at the end of the unprecedented disaster of the "cultural revolution" when Deng Xiaoping took charge of state affairs and embarked on arduous "rectification work," calling on the nation to "respect talented people and respect knowledge."

At that time, a general physical check-up showed that many of the 650 researchers at the Institute of Mechanics of the Chinese Academy of Sciences were in poor health. In a research department of 32 people, for instance, seven were suffering from hepatitis, four from cancer, and still others, from arthritis as well as heart disease and throat problems. These people mainly were key researchers in their 40s and 50s. Obviously, many gifted people would die young unless they received better health care and physical conditioning. Under these circumstances, the Zhongguancun Taijiquan Coaching Center was founded.

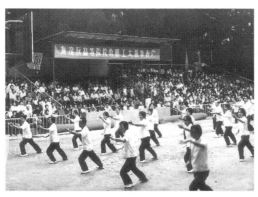

Faculty members at Renmin University perform Taijiquan at a gathering at the university in Beijing's in Haidian District, 1962.

At first, the Zhongguancun Taijiquan Coaching Center attracted only a few Taijiquan practitioners who gathered for exercise on the playground of a primary school. Among them was Cao Yimin, an architect who became a Taijiquan devotee during his recovery from a bout of hepatitis 10 years earlier. Gradually, as more people joined and the group got support from the Trade Union of the Chinese Academy of Sciences as well as the Sports Association of Haidian District, Zhongguancun area saw a wave of popularity for Taijiquan. In this "city of science" of some 100,000 people, the Taijiquan Coaching Center over the past 20 years has trained over 40,000 Taijiquan practitioners.

Many of these people have testified to a marked improvement in the health through Taijiquan. For instance, Bian Yingui, a senior researcher who studied in the United States, credits Taijiquan with helping improve a heart condition. He also is grateful for having formed the good habit of getting up early in the morning and for not getting cold so easily in winter. He tells people, "After doing Taijiquan in the morning, I don't feel tired even if I get very busy."

And Ms. He Weilang, an instructor at the center and a researcher in the Institute of Mechanics of the Academy, once told me:

"I used to be very weak. When I began to learn Taijiquan, I felt dizzy even after a few movements and had to take a rest against a tree. Now I can do three to four forms of Taijiquan continuously without feeling tired. Two years ago, I had a major five-hour operation on the abdomen. But I recovered quickly and could work normally after three months."

Today my old friend Cao Yimin, now 74-years-old and chairman of the Martial Arts Association of the Chinese Academy of Sciences, can look at many stellar accomplishments of the Zhongguancun Center. Zhongguancun Center's contingent of 300 people led the 10,000-person Taijiquan demonstration in Tian'anmen Square in 1988 for the 10th anniversary of Deng Xiaoping's 1978 inscription "Taijiquan is Wonderful;" a thesis entitled "Scientific Research on Physical Fitness and the Movements of Taijiquan" won first prize at the National Conference on the Scientific Research of Martial Arts; and in recent years several athletes from the center have medalled at the National Taijiquan Competition.

Government Support

Since the founding of the People's Republic of China in 1949, Taijiquan has received support from the highest levels of the Chinese government. In June 1952, Mao Zedong, chairman of the Central People's Government, issued a call to "encourage all people who can to engage in exercises, ball games, running, mountain climbing, swimming and practicing Taijiquan." In 1978, Chinese Vice Premier Deng Xiaoping inscribed in his calligraphy the Chinese characters: "Taijiquan is wonderful" (太极拳好). With the support of national leaders, Taijiquan thrived even in the early years of the People's Republic of China as well as in the difficult years after the "cultural revolution." The State Martial Arts Administration established a ranking system with corresponding instructional materials for evaluation of different levels of the martial arts. The month of May was set as National Martial Arts Health month, a time during which Taijiquan is taught free to the public nationwide in China with celebrations and activities that have attracted thousands of amateur Taijiquan practitioners. Since 1959, the martial arts — including Taijiquan — have been included as a formal event in China's top national sports meet, held every four years where the martial arts events until today are the only ones not included in the venue of the Olympic Games.

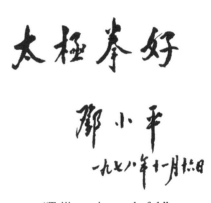

"Taijiquan is wonderful."
Deng Xiaoping
1978

Among all these activities, Taijiquan competition has received the most attention, without a doubt. Throughout martial arts history, contests have been held to compare the "gongfu" or prowess of competitors that have allowed the most powerful competitor — the champion — to appear. Contests in Taijiquan also have been conducted through push-hands between two competitors, with the more skillful regarded as the winner. Following the listing of Taijiquan as a recognized national sport in China, competition in Taijiquan came to include, in addition to push-hands, the many forms or set routines of Taijiquan.

At first, judges gave on-the-spot evaluations and accorded marks according to the display of individual skills. However, because traditional Taijiquan routines are rather long — an average of 80-100 routine movements with many repetitions — it takes at least 20 minutes to finish one form. This was hardly acceptable to the audience or event organizers of modern-day sports competitions. Besides, it is difficult to make a judgment about traditional Taijiquan because of the differences in standards and ways of practice among different regions, schools and masters. So to make Taijiquan suitable as a spectator sport, the rules for Taijiquan competition had to change — and they have gone through several revisions.

In the 1960s and 1970s, specific rules were established for Taijiquan competition. A time limit was set at five or six minutes for each Taijiquan routine. Athletes could choose their own routines for competition, but the routine had to include four different kicks and six movements from different categories of movements. The rules included specific guidelines on technical requirements as well as movement categories. Meanwhile, five standards were set for evaluation of different competition routines selected by athletes themselves.

In the 1990s, the Chinese Martial Arts Association established competition guidelines for the five major schools of Taijiquan — Chen-style, Yang-style, Wu (吴)-style, Sun-style, and Wu (武)-style Taijiquan, as well as for the combined-form of 42-step Taijiquan and Taiji sword, that provided standardized forms to make Taijiquan more suitable for competition.

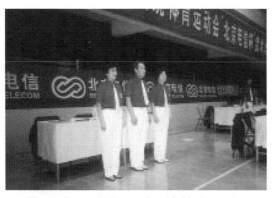

The author (middle) as the chief judge at the National Martial Arts Competition at Beijing Olympic Sports Center in 1999.

In the 21st century, more specific scoring system rules have been added related to quality and degree of difficulty, improving Taijiquan sports competition by encouraging performances that are both more elegant and up to date. The rules stipulate that judges must take into account these three aspects in their scoring: Quality of movement, performance ability and technical difficulty. These rules have made Taijiquan competition more exciting, focused and accurate.

Taijiquan competition today in China can be divided into three kinds: Optional routines, compulsory routines, and routines that can have extra credit according to the levels of technical difficulties.

Among the myriad of competition routines, one stands out — Simplified or 24-Step Taijiquan. (See Chapter VI) It appears everywhere, from grass roots competitions to national Taijiquan conferences and competitions — even at the Annual International Taijiquan Convention and Competition held in Wenxian County in Henan Province, the birthplace of traditional Taijiquan. Why has the modern 24-Step Taijiquan, one small flower in the garden of Taijiquan, attracted so much care and attention?

Not long after Mao Zedong issued a proclamation to promote physical education, a national meet featuring Chinese sports was held where Taijiquan appeared at a national sports meet for the first time in the history of the People's Republic of China. During that gathering, Marshal He Long, director of the State Physical Culture and Sports Commission, urged extensive research into the traditional martial arts to make them more scientific with the hope that the martial arts might become a modern-day sport and as such play a bigger role in the physical fitness of the nation.

In response to this significant challenge, Taijiquan lead the way. In 1956, a group of Taijiquan experts organized by the State Physical Culture and Sports Commission created the Simplified 24-Step Taijiquan based on Yang-style Taijiquan, making a complicated form simple and concise, and removing repetitions. The 24-Step Taijiquan then became the first set of martial arts material published by the national government. It was an epoch-making event. From that moment, martial arts in China went beyond the bounds of the traditional way of teaching passed on by word of mouth from master to disciples. Instead, Taijiquan entered into schools, factories, hospitals and the daily life of the ordinary people — truly carrying Taijiquan forward into modern times.

This was not welcomed in some conservative and sectarian martial arts circles where the new form was criticized as "departing from tradition" or for "losing the nobility of tradition." However, Simplified 24-Step Taijiquan in fact neither changed the traditional ways of practice, nor did it lower the standards of Taijiquan. What it did do was provide a step for beginners to enter the door, leading many to continue to probe ever deeper as they constantly worked to improve their Taijiquan techniques. Many life-long followers of Taijiquan first began to know and love Taijiquan through the 24-Step form.

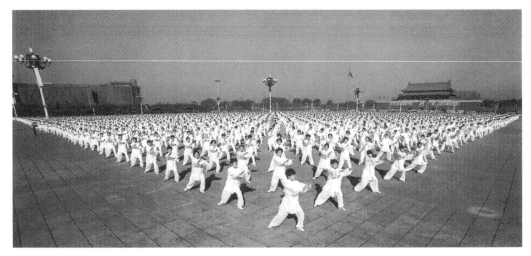

A 10,000-person performance of 24-Step Taijiquan in Tiananmen Square, Beijing in 1998.

Today 24-Step Taijiquan has answered all its critics by becoming the most popular form of Taijiquan in China, and the world. Both Beijing and Shanghai have held 10,000-people performances of 24-Step Taijiquan. It is among the required physical education classes at Beijing University and many other universities, and tens of thousands of students every year are practicing the simplified form of Taijiquan. It is estimated that the simplified Taijiquan has spread to more than 100 countries, and several hundred millions of people have practiced it. Take the Japanese Federation of Martial Arts and Taijiquan, for example, where some 90 percent of its 10 million registered members have practiced 24-Step Taijiquan. This simplified Taijiquan has played an enormous role in promoting Taijiquan, which is why this little flower is so treasured by so many people.

International Host

Every year throughout China, Taijiquan competitions and public demonstrations are held at every level, sponsored by many different organizations. Conventions also are held where prominent Taijiquan masters and experts lecture and transmit their skills through seminars, training classes and technical level assessments of all kinds. As an example, I will briefly note some of its highlights of the International Taijiquan Health Conference I attended as a Taijiquan expert in March 2001 in the beautiful Chinese city of Sanya on Hainan Island.

Some 3,000 people from all over the world attended the conference, and it was an impressive sight to see many of them practice 24-Step Taijiquan together in the morning, along with local people, in a group that stretched several miles along the Pacific shore. Bathed in the morning sun and cool ocean breeze, this diverse group came together to perform slowly to the rhythm of music in harmony under the blue sky and white clouds. The natural and harmonious spirit of Taijiquan was fully present in this flowing magnificent scene.

Invited guests included 90-year-old Sun Jianyun, daughter of Sun Lutang—founder of the Sun-style Taijiquan; Chen Zhenglei, the 11th generation disciple of Chen-style Taijiquan from Chenjiagou in Henan Province; Yang Zhenduo, great grand-son of Yang Luchan—founder of the Yang-style Taijiquan from Shanxi Province; Qiao Songmao, the fifth generation disciple of the Wu (武)-style Taijiquan from Hebei Province; Li Bingci, the fourth generation disciple of the Wu (吴)-style Taijiquan from Beijing; Zhao Zengfu, follower of the Zhaobao Taijiquan from Henan Province; Zeng Nailiang, one of the top-10 martial arts coaches in China; Men Huifeng, one the top-10 martial arts professors in China; Xia Paihua,

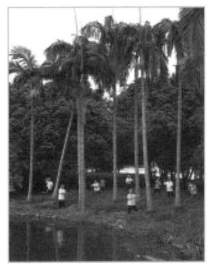

Practicing Taijiquan in the peace and beauty of nature.

researcher in the Chinese Martial Arts Research Institute; and Chen Sitan and Wang Erping, both champions in National Taijiquan Competitions. These experts and masters of Taijiquan selflessly presented their skills and valuable experiences accumulated over the years to people who love Taijiquan.

Among the many exchanges and demonstrations of Taijiquan at the conference were competitions in 42-Step Taijiquan and 42-Step Taiji sword, evaluations of traditional and optional forms of Taijiquan, Taiji push-hands competition, group Taijiquan performance competition, and all kinds of performances with weapons.

In traditional Taijiquan competition and performance, the styles included such popular ones such as the Chen-style, Yang-style, Wu (武)-style, Wu (吴)-style, and Sun-style, as well as those forms known locally such as the Zhaobao, He-style, Li-style, Fu-style, and Bagua-style of Taijiquan. Modern Taijiquan forms included Hunyuan, Siwei, Dongyue, the 36-Step Chen-style, the simplified Sun-style, the 13-Step Wu (武)-style Taijiquan, as well as Taiji club, Taiji spear, Taiji fan, Taiji ball, and Taiji stick. The office staff of the central government office from Beijing and the Macao Martial Arts

Association both were given special awards for their group performances. Young athletes from Guangdong Provincial Martial Arts Team won a special award for their group performance of Taijiquan that expressed solid basic skills, a high degree of technical difficulty, and dazzling choreography and artistry.

Among the modern forms of Taijiquan, those considered as the official standard are those created, designed, examined and approved by the experts organized by the State Martial Arts Administration. Often referred to as prescribed Taijiquan, these standard forms include the 24-Step Taijiquan, 48-Step Taijiquan, 88-Step Taijiquan, 32-Step Taiji Sword compiled under the direction of the State Physical Culture and Sports Commission; as well as all kinds of competition forms for Taijiquan and Taiji push-hands compiled under the direction of the Chinese Martial Arts Association.

The martial arts grading system under the State Administration of Martial Arts consisting of three grades and nine levels was presented at the conference through a demonstration of the beginning levels of instruction for Taijiquan — 10-Step Taijiquan at the first level, the 16-Step Taijiquan at the second level, and the 24-Step Taijiquan at the third level. Based on the Yang-style Taijiquan, these instructional materials help teach and assess those applying for beginning levels through concise and clear instructions suitable for people of all ages with different physical abilities.

The conference also heard reports on special topics given by experts on such topics as "The Development of Taijiquan," "The Basic Physiological and Health Care Element of Taijiquan," "The Teaching and Training of Taijiquan," and "The Cultural Implications of Taijiquan." In response to these lectures, audiences asked for even more reports, so extra night sessions of the lectures were added on demand.

Beyond all the official activities, this international gathering offered Taijiquan practitioners many other ways of getting together, such as sightseeing. People took walks on the beaches among the coconut trees or visited nearby temples and mountains, fully enjoying the beauty of nature in the company of friends looking toward a bright future — truly a manifestation of an international community dedicated to health, peace and harmony.

CHAPTER II
FOUR GENERATIONS OF
A TAIJIQUAN FAMILY

Our family traces its roots to central Hebei Province, where our ancestors engaged in farming until Li Yulin (1885 - 1965) changed the family's destiny. Before Grandfather, land was an inseparable part of my family; after him, it was Taijiquan. More than 100 years have passed since my family first became engaged in practicing martial arts and teaching Taijiquan, and today a new generation continues a legacy passed on through my grandfather to his sons, my father Li Tianchi (1913-1989) and my uncle Li Tianji (1914-1996) and their children including myself, Li Deyin (1938-).

My Grandfather Li Yulin

Li Yulin began studying martial arts as a boy in Quantou Village (formerly in Renqiu County in Hebei Province, now a part of Anxin County in Hebei, about two hours from Beijing). When my grandfather lost his father at the age of three, his young mother was highly protective of him, especially accepting as she did the Confucian belief that "of the three unfilial acts, leaving no heir is the greatest." As Li Yulin was her only son, she did not want to be left facing the ancestors of the Li Family with a guilty conscience. So to assure her son's strength and health, she sent Grandfather to study with a prominent martial arts master in the village named Hao Enguang.

My hometown was famous for martial arts. Many peasants worked in the fields during the day and practiced martial arts at night. Every year during Chinese New Year's, the village celebrations, along with lion dances and dramatic performances, included dynamic martial arts demonstrations.

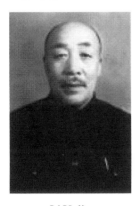

Li Yulin

17

As my grandfather matured, he grew more and more fascinated with martial arts until he himself became a highly respected martial arts instructor.

Grandfather became not just physically strong, he also came to hate injustice like poison. He was not even afraid of ghosts and gods that were held in awe by others. One story about Grandfather, "Li Yulin Gives the Buddha a Whipping," is still told by the old folks in Quantou Village. His son — my father — was sickly shortly after his birth. My great grandmother went to the village temple everyday to kowtow, burn incense and pray to Buddha for her grandson's safety. However, none of that worked. My father didn't recover. To make matters worse, my great-grandmother also fell ill from anxiety. This made my young and impetuous grandfather mad. In the still of night, he ran to the temple and punched and kicked the statue of the Buddha, shouting:

"I'm not going to make a fuss about my son's death or danger. But if anything should happen to my mother, I'll never let you off."

Unexpectedly, my father's situation started day-by-day to take a turn for the better, which also set my great grandmother's mind at ease. Because my grandfather's beating of the Buddha happened to have been witnessed by a peasant in the neighborhood, the story got around. The villagers said, "Even ghosts and gods are afraid of martial arts masters."

At the age of 30, Grandfather lost Hao Enguang when his martial arts teacher was shot and died at his post during a fight with bandits in what was then Rehe Province, an area composed of parts of Hebei Province, Shanxi Province and the Inner Mongolia Autonomous Region. In deep mourning, Grandfather sold off his property and embarked on a long trek to bring his teacher's body back to his hometown. When they passed the city of Tianjin, friends in martial arts circles held a memorial service for Hao Enguang. Everyone had great respect for Grandfather's loyalty. Sun Lutang — a master of Taijiquan, Baguaquan [Eight-Diagram Boxing] and Xingyiquan [a kind of martial arts based on the fighting movements of 12 different animals] — was so moved by Li Yulin's action that he decided to take Grandfather on as a disciple. Sun Lutang then became my grandfather's second teacher. Grandfather left his hometown from that time on to follow Sun Lutang to Tianjin and Shanghai and to practice and teach martial arts. Ten years later, he had advanced in his Taijiquan skills to become "senior disciple" among Sun Lutang's followers, and also the first generation full-time martial arts master in our family.

In 1930, Grandfather became Dean of Studies at the Shandong Provincial Martial Arts School, established by Li Jinglin who was skilled in Yang-style Wudangjian [Wudang Sword] and Taijiquan. Li Jinglin had been in the military for a long time, serving as Military Supervisor of Hebei Province, equivalent to the rank of provincial military commander. After retiring from military service, Li Jinglin became a leader in martial arts circles. Appreciating Grandfather's skills and character, Li Jinglin became Grandfather's third martial arts teacher.

After the War of Resistance against Japanese Aggression broke out in 1937, Grandfather's focus on teaching Taijiquan in the northeastern provinces earned him the title, "Northeast China's Taijiquan Pioneer." People in this border area were not then familiar with Taijiquan but considered it as an activity for the old, weak, sick and disabled. One tall and strong man Grandfather met when he first arrived in Harbin, the capital city of Heilongjiang Province, said, "How can this soft skill be called gongfu?"

Grandfather answered, "If you can shove me away from where I'm standing, you can be considered a gongfu master."

The tall man made every effort, but failed. Grandfather said: "Believe it or not, I can throw you with one hand."

The tall man didn't believe it. Grandfather grabbed him and pushed while the tall man resisted with all his strength. Suddenly, grandfather relaxed his grip. The man lost his balance, moving quickly backwards. Grandfather took advantage of the chance, actually making the tall man's feet lift into the air before he fell. This convinced the man, who then became one of grandfather's earliest Taijiquan followers in Harbin. Grandfather had a lot of Taijiquan disciples, many of whom later became famous local or even national Taijiquan masters. Among them was Zhang Jixiu, one of the Top 10 National Martial Arts Masters, who lead the group of masters responsible for compiling the Taijijian [Taiji sword] form for competition.

Grandfather spent his last years in researching Taijiquan for the elderly and for people suffering from chronic diseases.

"Helping old people live longer and patients recover is a big issue for society, also a big task for Taijiquan," he said. For this reason, he also studied traditional Chinese medicine and osteopathy. Among the visitors to our home were not only people coming for advice in martial arts, but also people seeking medical treatment and medicine.

My Uncle Li Tianji

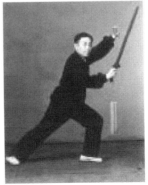

The author's father, Li Tianchi, applied his knowledge of Taijiquan in his medical practice.

My father, Li Tianchi, honored his father's wish that he combine martial arts with medical skill. When Father became a medical doctor in the hospital attached to Harbin Medical University, he applied with success Taijiquan, qigong and massage in clinical treatments for ailments such as chronic bronchitis as well as diseases related to old age.

But it was my uncle Li Tianji — known in Chinese martial arts circles as "Longfei" or "Flying Dragon" — who made his name in the martial arts. A graduate with honors from Shandong Provincial Martial Arts School, he became a martial arts lecturer at Harbin Industrial University and coach of the martial arts team at the Central Institute of Physical Education. That team was actually the first national martial arts team of the People's Republic of China, one that trained many talented martial artists. In 1954, my uncle was transferred to the State Physical Education and Sports Commission and China Martial Arts Association, where he became engaged in researching and classifying the martial arts. A member of the group that compiled the first national martial arts textbooks in China, he wrote Simplified Taijiquan and 32-Step Taijijian [Taiji Sword]. He also classified and published various instructional materi-

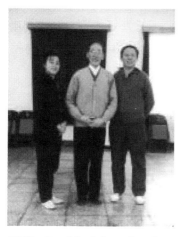

als on traditional martial arts such as Xingyiquan, Baguazhang, Wudangjian and Shaolinquan. He was acknowledged as a "People's Republic of China Sports Pioneer" and one of China's "Top 10 National Martial Arts Masters."

Li Tianji also pioneered international communication in Chinese martial arts through his teaching of Taijiquan to Japanese. After Premier Zhou Enlai in 1959 introduced Taijiquan to some visiting Japanese friends on the occasion of 10th anniversary of the founding of the People's Republic of China, my uncle was entrusted by the Chinese leadership on several occasions to teach Japanese friends Taijiquan. Li Tianji's teaching had a significant impact on the development of Taijiquan in Japan. When my uncle

Li Tianji — "the father of modern Taijiquan" — with his daughter, Li Defang, and nephew, Li Deyin.

passed away in 1996, friends from Japanese martial arts circles expressed their heartfelt condolences and set up a monument to his memory on which the former Japanese Prime Minister Hata Tsutomu wrote an inscription, respectfully referring to my uncle as "the father of modern Taijiquan."

My Taijiquan Career

As for myself, the third generation, I served some 40 years as a Taijiquan instructor at Renmin University in Beijing. During that time, I became a professor in physical education, was recognized as one of the Top 100 Chinese Martial Arts Masters, achieved national ranking as a community physical education instructor, was awarded the 8th level in Chinese martial arts, became an international martial arts judge and so on. My cousin, Li Defang who is Li Tianji's daughter, has been teaching at the Sino-Japanese Friendship Association's health center in Tokyo for 10 years where she established the Japanese Longfei Taijiquan Association.

As a boy, I grew up on a steady diet of the martial arts and Taijiquan. When an adult was doing a leg lift, he would perch me on his leg to add weight. When my elders practiced, I followed along imitating their actions. When they took breaks from practice, they told me stories about Bodhidharma [the legendary Indian Buddhist monk who is said to have brought the martial arts to the Shaolin Temple in Henan Province]; Zhang Sanfeng [a semi-legendary Daoist priest from the Song Dynasty (960-1279), associated with the origins of Taijiquan]; Guan Yu [160-219, a famous warrior of the ancient Three Kingdoms period in China] and Yue Fei [1103-1142, patriot and national hero of the Southern Song Dynasty].

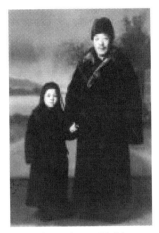

The author with his grandfather.

When I was eight, Grandfather began formal instruction in the martial arts for my older and younger brothers and me. We did leg squats, kicks and standing qigong (techniques to develop the legs) in the yard every day after school. Grandfather's teaching was strict and rigorous. He told us that the ancients "read books during the day and practiced martial arts at night," as he kept us practicing the same simple beginning positions of Xingyiquan and Taijiquan over and over again for weeks. He never granted requests for something new. I actually was able to imitate some other movements, but I didn't dare show him unless he asked. So a single Taijiquan form took us more than a year to learn. We spent three years in practicing the five movements of Wuxingquan (five-element boxing) over and over again. As a result, thick calluses appeared on the soles of our feet, but still Grandfather was not satisfied.

"My chief instructor spent eight years on Bengquan [short-punch or smashing fist]. What you've done is far from enough," he said. Only when practicing push-hands did we become excited. Grandfather was always the target, asking us to attack him any way we liked. In the end, it was always us who were sent flying right and left.

In 1957, I passed the Beijing Renmin University entrance examination to become the first university student in our family's history, which pleased the whole family. I majored in industrial economics with the goal of working in modern industrial management. I did quite well at the university where I also was enthusiastic about sports. But although I remained devoted to Taijiquan, there was almost no Taijiquan activity at the university. So I had to choose other sports including track and field in which I broke the university's record in the 400-meter hurdles — an accomplishment I attributed to my martial arts practice.

Finally, an opportunity came when news spread to Renmin University about a Beijing University Students Martial Arts Competition. Student union leaders at Renmin University were anxious to know where they could find martial arts athletes to compete. My offer to take up the challenge surprised them: How could a track and field athlete do Taijiquan? All doubts vanished when I came back with a Taijiquan championship medal. Soon more and more schoolmates began to learn Taijiquan from me. They realized that this ancient sport is not only good for the health, but is full of underlying Chinese cultural implications. Taijiquan cultivates both the body and the mind, representing Chinese civilization and a standard of conduct. The enthusiasm of these students for Taijiquan caught the attention of university officials. The dean of the Physical Education Department asked me to work as martial arts instructor at the university after graduation. My grandfather, father and uncle also encouraged me to carry on our family's tradition to be the third generation professional martial arts teacher. So I gave up my original goal and started to devote my life to Taijiquan.

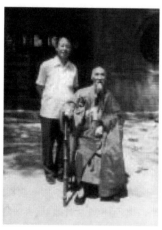

Li Deyin's studies included a visit to the Shaolin Temple in Henan Province.
He is shown here with the abbott, De Chan.

After I became a teacher at the university, I worked to realize my goals to make Taijiquan a popular sport for university students and to integrate this ancient national sport into a modern university education. To this end, I attended the Institute of Physical Culture to take all the foundation courses required for a physical education major; consulted several senior martial artists including Sun Jianyun, Xu Zhiyi, Li Jingwu and Hao Jiajun; visited monks and Taoist priests at the Shaolin Temple and on Wudang Mountain to seek understanding of the historical path of development of the martial arts; studied the teaching experiences of other instructors and coaches; and got instruction and support from my grandfather, father and uncle.

After three years' hard work, a promising sports presence took shape on the campus of Renmin University centered around "doing exercise, practicing Taijiquan, and running. " Taijiquan became a required university physical education course. Every morning and during class breaks, Taijiquan music was heard with students performing Taijiquan on the campus. The student martial arts team I coached won 13 gold medals and first place in group scores at the Beijing University Students Martial Arts Competition.

My first experience on the international level came when the Beijing International Club opened a Taijiquan training class for foreign friends who were living in Beijing. As a young martial arts instructor at Renmin University, I was asked to take charge at the club where more than 600 diplomats, foreign specialists, business people and their families from over 40 countries at some time participated in the Taijiquan club. Among them was Barbara Bush, mother of U.S. President George W. Bush [42nd President of the United States] and wife of President George Bush [40th U.S. President] who served from 1974 to 1976 as the top diplomat to the People's Republic of China as head of the U.S. Liaison Office. Thanks to her rapid progress, Barbara Bush was elected class representative for the United States to give a demonstration at graduation ceremonies. Her performance of 24-step Taijiquan drew enthusiastic applause from the audience.

At that time, China had not yet adopted the policy of opening to the outside world, so that was the first time for me to have contact with people from other countries. At first, it was hard not to be nervous. But gradually I came to realize that Taijiquan worked as a bridge of friendship among people from different countries. Deep and lasting relationships evolved between me and my foreign students.

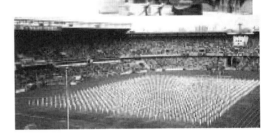

The ambassador from Madagascar was reluctant to leave his post in Beijing. He told us during a dinner before departure:

"Taijiquan is a splendid cultural heritage. In the past, Chinese lychee was carried to my country and became people's favorite fruit. Today, I return with Taijiquan with the hope that it will become our people's favorite sport."

In 1990 when the 11th Asian Games were held in Beijing, I was asked to take on some significant tasks. For this major

Directing the Sino-Japanese Taijiquan performance at the opening ceremonies for the 11th Asian Games in Beijing.

international sports event, I trained some 1,500 Taijiquan practitioners from China and Japan to perform at the opening ceremony, marking the first time for any Taijiquan group performance to appear at an international sports meet; I gave an instructor's training class to members of this Sino-Japanese group; I conducted classes on international judging and finally I served as Taijiquan coach for the 20-member Chinese martial arts team. After rigorous training of the assembled athletes of the Chinese team, I finally picked four official Taijiquan competitors, and China placed first at the 11th Asian Games in both the men's and women's divisions of Taijiquan.

The opening Asian Games Taijiquan performance turned out wonderfully well — so much so that some participants actually wept with emotion. Some 750 Japanese performers from 27 provinces and cities in Japan participated with Chinese performers

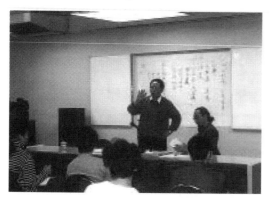

who came from more than 50 Beijing Taijiquan groups. With so many people from so many different backgrounds, styles and places of Taijiquan practice, it had been a difficult task to organize group training. But I managed to work out a training routine that assured success by emphasizing uniform movements, steps and formations. The average age of participants was 42.

Lecturing on Taijiquan theory.

For the instructor's training class, I emphasized 10 technical mistakes to guard against to assure that Taijiquan is performed correctly, not just as a show of gymnastics. These mistakes are:

1. The chest is thrust out, the waist sinks in, and the limbs are stiff.

2. Movements are too soft and weak so that they look old and feeble.

3. The body leans forward or backward into unnatural postures.

4. Movements are sloppy, and the feet lack roots.

5. Strength or energy is applied erratically and ineffectively, without coordination between the limbs and torso.

6. Hands and feet are not coordinated, and the timing is off.

7. Movements begin and end too abruptly or stiffly without a continuous flow.

8. No distinction is made between substantial and insubstantial, lacking related changes in rhythm and applications of force.

9. Breathing is not regular nor is it coordinated with the use of strength.

10. The movements appear dispirited, lacking external grace and internal vitality.

As for the class on international judging, I gave a detailed explanation of competition rules and standards that require every judge to be fair and accurate. Someone suggested that in the spirit of "friendship first, competition second," special consideration and gold medals should be given to athletes from countries that had made great contributions to Taijiquan development as well as to countries undertaking the next games. I firmly disagreed.

I explained that while it is absolutely correct that a martial arts competition should first of all promote a spirit of friendship with an emphasis on participation rather than winning — for judges, it is their fairness and accuracy that will guarantee and manifest that spirit. Athletes from different countries and different levels must be treated equally. No matter what reaction and applause athletes receive from the audience, no matter if athletes are known or not known to the judges, no matter what sort of previous impression judges may have, athletes must be treated equally. Anything less would make martial arts judges — and their work — untrustworthy. Only when judges work fairly and accurately during a competition can friendship and unity prevail.

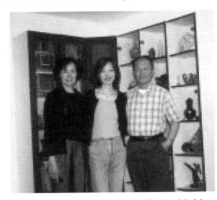

The author at home in Beijing with his wife, Fang Mishou, and their youngest daughter, Li Yue.

Since my retirement from Renmin University in 2000, I have not lost my love and pursuit of Taijiquan. I continue to teach both in China and abroad, serve as vice-chairman of the Beijing Martial Arts Association, and have compiled many books and videos on Taijiquan, hoping to help beginners. Every morning I practice Taijiquan with my wife, Fang Mishou. Not long ago, she and I created "Taijishan" or "Taiji Fan" together, which was performed by 2008 middle-aged and older Taijiquan friends at Tian'anmen Square as part of Beijing's successful effort to become host of the 2008 Olympic Games.

As for the new generation, my daughter, Li Hui (Faye Yip), established the Deyin Taijiquan Institute in Britain to become the fourth generation Taijiquan martial arts master in my family. My youngest daughter Li Yue, who lives in Houston, Texas in the United States, decided to pursue a medical career, but she and her husband were members of my martial arts team at Renmin University where both were champions in the Beijing University Students Martial Arts Competition.

CHAPTER III
ESSENTIALS OF TAIJIQUAN

Its History — Its Name — Its Nature as a Martial Art — "Treatise on Taijiquan" and "Song of the 13 Methods" — The Health Benefits of Taijiquan

Origins and Development

Various ideas exist as to the origins of Taijiquan, some of them shrouded in mystery. One popular story credits Zhang Sanfeng, a Taoist who lived on the famous Wudang Mountain [a Taoist center in Hubei Province], with creating Taiji in the Song Dynasty (960-1279): Summoned to an interview by the Emperor, Zhang Sanfeng was held up by bandits on his way to the capital. That night, he dreamed of being taught some skills in unarmed combat that enabled him to defeat over 100 bandits, and thus to create Taijiquan.

Another version holds that Zhang Sanfeng was born at the end of the Yuan Dynasty (1271-1368) or early Ming Dynasty (1368-1644). While practicing Tao-ism and making pills of immortality on Wudang Mountain, he observed how snakes and sparrows fought each other and tried to discover the secret of why turtles and cranes live so long. From this, he created Taijiquan. On Wudang Mountain, Zhang Sanfeng cultivated himself and perfected his skills with the sword. He also traveled to Gansu and Yunnan provinces and was well known in these places, too. However, according to all available historical records, no evidence exists connecting Zhang Sanfeng to Taijiquan. So the popular belief that Zhang Sanfeng created Taijiquan has not been proved and remains an open question in martial arts history.

Others believe that Taijiquan began with Xu Xuanping of the Tang Dynasty (618-907) or Chen Bo of the early Ming Dynasty. But this is mentioned only in hand-copied genealogies of Song-style and Chen-style Taijiquan. Without other evidence, it is hard to accept as fact.

According to modern history, Taijiquan was practiced along the Yellow River in Henan Province at the end of the Ming and early Qing Dynasty (1644-1911) in an area centered around Chenjiagou and Zhaobaozhen in Wenxian County, with Chen Wangting and Jiang Fa as its major exponents. Tang Hao, the martial arts scholar, bases his assertion that Chen Wangting was the creator of Taijiquan on genealogies of the Chen clan and Chen-style Taijiquan as well as on poems composed by Chen Wangting. Records on Taijiquan available in Zhaobaozhen show that Jiang Fa went to Shanxi Province to learn Taijiquan at the age of 22. He came back seven years later and began to teach Taijiquan, working to introduce it in Henan Province.

Judging from all of the above, the origin of Taijiquan has yet to be ascertained. However, what we can say is:

1. Chenjiagou and Zhaobaozhen are the earliest known places where Taijiquan was practiced, and Chen Wangting and Jiang Fa were the most influential masters of Taijiquan of the place and time.

2. Jiang Fa was born in 1574, the second year of the Wanli reign of the Ming Dynasty. He returned from his study trip to Shanxi Province back to his hometown Wenxian County in Henan Province to teach Taijiquan in 1603. Chen Wangting was a government student at the end of the Ming Dynasty. He was appointed as township militia commandant of Wenxian County in 1621. These facts prove that Taijiquan has a history of at least some 400 years.

3. A continual and long process that incorporated whatever was available formed Taijiquan. Whether in Chen Wangting's creation or in Jiang Fa's introduction, Taijiquan drew from the wisdom of a long ancestry and included many different unarmed combat techniques developed among the ordinary people. From the genealogy of Chen-Style Taijiquan, we can see that many of the names of the methods and the songs of Taijiquan are the same as the "32-Step Changquan (Long Fist)" designed by the Ming Dynasty general Qi Jiguang. The "32-Step Changquan" of Qi Jiguang, in turn, was created by absorbing the best of 16 kinds of folk "fist" or unarmed combat techniques.

4. The yin-yang theory of ancient Chinese philosophy, the meridian doctrine or the theory of channels and collaterals of traditional Chinese medicine and the Taoist theories related to maintaining good health provide the foundation on which Taijiquan was created.

Originally called the 13 Methods, Taijiquan contains the meaning of the eight trigrams [eight combinations of three whole or broken lines formerly used in divination] and the five elements [metal, wood, water, fire and earth]. Huangtingjing, one of the Taoist classics on cultivating life and strengthening vitality through breathing practice, is referred to by Chen Wangting in his poem in a line that states:

"The *Classic of Huangtingjing* is always by my side." Many Taijiquan methods are consistent with ancient Chinese theories and techniques of expiration and inspiration for promoting health and curing diseases through combining regulated, controlled breathing with physical exercises.

For a long time, the practice of Taijiquan was limited to the rural areas of Henan Province. In the early 19th century, Yang Luchan, a native of Yongnian in Hebei Province, became an apprentice of Chen Changxing in Chenjiagou. After learning Taijiquan, he returned to his hometown in Hebei Province and then later taught in Beijing, thus initiating the spread of Taijiquan throughout the whole country.

In the last century, Taijiquan developed as never before, with skills changing and techniques improving all the time. Many schools gradually appeared, and the major ones are:

Yang (杨)-style Taijiquan, created by Mr. Yang Luchan and refined by his grandson Yang Chengfu. Yang style is performed with a poised upright body and a slow even speed, with rather extended movements done in a smooth, rounded way. Yang style is the most widely practiced Taijiquan style in and outside China.

Chen (陈)-style, the oldest among all the schools of Taijiquan. Chen style retains the ancient way of discharging internal energy, with jumping and stamping of the feet. Its execution demands more energy as it is performed in a less uniform rhythm, often intertwining its movements in coiling motions that temper toughness with gentleness.

Wu (吴)-style Taijiquan, composed by Quan You and Wu Jianquan, father and son who once followed the Yang Style. Wu (吴) style is noted for its refined, gentle and circular movements, which are performed in a measured way in leaning postures but with the body held straight.

Wu (武)-style Taijiquan, designed by Wu Yuxiang on the basis of the Taijiquan popular in Zhaobaozhen in Henan Province. Wu (武) style is concise and compact, simple and elegant. With the body upright, its movements are slow and gentle, less extended compared to the other styles.

Sun (孙)-style Taijiquan, composed by Sun Lutang, a renowned master of Xingyiquan and Baguaquan on the basis of the Wu (武)-style Taijiquan in the early years of the Republic of China (1911-1949). Its movements are short, with agile foot work. With quick steps that closely follow an opponent's, Sun Style Taijiquan is also known as "nimble foot work or nimble step Taijiquan."

After the founding the People's Republic of China in 1949, Taijiquan gained its prominence as an important component of the martial arts. Today public Taijiquan learning centers are open throughout China; many Taijiquan books, charts, audio tapes and videos have been published; research and theoretical discussions on Taijiquan go on continuously; nationwide and regional Taijiquan competitions are held every year that attract large numbers of people from abroad, helping to spread Taijiquan worldwide.

To meet the demands of the times, the State Physical Cultural and Sports Commission organized systematic studies and classifications of Taijiquan, and it compiled a series of standardized textbooks including the 24-Step Simplified Taijiquan, the 48-Step Taijiquan, Taiji push-hands and routine competition rules for different forms of Taijiquan. These have enriched Taijiquan, promoting its practice both generally and in competition while paving the way for Taijiquan to develop in a modern and standardized way on the solid basis of its various traditional schools.

Meaning of the Name

In Chinese "Tài 太 " means the highest or supreme, as in describing the highest heaven or the supreme ruler. "Jí 极" means the last or the ultimate. The word "Tàijí 太极 " first appeared in *The Book of Changes*, which was written more than 3,000 years ago, in a reference to the most primitive state of the universe, the origin of all changes, or the highest realm of existence.

*The Book of Changes (*Yìjīng 易经) is composed of two parts, the Text (Jīng 经) and Commentaries (Zhuàn 传). The Text deals mainly with divination and an integrated system of trigrams or hexagrams (guà 卦). As symbols of divination, the eight trigrams are formed in various ways to tell fortunes according to interpretations of the lines of the trigrams. Legend has it that the classic Text was written by the King Wen of the Zhou Dynasty (11 century- 256 BC). The Commentaries include an interpretation or discussion of the Text, composed of philosophical essays by many different people that express their world outlook based on the theory of yin and yang. In "The Great Interpretation" essay in the Commentaries section of *The Book of Changes*, Taiji was first mentioned as follows:

"Yì (易) contains Tàijí (太极) which gave birth to the two basic elements; the two basic elements gave birth to the four symbolic figures; the four symbolic figures then gave birth to the eight elementary trigrams (bāguà 八卦) that can predict fortune and misfortune, which enables great accomplishment."

Here Taiji refers to the origin of changes, the most primitive state from which everything evolves. It is the highest state of existence. Throughout the ages, Chinese scholars have offered different philosophical interpretations of the world based on the Taiji yin-yang theory. For example:

"Before Heaven and Earth were divided, the primal fluid—primary elements that form Heaven and Earth—were combined into one. That is the beginning of the great Unity of Tai or the great oneness of Tai."

— Kong Yingda of the Tang Dynasty (618-907)

"Taiji was the primeval chaotic and primitive state of the universe before Heaven and Earth were formed."

— Wang Tingxiang of the Ming Dynasty (1368-1644)

"When Taiji moved, it gave birth to yang. When the movement reached its peak, it quieted down into motionlessness to become yin. At its extreme point, yin began to move and turn toward yang. The polarized motion and stillness or yang and yin produce and promote one another. The theory of the five elements (wǔxíng 五行) came from yin and yang; Yin and yang came from Taiji."

— Zhou Dunyi of the Song Dynasty (960-1279)

"Taiji covers everything in the universe."

— The Song Dynasty philosopher Zhu Xi

"Taiji is the heart and mind." And: "Taiji is the Dao (Way)."

— Shao Yong of the Song Dynasty

The Taiji yin-yang theory that is such an important part of ancient Chinese philosophy serves as the theoretical basis of Taijiquan. But only in modern times did the Taiji name become associated with a kind of unarmed method of combat [quán 拳, literally, "fist"].

Taijiquan (太极拳) or "Taiji Fist" was first called the "13 Methods (eight techniques plus five stances)." It was also called Changquan (long fist), referring to its long and continuous form; Ruanquan (soft fist), Rouquan (gentle fist), and Zhanmianquan (adhering fist). The name of Taijiquan formally came into being in the "Treatise on Taijiquan" written by Wang Zongyue, a martial arts master of the Qing Dynasty (1644-1911). Wang Zongyue named Taijiquan after the Taiji yin-yang theory to signify that Taijiquan is based on this fundamental principle of the universe as well as on the belief that people are an integral part of nature. The name also represents Taijiquan's combining firmness with gentleness. Unfathomable and unpredictable through its interplay of the insubstantial and the substantial (empty and solid), Taijiquan is invincible.

Taijiquan and the Martial Arts

Taijiquan as a martial art is noted for its relaxed, calm and gentle movements that are performed slowly and continuously.

An ancient treasure of China's cultural heritage, the martial arts above all are characterized by offensive and defensive techniques. In precise movements performed for technical training or for competition, martial arts provide an exercise for both the mind and the body through practice as a way to keep fit, to cultivate oneself and for self-defense.

The earliest martial arts were created in China by people in the remote past who had to fight with wild animals to stay alive. With the development of society, martial arts evolved from a means of survival and of warfare into a kind of athletic activity for physical and mental fitness, gaining some artistic and recreational features. Nevertheless, Taijiquan still retains its original offensive and defensive meaning in each movement, which makes it stand apart from other recreational sports such as gymnastics, dancing and qigong.

With such a long history and rich heritage, some 129 kinds of Chinese combat styles have survived with definite origins, systematic theories and unique styles, according to a nationwide survey of the Chinese martial arts conducted in the 1980s. And of these, Taijiquan is one of the most important.

Many find it hard to understand how Taijiquan could be related to the intrepid fighting styles of the martial arts. In fact, all martial arts involve different techniques of offense and defense, advance and retreat, hardness and softness, emptiness and solidity, motion and stillness. It is the ability to make a correct assessment of a situation and to respond with the right strategy and technique that enables a martial artist to defeat an opponent — even a stronger opponent — by turning the tide. For instance, some forms of unarmed combat stress fast attack through so-called "starting out like a wind, landing like an arrow, accelerating speed even if the opponent is beaten." Some move in a roundabout way by "drawing in the opponent" or "avoiding the front to attack the side." Some find success by "initiating a strong offense with a direct strike that eliminates the need to ward off any blows." Others encourage "a shorter, smaller, lighter, softer yet unbroken and skillful" force and then win by "deflecting 1,000 pounds with a force of four ounces." Some martial arts are especially good at hand techniques by "hitting with fists that land as dense as raindrops with a sound like a string of firecrackers." Some stress the use of the legs as described in: "The hands are as gates while attacks are the domain of the legs." Some use "the strategy of delay to further an attack;" while others "follow the opponent closely and strike directly." Some hold that "to advance is the only way to survive," while others advise "to keep still if the opponent doesn't move." A great variety of schools, each with its own strategic and tactical features, make up Chinese martial arts as a whole.

As for Taijiquan, successful strategy and technique requires the mastery of four important points or skills: Feeling, neutralizing, controlling, and attacking.

Feeling (tīng 听) means to wait and sense the opponent's attack and to strike only after the opponent has struck. It means to react swiftly to an opponent's shifts by judging correctly the oncoming force from the opponent.

Neutralizing (huà 化) means to yield to the oncoming attack. Instead of confronting the opponent with force, neutralize the attack as it comes in by moving around with agility and strategy to lead the opponent's force and direct him or her to emptiness, thus breaking down the opponent's offensive.

Controlling (ná 拿) means to dodge the opponent's main force. It means to keep the opponent under control by targeting his or her weaknesses, thus putting oneself in an advantageous position over the opponent.

Attacking (fa 发) means to break through at the opponent's weak points, to take advantage of his or her lack of readiness, and to attack with both one's own and the opponent's force to achieve the best result.

From these four points, we can see that Taijiquan as a martial art emphasizes waiting in stillness to allow the opponent to initiate movement and then to get the better of the opponent through a faster and earlier strike. Soft as it appears, Taijiquan can defeat a powerful opponent through its various strategies and techniques. Since Taijiquan basic training emphasizes keeping calm, relaxed, gentle and steady — Taijiquan naturally developed into a calm and relaxed sport characterized by slow, steady, rounded and flexible movements. Sudden strong and quick discharges of energy, jumping, stamping and kicking are preserved only in limited number of Taijiquan routines.

Because of its appearance, Taijiquan has been regarded by some as a kind of qigong or an advanced form of breathing exercise for good health. But this is not correct.

Throughout their long historical development, both Taijiquan and qigong have been deeply influenced by classical Chinese philosophy in such fundamental theories and techniques as the unity of the universe and human beings, the mutual influence and opposition of yin and yang, the concept of keeping fit by combining movement with tranquility, and the idea of cultivating oneself internally and externally. Both stress the ideas of "keeping the mind calm and body relaxed," "keeping the body naturally upright and comfortable," "sinking the vital life energy (qì 气) to the field of elixir

(Dantián 丹田)," "initiating movements by the mind and heart," and "seeking stillness in movement." Both strive to find internal and external balance, while adjusting the mind and qi. Therefore, they have much in common that mutually influence each other.

However, we cannot disregard that Taijiquan and qigong belong to different categories. Because they differ in aspects of origin, content and form — each with its own characteristics and features — we cannot take them as the same.

First, as a martial art, Taijiquan has distinctive offensive and defensive movements with specific hand and foot techniques for applying force to certain points. The applications in Taijiquan are obviously for offense and defense. As a sport, the aim of Taiji push-hands is to win. But the movements of qigong are meant neither as offense or defense, and qigong is not a competitive sport.

Second, a major part of Taijiquan is movement, although it is performed gently and slowly with tranquility. So Taijiquan is rather demanding in regard to body strength, balance, coordination, and flexibility. Qigong, on the other hand, is mostly done without any movement, as it seeks motion in stillness, so it does not require much in terms of physical development and is easier for people to practice who are not physically strong or who are in the recovery stage of illness or injury.

Third, in Taijiquan, the mind and breath are closely related to the movement so that the mind's intention, strength and qi unify in focusing on the movement. For instance, when the hands stretch forward, the state of solidity or emptiness of the mind may be different, or even opposite, according to purposes such as pushing out the hands or drawing in the hands. Whereas in qigong, the mind focuses on a certain acupuncture point or on the main and collateral channels. Breathing should be kept natural and smooth, both even and deep. The movement follows and tries to support the focus of the mind and adjustment of the breath.

"Treatise on Taijiquan" and "Song of the 13 Methods"

In the 1950s, an important work on Taijiquan, *The Genealogy of Taijiquan* by Wang Zongyue was discovered in Wuyang County, Henan Province. Although no information on the writer is contained in the work itself, other sources report that Wang Zongyue was born in Shanxi Province and traveled to Henan Province where he taught from 1791 to 1795 in the Qing Dynasty. As a good master of the martial arts, he also was well versed in literature, history and philosophy, Taoism and military strategy. *The Genealogy of Taijiquan* was preserved and passed down by Wu Yuxiang, founder of the Wu (武)-style Taijiquan, as the most highly valued classic on Taijiquan. Widely read by people who practice Taijiquan in and outside China, the work has had a deep influence on the Taijiquan theory and practice over the past century.

The classic includes two articles, "Treatise on Taijiquan" and "The Name of Taijiquan," as well as two folk ballads, "Song of the 13 Methods" and " Song of Push-Hands." The following presentation of "Treatise on Taijiquan" and " Song of the 13 Methods" is offered to help readers further understand Taijiquan.

1. Treatise on Taijiquan — The Text

"Supreme Ultimate (tàjí 太极) is born of Formless Void (wújí 无极). Taiji is the mother of yin and yang. In motion, yin and yang separate; in stillness, they combine."
太极者，无极而生，阴阳之母也。动之则分，静之则合。
Note: The term "Wuji" — referring to the original shapeless state of the universe — comes from "Return to Wuji" in the Taoist classic, *The Book of Lao Zi* [also named *The Scripture of Ethics*, thought to have been written in the late Spring and Autumn Period (770-476 BC)]. The term does not appear in works of the Confucian school or *The Book of Changes*. Zhou Dunyi of the Song Dynasty (960-1279) put forward the idea that "Taiji comes from Wuji" in his Explanations of the Taiji Chart, reflecting the Taoist idea: "Everything comes from being, being comes from non-being." The reference to Taiji as the mother of Yin and Yang comes from Zhou Dunyi's Explanations of the Taiji Chart of the Song Dynasty.

"Never overextend or under-extend, follow bending with expanding."
无过不及，随屈就伸。
Note: In the phrase 无过不及 (wúguò bùjí), the Chinese 过 (guò) means too much, 不及 (bùjí) means not enough. The phrase means never overdo or under-do anything.

In the Chinese phrase 随曲就伸 (suíqū jiùshēn) — literally, follow bend, adapt stretch — follow (suí 随) means the same as adapt (jiù 就). The phrase refers to adapting to or following an opponent.

"Faced with a stronger opponent, I yield; then when I have the advantage, I maintain control by sticking to the opponent (nián 粘)."
人刚我柔谓之 "走"，我顺人背谓之 "黏"。
Note: In the last phrase 我顺人背 (wǒshùn rénbèi) in which I have the "advantage" (shùn 顺), the opponent is described as being controlled in a "passive state" (bèi 背).

"Respond quickly if the opponent's movement is quick; follow slowly if his or her movement is slow. Throughout numerous variations, the principle remains the same."

动急则急应，动缓则缓随。虽变化万端，而理唯一贯。

"As practice leads to a high level of skill, one comes gradually to achieve 'understanding of inner power' (dǒng jìn 懂劲) to begin to enter the realm of freedom. Without continuous and diligent practice, one cannot become enlightened."

由着熟而渐悟懂劲，由懂劲而阶及神明。然非用力之久，不能豁然贯通焉！

Note: In the Chinese expression for "skilled" (zhao shú 着熟), the character 着 refers to both offensive and defensive techniques. "Understanding of inner power" (dǒng jìn 懂劲) is a special martial arts term, meaning mastery of the principles and techniques of the changes in the application of inner strength.

"Walk onto the steps of the kingdom of freedom" (阶及神明) refers to achieving god-like powers.

用力 (yòng lì) — That is, to work hard.

The word huòrán 豁然 comes from a phrase used in *The Legend of the Peach Garden* by Tao Qian — 豁然开朗, meaning a sudden change from a narrow, dark place into a bright and open one.

"Let the inner power (jìn 劲) rise to the top of the head, and the qì (气) sink to the Dantian."

虚领顶劲，气沉丹田。

Note: In 虚领, 领 (lǐng) means to raise one's spirits and 虚 (xū) refers to the state of being light and natural.

Dantian (丹田 field of elixir) in acupuncture refers to the Qihai point below the navel; in martial arts, it refers to the abdominal area just below the navel. The term "field of elixir" refers to the place where Taoists attempted to produce an elixir of immortality.

"Do not lean in any direction or show any sign of substantial or insubstantial to your opponent. Suddenly appear, suddenly disappear."

不偏不倚，忽隐忽现。

Note: 不偏不倚 — 偏 (pian) and 倚 (yǐ) both mean off to one side and out of balance.

"When an opponent presses on your left side, empty the left side; if your right side is pressured, let the right side disappear without a trace."

左重则左虚，右重则右杳；

Note: 杳 (yǎo) — leaving no trace.

"If the opponent stands tall, you stretch taller; if the opponent bends down, you go lower. When the opponent advances, make him or her feel as if the distance is increasing; when the opponent retreats, let the opponent feel the distance has become short. The body is so sensitive that it can feel a feather's weight, so supple that a fly cannot alight on it."

仰之则弥高，俯之则弥深；进之则愈长，退之则愈促，一羽不能加，蝇虫不能落；

"The opponent cannot discover your intentions, but you can detect the opponent's. If you have these abilities, you are invincible."

人不知我，我独知人。英雄所向无敌，盖皆由此而及也。

"There are many other boxing arts. Although they differ in forms, they never go beyond the stronger dominating the weaker, and the swifter defeating the slower. Natural ability enables this, not well-trained skills. 'A force of four ounces deflecting 1,000 pounds' is obviously not done through strength. How can it be speed that allows an 80- to 90-year-old to defeat a great number of men?"

斯技旁门甚多，虽势有区别，概不外乎壮欺弱，慢让快耳！有力打无力，手慢让手快，是皆先天自然之能，非关学力而有为也。察"四两拨千斤"之句，显非力胜；观耄耋能御众之形，快何能为？

"Stand like a poised scale and move like a turning wheel."
立如平准，活似车轮。
Note: The term for scale (píngzhǔn 平准) originally was the title for an official in the Han Dynasty in charge of setting prices. When local people paid tributes to the central government, this official calculated the worth of the tributes. Here it means being just, fair and precise. Some believe it means being as accurate as a scale.

"Placing the center of gravity to one side allows you to rotate easily; spreading your weight on both feet makes it hard to move. Many people have practiced Taijiquan for years but still cannot control and move the body in a Taiji sphere: They are always controlled by the opponent because they fail to recognize the flaw of double-weightedness."

偏沉则随，双重则滞。每见数年纯功不能运化者，率皆自为人制，双重之病未悟耳！

"To avoid being double-weighted, you must understand the relationship between yin and yang. To control the opponent by adhering to him or her (nián 粘) contains something of retreating with a soft movement or appearing to yield (zǒu 走), and so does yielding contain something of adhering. Yin is inseparable from yang, and vice versa. When you come to see that yin and yang complement each other, you can come to understand inner power (dǒngjín 懂劲). With this understanding, the more you practice, the higher your skill. Commit this to memory and think about it time and again. Gradually you will be able to accomplish anything you want."

欲避此病，须知阴阳。黏即是走，走即是黏。阴不离阳，阳不离阴，阴阳相济，方为懂劲。懂劲后愈练愈精，默识揣摩，渐至从心所欲。

"Forget about yourself and yield to others. Many err in seeking the far over what is near. Practitioners must be careful to study techniques correctly, for 'missing by a little will lead one 1,000 miles astray.'"

本是"舍已从人"，多识"舍近求远"！所谓"差之毫厘，谬之千里"，学者不可不详弁焉！

Note: The phrase "missing by a little will lead one 1,000 miles astray" comes from the book *Biography of Dongfang Suo* of the Han Dynasty.

"That is all of the treatise."

是为论。

Analysis

Brief and concise, the treatise expounds on the following concepts:

1. The name of Taiji originated from the ancient Taiji theory of the yin and yang, reflecting simple dialectics. Having been influenced by Zhou Dunyi, a Confucian idealist philosopher of the Song Dynasty, the author Wang Zongyue held philosophical views that combine Confucianism and Taoism.

2. Taijiquan is a kind of martial art since its techniques express the rules of offense and defense. Despite Taijiquan's having become slower and softer in recent years to play a larger role in healing and physical fitness, its movements are still a means of offense and defense for combat. Taijiquan belongs to a different category from qigong and daoyin (an ancient martial art for promoting health and curing diseases through combining regulated, controlled breathing with physical exercises), with a different origin and path of development.

3. The main principle behind the fighting techniques of Taijiquan is to "defeat hardness with softness" and to "forget oneself to yield to others." Technically, the principle opposes rash action and confrontation but seeks to respond like the Taiji sphere, diverting and changing the direction of the applied force and to "seek the straight in the curve." The

response keeps the body balanced and the qi sinking down to the dantian. The opponent cannot discover your intentions, and only you can detect the intention of the opponent. These principles constitute the features of Taijiquan as an exercise performed with a calm mind and a relaxed and upright body in gentle, continuous and flexible movements.

4. The techniques of "deflecting 1,000 pounds with a force of four ounces" and "responding quickly if the opponent's movement is quick; following slowly if the opponent's movement is slow" are typical of Taijiquan that can use a small force to defeat a strong opponent and that always greets motion with stillness. These ideas are also important in all other competitive sports and in military tactics. Yet the treatise holds that conquering the weak by the strong and defeating the slower by the swifter are something of a natural endowment and should be excluded from the techniques and tactics of offense and defense. That is a narrow and incorrect judgment.

2. Song of the 13 Methods

With 13 basic methods, Taijiquan is also known as The 13 Methods, and the song is also called "The Song of Taijiquan."

The 13 Methods should never be treated lightly.
The source of strength of the body and spirit is in the waist.

Pay attention to the changes between empty and solid;
Make sure that qi flows freely throughout the body.

Feel movement in stillness and seek stillness in movement;
Fill the opponent with wonder with your unpredictable responses.

Make a thorough study of the meaning and purpose of each movement.
This will make it easy to achieve the goal.

Always keep the mind centered in the waist;
When the abdomen is relaxed and at ease,
The qi can rise without hindrance.

Keep the tailbone straight to let "spirit of vitality" rise to the top of the head;
Then the whole body is relaxed and light,
The head is upright as if suspended on a string.

Research techniques deep to their roots,
Bend—extend, open—close, all will be done with high skill.

When entering the door, you need a teacher to lead the way;
Then you have to practice unceasingly and to study on your own.

What is the principle of Taijiquan that guides its application?
The mind and qi are king, and the bones and muscles are the subjects.

Think carefully what the ultimate aim of Taijiquan is:
To prolong life and maintain youth.

Every word in this song of 140 characters is true and accurate;
No important meaning of Taijiquan is left behind.

If you don't follow the song closely,
You will waste time and come to regret it.

十三总势莫轻视，　命意源头在腰隙。
变换虚实须留意，　气遍身躯不少滞。
静中触动动犹静，　因敌变化示神奇。
势势存心揆用意，　得来不觉费功夫。
刻刻留心在腰间，　腹内松静气腾然。
尾闾中正神贯顶，　满身轻利顶头悬。
仔细留心向推求，　屈伸开合听自由。
入门引路须口授，　功夫无息法自修。
若言体用何为准？　意气君来骨肉臣。
详推用意终何在？　益寿延年不老春。
歌兮歌兮百四十，　字字真切意无遗。
若不向此推求去，　枉费功夫贻叹息。

Analysis

Also called "Expositions of Insight into the Practice of the 13 Methods (Shísan Zŏngshì 十三总势)," the Song of the 13 Methods was composed to help in the practice of Taijiquan, and the 13 methods refers to the eight basic hand techniques and five basic stances: péng (棚 ward off), lǚ (将 roll back), jǐ (挤 press, squeeze), àn (按 push forward), căi (采 pull down), lio (捌 split), zhŏu (肘 elbow strike), kào (靠 shoulder/lean), and five basic foot techniques of jìnbù (进步 step in), tuìbù (退步 step back), zuǒgù (左顾 move to the left), yòupàn (右盼 move to the right), and zhōngdìng (中定 keep to the central position). Since it is written in colloquial Chinese, the Song might have been compiled based on Taijiquan folk songs and other works collected by Wang Zongyue from anonymous sources.

Wu Yuxiang (1821-1880) who preserved and passed down *The Genealogy of Taijiquan*, began learning Taijiquan from Yang Luchan, founder of the Yang Style Taijiquan. Then he went to Zhaobaozhen in Wenxian County, Henan Province to learn Zhaobao Style Taijiquan from Chen Qingping. He combined the two styles to create Wu Style Taijiquan. Wu Yuxiang made a thorough study of the Treatise on Taijiquan by Wang Zongyue. Whenever he came to understand something, he wrote his idea on a slip of paper and stuck it on the wall or added it to the song. People later collected these ideas into an article, entitled Insights into the Practice of the 13 Methods. The Song of the 13 Methods with Wu Yuxiang's insights on the methods have greatly promoted the development of Taijiquan.

Although it contains only 140 characters, the song is rich in content:

The Song points out that the mind and qi are inner and primary, the body is outer and secondary. The internal and the external form a harmonious whole with the mind and qi as the source, the bones and muscles as their application. All movements are motivated by qi and directed by the mind. Wu Yuxiang drew a vivid analogy: The mind (xīn 心) is the commander, vital life energy (qì 气) is the banner; the spirit of vitality (shén 神) is the general, and the body (shēn 身) is the one who follows orders. In saying that the source of strength of the body and spirit is in the waist (yāo 腰), the term used is yāoxī 腰膝, a place in the lumbar region of the spine that here refers to the acupuncture point of Mìngmén 命门. Traditional Chinese medicine holds that Mingmen is the root of vitality, or the root of the internal organs and the 12 channels and collaterals. The term for waist (yāojiān 腰间) in the 9th line refers to the lumbar vertebrae — the part of the spine that connects the upper and lower body and supports the trunk and that martial arts masters deem very important. A martial arts proverb says, "The waist (yāo 腰) is the trunk, and the limbs are the branches." Taijiquan masters put it as: "The waist and spine dictate to all," and "the waist is the axis."

The song stresses that while paying attention to the key points of the 13 methods, it is more important to keep in mind the source of strength of body and spirit (mìng yì yuánteu 命意源头) to allow qi to circulate throughout the body. In a nimble and well-coordinated body, let the spirit of vitality reach the top of the head so that the whole body is energized with qi. In short, the Song tells people that Taijiquan trains both the body and the mind, with the latter as the more important. Never practice Taijiquan by merely imitating the form. [Qi itself can be divided into inner and outer types. The outer qi refers to the air that we breathe. The inner qi refers to the vital energy flowing in the channels and collaterals, which is also called in traditional Chinese medicine primordial qi (元气) or central qi (中气). As to the essence of qi, some people say that it is biological electricity, while others say it is a life energy or the carrier of life functions. All this needs to be further studied.]

The Song of the 13 Methods also discusses form and techniques for both offense and defense. Strategies of attack and defense should be able to adapt quickly to an opponent's changes. Practically speaking, Taijiquan uses stillness to control movement and moves with tranquility.

The Song emphasizes that one must follow the key points of each position correctly, and "study techniques to their roots." It also stresses that a master can only show you the way to enter the door. You must keep practicing and studying on your own to be successful. If you are content with some superficial knowledge or rely on the teacher for all without any creativity or the use of your intelligence, you will never reach the realm of freedom.

The Song makes it clear that the purpose of learning Taijiquan is to maintain good health, extend the years of one's life and preserve youth. Ever since the martial arts came into being, their main purpose has been for keeping fit and combat. With the development of military technology, the combat aspect of martial arts has been reduced while the athletic aspect has increased. The practice of Taijiquan requires a calm mind and a relaxed body, with all the movements motivated by qi and directed by the mind. It is a typical way in Chinese culture to combine motion and stillness and to cultivate the mind and the body together to maintain good health. Therefore, the practice of Taijiquan has been a highly valuable way of physical exercise ever since its creation.

Today, the emphasis of Taijiquan should be on promoting universal good health. Any other approach would be contrary to the principles of sports and the teachings of the forefathers of Taijiquan.

Health Benefits

As both experience and scientific research have shown, Taijiquan is a physical activity that helps keep both the mind and body healthy. Combining motion and stillness, Taijiquan embodies Chinese cultural approaches to maintaining good health: Motion keeps the body fit while stillness nourishes the mind.

1. How Taijiquan Works on the Nervous System

When practicing Taijiquan, your mind should be calm with all movement initiated and directed by the mind (yì 意). The cortex of your brain should be in a protective state of rest. This is a kind of active rest for people who use their brains a lot at work, a helpful treatment for the modern sickness caused by too much tension and lack of exercise. Experiments show that the brain consumes 1/8 to 1/6 of the energy needed by the human body. Too much tension not only consumes a lot of energy but can also lead to a lack of coordination in the sympathetic and parasympathetic nervous systems, causing disruptions in the brain cortex and thus inviting many diseases. The practice of Taijiquan can dispel tension and fatigue in the nerves of the brain, refresh the mind, and activate the spirit. It can help regulate the nervous system and help cure some chronic diseases, promoting hormonal balance and improved immunity. Also, because Taijiquan requires the use of the mind, the brain continuously sends out benign signals to cause the qi, blood and energy to focus on the intended parts of the body in a way that can invigorate the body's metabolism and increase blood circulation by some 30 percent. Doctors sometimes use "biofeedback" to describe this phenomenon. Buddhist meditation, the ancient Chinese method of expiration and inspiration, and qigong in modern times are all examples of trying to cause physiological changes by using the mind and will. It is through "leading the body with the mind" (yǐ yì dǎotǐ 以意导体) and the "focus of the mind" (yìniàn guànzhù 意念贯注) that Taijiquan can assist the smooth circulation of blood and energy throughout the body.

2. How Taijiquan Works on the Cardiovascular System

The gentle and coordinated movements of Taijiquan can make the blood vessels more "springy" and the nerves steadier, thus more adaptable to changes in temperature and unexpected trauma. Not an intensive or aerobic exercise, Taijiquan can decrease blood pressure so that its faithful practice can help prevent high blood pressure and hardening of the arteries. Experiments have shown that constant intensive movement makes animals prone to high blood pressure, while gentle and moderate exercises can keep the blood pressure stable. Taijiquan is just such a moderate exercise. According to research, elderly people who practice Taijiquan on a regular basis enjoy normal blood pressure, a strong pulse and rarely suffer from arteriosclerosis.

3. How Taijiquan Works on the Respiratory System

To allow qi to sink down to the dantian, Taijiquan uses deep abdominal breathing in a way that intensifies the exercise of the diaphragm. Beyond increasing depth of breathing, this exercise of the diaphragm also stimulates the movement of the bowels, thus enhancing digestion as well as blood circulation in the abdomen.

4. How Taijiquan Works on the Bones and Muscles

To practice Taijiquan, one needs to keep the body upright, the feet steady and the joints flexible. The exercise will enable the practitioner to keep in good shape, have strong legs, and an agile, pliable, energetic and well-coordinated body. It truly helps to extend life while preserving a youthful appearance and attitude.

CHAPTER IV
TAIJIQUAN TRAINING

The Key Points — Stages of Practice — Tips for Beginners

Key Points

In performing Taijiquan, the body should be poised, naturally upright, relaxed, agile and steady. The Rules for Taijiquan Competition provide standards for postures (the stance as well as the positioning of the hands and feet) and movements (of the torso, hands, feet and sword) that also can serve as key points for the general practice of Taijiquan:

1. Push the Head Up; Be Calm and Natural (Xuán Dǐng Zhèng Reng 悬顶正容)

Keep the head and neck naturally straight to allow qi to rise to the top of the head. Imagine that the top of the head is being suspended from above. This is called "pushing up with the head without using strength." It helps to make a stance stable, invigorates the spirit and promotes the smooth flow of qi throughout the body as described in the Song of the 13 Methods:

"Keep the tailbone straight to let the spirit of vitality (shén神) rise to the top of the head; then the whole body is relaxed and light, and the head is upright as if suspended on a string."

Some people who practice Taijiquan let their heads and necks become too lax, giving them a weak and dispirited look. Or, they allow their heads to move back and forth or they lower their heads and bend at the waist. None of these is correct. Of course, don't force your head and neck so that they become tense and stiff. If you do, you are not "pushing up with the head without using strength." People who practice Taijiquan should just look natural as they are, calm and poised. Never become affected or put on airs.

2. Keep the Shoulders and Elbows Down (Chén Jian Zhuì Zhǒu 沉肩坠肘)

Keep the shoulders down and relaxed. Don't shrug the shoulders, arch them or stretch them back. When bending the elbows, bend them naturally with a feeling as if they are hanging slightly down. Never raise the elbows or stretch them out too straight. In this way your postures will look natural and your movements steady and gentle.

3. Stretch the Arms with Empty Armpits (Zhǎn Bì Xū Yè 展臂虚腋)

When practicing Taijiquan, the arms are filled or inflated with springy energy no matter if they are bent or straight. This quality is known in Taijiquan as Péngjìn (掤劲). When bent, the arms should not be soft or lax, nor should they be held too tight to the body or bent too much. Instead, keep the arms held in a curve and extended outward. When stretched straight, the arms should feel as if being pulled towards both ends, with the elbows sinking down but still bent slightly to form a curve. In this way, the arms will be gentle and natural as well as solid and full of strength. The "empty armpits" refers to keeping an empty space under the armpit rather than pressing the arms too tightly against the ribs. This way the movements look lively, round and natural.

4. Relax the Fingers and Lower the Wrist (Shū Zhǐ Ta Wàn 舒指塌腕)

Separate the fingers naturally in practicing Taijiquan and let the wrists sink to send strength into the palms, wrists, and all the joints of the fingers. Of course, the strength in the hands keeps changing in the interchange of movements from substantial to insubstantial. Also, different techniques and movements require different points to which force is applied in the hands. Yet no matter how the hands change, the fingers and the wrists should be neither too soft and relaxed nor too stiff. It is incorrect either to have the fingers bent and the wrist too loose or to hold the fingers close together and the wrist tense.

5. Sink (Bow in) the Chest and Broaden the Back (Hán Xiōng Bá Bèi 含胸拔背)

Sink the chest simply means that the chest should not stick out but rather be kept relaxed and comfortable in a natural way. Broadening the back makes it easier to move in a gentle, relaxed, circular and flexible way in Taijiquan. This is different from the other sturdier types of unarmed combat that require an expanded chest, tight back, and contracted abdomen. The important point in sinking the chest and broadening the back is just to be natural and relaxed, not to hunch the back or shrink the chest. Never sink the chest at the expense of being poised and natural.

6. Relax the Waist and Straighten the Spine (Sōng Yao Zhèng Jí 松腰正脊)

This is crucial for keeping the muscles of the waist and lower back relaxed and the body upright. Once the muscles of the waist tense up, movements cannot be agile and natural. Straightening the spine requires the spine to be upright and relaxed. Although some downward movements like Needle at the Bottom of the Sea may make the body lean slightly forward, still the spine should be straight, neither twisted nor contracted.

7. Keep the Hips and Buttocks Down (Suō Kuan Liǎn Tún 缩髋敛臀)

Most of the movements in Taijiquan are done by bending the legs into a half squat. Don't stick out the buttocks or hips, which distorts movement by causing the torso to lean forward or backward into a posture that is not upright. The correct way is to tuck in the hips and lower the buttocks to enable the torso to sit straight on the legs.

8. Lift Up the Perineum and Keep the Abdomen Firm (Tí Gang Shí Fù 提肛实腹)

To practice Taijiquan, one needs to sink the qi down to the Dantian — to exhale deeply when finishing a movement and to tense the abdominal muscles to increase pressure in the abdomen. At the same time, the muscles of the perineum (internal anal sphincter) are contracted and pulled up to keep the legs steady, firm and full of strength. The result cannot be achieved if the muscles of the abdomen and the perineum are too lax.

9. Bend the Legs and Drop the Hips (Qū Tuǐ Luò Kuà 屈腿落胯)

The movements of Taijiquan often require the bending of one leg, with that leg then carrying most of the body weight. The lower the posture and the more the leg is bent, the more physically demanding. To have a steady posture and correct movements, consciously keep the legs bent and the hips down. Either because of weak legs or a poor understanding of the key points, some people allow their center of gravity to go up and down; they don't bend their legs enough or straighten them up with a swaying or sticking out of the hips. All this should be corrected.

10. Keep the Knees Flexible and the Feet Solid on the Ground (Hue Xī Kòu Zú 活膝扣足)

Only when the knees are relaxed, agile and strong can the legs bend and stretch freely. So even when the leg is straight — for example, as in the back supporting leg of bow stance as well as in one-leg stance — the knee should never be tense or stiffly straight. Always keep some room ready for movement. Having the feet solid on the ground means to stand firmly and completely on the ground, with a steady center of gravity. For instance, in bow stance and crouch stance be careful not to raise the heels or the outer sides of the feet.

Stages of Practice

Taijiquan normally is divided into three stages of learning. In the first stage, practitioners must become familiar with the movements and have a good mastery of the form. In the second stage, practitioners need to improve their techniques through learning the mechanics of each posture and the principles behind various applications of intrinsic strength (jìn 劲). In the third stage, practitioners need to be able to combine qi with physical strength to reach a state of awareness in which they can do Taijiquan freely with grace and spirit. This is summarized in The Treatise of Taijiquan by Wang Zongyue:

"Through practicing toward proficiency, one gradually understands jìn (劲) . Through understanding jìn (劲) one begins to enter the realm of freedom."

1. The First Stage: Basics

In the basic stage of learning Taijiquan, most important is mastery of correct body position and movement, arm and hand techniques, stances and footwork, kicks and use of the eyes. All movements and techniques should be performed correctly. Also important is building up physical fitness through strength and conditioning exercises to prepare for the next stage of improving technical ability. In the basic stage, key points are:

(1) Relax the Body and Calm the Mind

Don't be tense or think about anything other than the Taijiquan exercise; gradually develop balance and self-control both physically and mentally. Taijiquan is a gentle and natural exercise that combines motion with stillness and cultivates both the body and mind. Some people think that to work hard at Taijiquan means to use more strength, but this idea only causes them to get tense and look flushed with effort. This is contrary to the philosophy of Taijiquan. Others can't seem to really relax during Taiji practice, which also prevents a good result because their minds are burdened with tensions and worries. A relaxed body and a calm mind are essential for the practice of Taijiquan. Only when the mind is at ease in a natural and relaxed state can one get focused into Taijiquan practice to "cultivate the mind in stillness and the body in motion."

(2) Keep the Body Upright

Keep the body comfortably upright, the head pushed up as if being suspended from above, the shoulders down and chest relaxed—a natural and dignified posture as seen in Buddhist meditation and qigong. Avoid any bad habits such as lifting the shoulders and hunching the back, or lowering the head and bending the waist, tensing up with a stiff and affected air, or leaning forward or backward. These should all be corrected.

(3) Correct Every Posture and Technique

Make sure to perform every movement correctly and exactly. Be clear about the rules and important points of all the postures and techniques. Even if at first you cannot meet the standard, understand clearly all instructions and guidelines. Don't rush to learn too much, or more than you can master. As the saying goes, "It is easy to learn but difficult to correct." Once an incorrect posture is learned, it takes much effort to correct it. The most effective and practical way to learn Taijiquan is to put quality before speed — to learn Taijiquan little-by-little correctly from the very beginning.

(4) Keep the Body Light, Agile and Steady

Most Taijiquan movements are performed with legs bent in a half squat with the body sitting upright on the legs. The stepping technique requires keeping one leg bent while in motion to support the center of gravity while, like a cat, moving the other leg lightly and landing it as if rooted in the ground. Although rather physically demanding, this is the characteristic of Taijiquan that makes movement agile, gentle and stable.

Strengthen the legs so that you can maintain a squat position without needing to stand up. Avoid an up-and-down, uneven movement. Some people just walk as they advance and retreat so that even after an hour's exercise they haven't managed to break a sweat, thus greatly reducing the effect of the exercise. Such people need more practice in basic footwork exercises like one-leg stance to strengthen their legs as well as more training in bending the legs and lowering the hips. Others make mistakes in the footwork or stances so that the torso sways or twists out of balance. To overcome these problems, these people need to work on their footwork and stepping techniques until they can meet basic technical standards.

(5) Be Relaxed, Natural and Flexible

Taijiquan postures and movements are not tense and stiff, nor are they soft and collapsed. Like blown up balloons, they are light yet filled with a springy inflated energy that extends outward to all directions. This is referred to in Taijiquan as Pengjin (péngjìn 掤劲), or firmness combined with flexibility. It is hard for beginners to master this skill, but aim for postures that are relaxed and natural, movements pliable but not soft, comfortable yet not stiff, appropriately firm and gentle. In short, present yourself in a natural way.

2. The Second Stage: Improvement

In this stage, students need to improve their techniques and perfect their mastery of the key points. Movements need to be well coordinated and continuous in a smooth flowing and natural circular motion without any break. In fact, the action of directing one's intrinsic strength (yùnjìn 运劲) and the action of the movement (yùndòng 运动) are two sides of the same thing. Sending intrinsic strength to the part of the body that is in motion ensures that movements are coordinated in a natural way. The application of intrinsic strength through appearing to yield (zhān 沾) and through adhering to keep control of the opponent and to stop him or her from getting away (nián 粘), and other techniques one after another forms continuity in the movements. So intrinsic strength and movements are closely connected and supplement each other. An important standard for technical improvement is mastery of the skills inherent in directing intrinsic strength in coordination with the techniques of the movements. In this stage, the major technical points are as follows:

(1) Coordinate Motion throughout the Whole Body

The practice of Taijiquan requires coordination of the movement of the hands, the eyes, the body and feet — a harmonious whole in which everything moves as one. For instance, in "Move the Hands like Clouds," as the waist and spine turn, the hands move like clouds while the arms cross each other in curves; meanwhile the center of gravity shifts from one leg to the other, the feet move sideways, and the eyes follow the hands as they rotate to the top of the curves, thus forming a non-stop movement involving coordination of the upper and lower parts of or the whole body. Beginners tend to pay attention to one movement and lose another, either the hands and feet are not in synch with each other or the hands and feet are not coordinated with the body so that movements appear mechanical and stiff — or as it is called in the martial arts: the movements have "a break in power" (duànjìn 断劲). Technical improvement in Taijiquan is marked by the ability to coordinate inner strength and physical movement.

(2) Move Smoothly and Naturally

The ability to move smoothly and naturally also demonstrates the level of skill of a Taijiquan practitioner. Just as in driving a car — which requires a good driver to keep the car moving steadily and evenly without sudden acceleration and veering to the left or right — the practice of Taijiquan requires smooth flowing movements that change naturally from one to another without any sudden forced interruptions. To achieve this, the turning of the waist and arms is very important. The waist should be like an axis that leads the movement of the four limbs. Meanwhile, the arms provide an axis for the hands so the whole motion "is rooted in the feet, controlled by the waist and manifested through the fingers."

(3) Move with Continuity

The movements of Taijiquan follow one another continuously without any obvious pause or break. To make it easier for students in the learning process, movements are often broken down for demonstration. But after learning the correct way to perform, all breaks in movement should be removed to ensure that "when postures change, the internal force is continuous; when the intrinsic strength changes the mind (yì 意) is not disturbed." Two movements are connected first by the will (yìniàn 意念) and qi, then by the waist and legs which lead the arms to change gradually from the internal to the external. Never start or stop a change in movement too stiffly or abruptly.

3. The Third Stage: Freedom

The goal of this stage is to achieve a union of spirit and form, internal and external, and qi and strength. Movements should be charged with intrinsic strength; vital spirit; rich expression of open or closed, empty or solid in a performance that inspires. The key points for training at this level are:

(1) Direct the Body with the Mind, and Make a Clear Distinction Between Substantial and Insubstantial

When practicing Taijiquan, the mind must be thoroughly concentrated. Most beginners can focus only on remembering the movements and technical points so that they concentrate on the hands and feet. After becoming familiar with the movements, one should concentrate on coordinating all parts of the body, with a focus on the waist and feet. With further improvement, turn to the differentiation of the substantial and insubstantial and the hard and soft applications of intrinsic strength, focusing on the direction of the mind. It is the same as when a good actor needs to impress the audience: He must present the inner world of the role by showing the inner feelings instead of merely the outer form. Taijiquan also emphasizes the mind (yì 意) over form (xíng 形).

Beneath its apparent steady and quiet appearance, Taijiquan is dynamic, full of changes as movements alternate between substantial and insubstantial, firmness and gentleness in internal energy, gathering and releasing of strength, and opening and closing the body. Generally speaking, every movement in Taijiquan has four stages: Beginning, continuing, landing and closing. Beginning and continuing are performed in the insubstantial stage as a technique turns from releasing to gathering with a rather gentle touch. The body should be open inside and closed outside. Landing and closing belong to the substantial stage as the technique turns from gathering to releasing with a steady and solid strength. The body should be closed inside and open outside, filled with a balanced and springy energy. These changes and applications of techniques are all directed by the mind, which is followed by the body. Only when the qi and the postures are in harmony can changes in technique be completely realized. Therefore, Taijiquan is never a pool of stagnant water; it is always full of vitality and change.

(2) Motivate the Body with Qi and Combine Strength with Qi

Beginners are required only to breathe naturally as needed; breathing need not be restricted by the movements. But as skills advance, consciously match breathing with movements to bring out a better result in both. This is called "posture breathing" (quánshì hūxī 拳式呼吸).

Generally speaking, when a movement turns into the substantial stage, start exhaling consciously to reinforce strength with qi. When a movements turns into the insubstantial stage, inhale consciously to help with the change of movement. As a classic of Taijiquan puts it: "Only when one knows how to breathe, can one become agile."

In fact, with or without our awareness, our daily breathing is coordinated with our body movements and use of strength. When movements are upward, rising, stretching and opening — the chest expands and we inhale. When landing, descending, contracting and closing — the chest contracts and we exhale. In short, inhale when gathering strength, and exhale when releasing strength. Taijiquan turns normal breathing to the conscious application of "posture breathing," so Taijiquan breathing is active and natural.

But to practice Taijiquan does not mean to replace natural breathing with "posture breathing." Since Taijiquan is not a breathing exercise, its movements are not based on breathing patterns but rather on techniques designed for combat. The number of inhalations and exhalations and the rhythm of breathing differs not only in different forms of Taijiquan, but even in the same form of Taijiquan depending on differences in physical conditioning, age and technical skills. The only requirement is to use "posture breathing" in the obvious opening or closing movements. In the transitional movements — or when breathing becomes difficult — we still need natural breathing or may need to adjust with some supplementary short breathing. So Taijiquan always combines "posture breathing" with natural breathing. At the same time, some short transitional breathing is also needed for adjustments to ensure the smooth cultivation of qi.

(3) Be Composed and Full of Spirit

The ultimate aim of Taijiquan is a purely natural and profound state in which a relaxed body and peaceful mind enjoy a free and elegant artistic expression. Therefore, classic Taijiquan theory holds that Taijiquan "uses the mind not power ... the strength lies not in postures but in the application of qi." In the practice of Taijiquan, we should gradually go beyond the exactness of the movements and technical points into the realm of spiritual expression and artistic skill. There are people whose understanding and study of Taijiquan stops at the form itself. They perform the movements up to standard, but lack vitality and spiritual expression. As in all art forms, "knowing and abiding by the rules" serve as a ladder for progress. Only by "going beyond the rules but still keeping the rules" can Taijiquan have boundless vitality and enter the "realm of freedom in which all the techniques can be used at will with expertise."

Tips for Beginners

1. Develop Self-Confidence

Some people think that Taijiquan is very abstruse, hence the saying in martial arts circles: "Taijiquan keeps one practicing at home for 10 years." Actually, that is only a variation on "there is no limit in art." As a gentle, relaxed and safe exercise, Taijiquan is easy for people to practice and master regardless of age and physical conditioning so long as they put some effort into it. For beginners, the greatest difficulty is that Taijiquan has so many movements that seem complicated and hard to remember and coordinate. But beginners will find they can perform Taijiquan fairly well in only a few months if they practice with confidence, study hard under the guidance of a teacher, follow the basic rules of Taijiquan, and don't try to learn too much, too fast without thorough understanding.

2. Practice Regularly

The way to learn Taijiquan is not "to spend three days fishing and two days drying nets." It takes a period of time, not just a few times, for Taijiquan to bolster fitness and health. Some people give up half way because they can't see immediate results, or they feel bored or discouraged because they fail to master the key points of Taijiquan. Other people may quit because of aches in the body from the exercise. But this is the process in which the joints and muscles are adapting to the demands of exercise, and it is common for people — particularly those who are not physically fit or who are not used to the exercises — to feel some pain in the joints and muscles after exercise, especially in the thighs. Keep practicing even if you have a few aches and pains, but let up accordingly on the intensity of exercise or straighten your legs a little bit. After a while, the pain will be gone.

3. Make Progress Step by Step

Some people want to learn quickly, so they make a detour by following along in all the movements perfunctorily with the thought of going back later to correct them. Others believe the more the better. They learn quite a few forms of Taijiquan, but not well, so they gain little from Taijiquan despite their seemingly impressive repertoire. As we know, the results of exercise are closely related to the quality of the performance. Without correct postures and movements, there will be no therapeutic benefits. Once an incorrect posture is formed, it is harder to correct that mistake than it is to learn a new posture. Also, if a movement is learned too quickly and in a perfunctory manner, the movement is easy to forget if not practiced for a few days. So Taijiquan must be learned slowly, step by step, little by little, but thoroughly. Only with a good foundation, can you achieve great results and quick progress.

4. Pay Special Attention to the Basics

Laying a solid foundation entails two things: First, it means to learn postures and techniques correctly up to standard, ensuring that every posture and movement is done perfectly. Second, it means to have solid basic skills, good physical conditioning and an ability to meet the specific physical requirements for Taijiquan. The belief that training in basic skills is necessary only for technical improvement — and that therefore beginners need not take on training in basic skills too early — is not right. We don't have to argue which comes first: Learning the form of Taijiquan or learning the basic skills of Taijiquan. What is important is that the two cannot be separated. Without basic skills, the form cannot be done right and its quality will be shaky. Without the form, basic skills will be aimless and fruitless. The best way is to combine the study of both skills and form at the early stage: Learn the form while doing the necessary specialized individual practices on skills like one-leg stance, stepping, leg-stretching, and various hand and foot techniques. This will help you master the key points of Taijiquan earlier and faster. Learning the form better with a correct start will mean making fewer mistakes, and avoiding a detour.

5. Practice in an Appropriate Way

If after doing Taijiquan you feel warm, relaxed, comfortable and in high spirits — you have practiced in an appropriate way in terms of time, height of posture, and precision of the performance. For instance, performing the postures at different heights puts different pressure on the legs with a subsequent difference on the amount of exercise involved. What the appropriate amount of exercise is varies from person to person. If the amount is insufficient, the lack of exercise will prevent the expected result. If the amount is too much, the exercise will make you tired and harm your health. Normally, when you feel warm and are sweating, that is enough. Those who are physically weak or are in the recovery stage of illness or injury should follow the advice of a doctor or teacher. For the elderly and those who are not strong enough, if they find it difficult to finish a whole set of movements, they can select basic parts of the movements. Those who cannot move their lower limbs can still do the basic waist and upper body movements, and if they follow the principles and practice regularly, they also will achieve good results.

6. Control Speed

Since beginners have to think about a movement before they can do it or while they are doing it, the speed of the exercise should be slow, and there can be some pauses in the process. For instance, doing 24-Step Taijiquan with proficiency normally takes about five minutes. But beginners can take eight to ten minutes to finish the form more slowly. At a slow pace, you can take care of the details of each step, check the movements and correct mistakes as they occur. A slow tempo makes it easier to calm the mind, relax the body and maintain a steady center of gravity. After becoming familiar with the movements, practice a little faster without any pause, trying to make the movements flow naturally in an even yet lively way. Different forms of Taijiquan can have different speeds owing to varying styles and number of movements. For example, the 81-Step Yang-style Taijiquan, with its smooth extended postures and simple and steady movements, takes 15-20 minutes to finish. The Sun-style Taijiquan — close-knit and agile, with constant changes in foot and hand techniques — normally takes eight minutes even though it has over 90 movements. Regardless of its form, every kind of Taijiquan requires a consistent flow of qi, with an even speed from beginning to end.

7. Select a Good Time and Place for Taijiquan

The best time to practice Taijiquan is in the morning or evening. Doing Taijiquan in the morning helps refresh the mind, work out morning kinks, and prepare one for the day's work and study. Doing Taijiquan in the evening helps get rid of fatigue with an active rest. As it is usually quiet in the morning and evening, it is easy to concentrate the mind. After the exercise, it's good to quiet down for a while from the stimulation of the exercise before taking breakfast or rest. Also, breaks during working hours and classes are a good time for Taijiquan exercise. An ideal place for practicing Taijiquan would be one with fresh air and a quiet environment such as a park, woods or yard without wind, dust, smoke or smog. Indoors, it is better to have some sunlight and good ventilation. When doing Taijiquan, it is better to wear loose, comfortable clothing or sportswear. Shoes with hard soles will hinder the exercise. Wear a hat and gloves if it is too cold. To avoid catching a cold, dry off sweat after exercise.

8. Do Warming-Up and Cooling-Down Exercises

Warming-up exercises for Taijiquan can include slow running, gymnastics, standing on one leg, stretching the legs, rotating the waist, etc. These preparatory exercises should be done seriously and sufficiently without too much intensity. Since Taijiquan is a gentle and slow sport, many neglect warming-up and cooling-down exercises. But it is well known that warming-up exercises are necessary to prepare people for athletic activity: If the muscles and joints of the body are stiff, and the mind is still occupied with something else, it is hard to get into a relaxed and calm state of mind for Taijiquan. Warming-up includes both mind and body. Warming-up the body removes sluggishness to get the body moving into an active state from a resting state; it gets stiffness out of muscles, joints, and ligaments; and it invigorates the spine and internal organs involved in athletics. Warming-up also reduces mental tension to help the mind calm down for its concentration on the exercise.

Cooling-down exercises at the end helps restore internal organs back to a resting state and to remove fatigue. They can be done through relaxing gymnastics, walking, games involving a light workout and massage to relieve tired knees and to work out any muscle tension. Some people have the habit of sitting down immediately or standing still to have a rest. These habits are not good — especially in that they could harm the knees — and should be corrected.

9. Seek a Balanced and Reasonable Training Program

Although Taijiquan is an exercise that helps maintain good health — like all other sports, it has some limitations. The most obvious limitation for Taijiquan is its lack of exercise for strengthening the arms and its lack of aerobic exercise for the body. For a comprehensive workout, those having the means and capabilities can select other appropriate sports to supplement and reinforce Taijiquan. To avoid over-fatigue and conflicts in practice, make reasonable arrangements of your time and strength for different kinds of sports. Some sports can be done at regular intervals with Taijiquan, while others may need to be done at some other time.

CHAPTER V

81-STEP YANG-STYLE TAIJIQUAN

Bāshíyī Shì Yángshì Tàijíquán 八十一式杨式太极拳

Introduction

Yang-style Taijiquan was created by Mr. Yang Luchan (1799-1872) of Yongnian County, Hebei Province, refined by his son Yang Jianhou (1839-1917) and completed by his grandson Yang Chengfu (1883-1936). The most widely practiced Taijiquan style in and outside China, Yang style is performed with a poised upright body and a slow even rhythm. It is noted for its smooth relaxed postures and gentle movements — soft but not weak, steady but not stiff. It naturally combines firmness with flexibility, with profound inner strength.

At first, Yang Chengfu set the number of steps of Yang-style Taijiquan as 81, but in his later years he changed the number to 85 by repeating the movement of "brushing aside over the knee in reverse forward stance," dividing the "turn around to tame the tiger left and right" into the left and right steps, and breaking "single bian [鞭] downward" into two movements, "single bian" and "push downward." The rest of the movements remain unchanged. Yang-style Taijiquan has variations such as the forms with 88 steps, 107 steps and 115 steps. These retain the basic movements while breaking some of them down into smaller and more detailed movements.

Li Yulin was dean of studies of the Shandong Provincial Martial Arts School when he was photographed in 1931 performing the complete set of the Yang-style Taijiquan in a project to provide teaching material for the school under the direction of Mr. Yang Chengfu [see above] and Li Jinglin, deputy head of the school he established in 1928. Tian Zhenfeng and Guo Shiquan directed the photography and edited the photographs into a textbook for which Li Jinglin wrote on the cover the title, *Textbook of Taijiquan*. This then became the most popularly accepted text in China on Taijiquan.

Li Jinglin was best known for his skills with the sword, known as the "Magic Sword." A student of Yang Jianhou [the father of Yang Chengfu, see above], he had a profound command of Taijiquan. Influential in martial arts circles, he also established in 1927 the National Martial Arts School in Nanjing with Zhang Zhijiang. After holding the National Martial Arts Competition in 1929 in Shanghai, he often discussed with Yang Chengfu how to summarize and popularize Yang-style Taijiquan. Li Yulin joined their work along with Chen Weiming, Wu Huichuan and Zhu Guiting.

The *Textbook of Taijiquan* features the typical Yang-style smooth, comfortable and upright postures, well-composed with gentle and steady movements. As some of the movements differ slightly from what Yang Chengfu taught, the 81-Step Taijiquan was referred to decades ago as the "Yang-style Taijiquan with Li-style Movements."

After the founding of the People's Republic of China in 1949, the 88-Step Yang-style Taijiquan was published by the State Physical Culture and Sports Commission, based on this set of Taijiquan.

Names of the Movements of 81-Step Yang-style Taijiquan

Pinyin Chinese (English)
1. Yùbèishì 预备势 (Ready Position)
2. Tàijí Qǐshì 太极起势 (Begin Taiji Position)
3. Lǎnquèwěi 揽雀尾 (Grasp the Peacock's Tail)
4. Dānbiān 单鞭 (Single Bian) *
5. Tíshǒu 提手 (Lift the Hands)
6. Báihè Liàngchì 白鹤亮翅 (White Crane Spreads Its Wings)
7. Lōuxī Àobù 搂膝拗步 (Brush Aside Over the Knee in Reverse Forward Stance)
8. Shǒuhuī Pípā 手挥琵琶 (Play the Pipa**)
9. Zuǒyòu Lōuxī Àobù 左右搂膝拗步 (Brush Aside over the Knee in Reverse Forward Stance — Left and Right)
10. Shǒuhuī Pípā 手挥琵琶 (Play the Pipa)
11. Jìnbù Bānlánchuí 进步搬拦捶 (Step In, Deflect, Block and Punch)
12. Rúfēng Sìbì 如封似闭 (Pull Back then Push, As if to Close)
13. Shízìshǒu 十字手 (Cross Hands)

---

* Dānbiān 单鞭 (Single Bian): "Dān" means single. "Biān" here refers to an ancient weapon, an iron rod that is either rectangular in shape or edged as in bamboo, or other patterns. Bian were often used in pairs, hence Danbian means Single Bian.

** Shǒuhuī Pípā 手挥琵琶 (Play the Pipa): A pipa is a pear-shaped Chinese four-stringed musical instrument made of wood, plucked, and usually held perpendicular with the body of the instrument on the performer's knee.

14. Bàohǔ Guīshān 抱虎归山 (Hold the Tiger and Return to the Mountain)
15. Zhǒudǐ Kànchuí 肘底看捶 (Fist Under the Elbow)
16. Zuǒyòu Dàoniǎnhóu 左右倒撵猴 (Drive the Monkeys Back Left and Right)
17. Xiéfēishì 斜飞势 (Diagonal Flying Posture)
18. Tíshǒu 提手 (Lift the Hands)
19. Báihè Liàngchì 白鹤亮翅 (White Crane Spreads Its Wings)
20. Lōuxī Àobù 搂膝拗步 (Brush Aside over the Knee in Reverse Forward Stance)
21. Hǎidǐzhēn 海底针 (Needle at the Bottom of the Sea)
22. Shàntōngbèi 扇通背 (Fan through the Back)
23. Piēshēnchuí 撇身捶 (Turn and Punch)
24. Jìnbù Bānlánchuí 进步搬拦捶 (Step In, Deflect, Block and Punch)
25. Shàngbù Lǎnquèwěi 上步揽雀尾 (Step Forward and Grasp the Peacock's Tail)
26. Dānbiān 单鞭 (Single Bian)
27. Yúnshǒu 云手 (Move the Hands Like Clouds)
28. Dānbiān 单鞭 (Single Bian)
29. Gāotànmǎ 高探马 (Gauge the Height of the Horse)
30. Zuǒyòu Fēnjiǎo 左右分脚 (Separate Feet Right and Left)
31. Zhuǎnshēn Zuǒ Dēngjiǎo 转身左蹬脚 (Turn and Kick with the Left Heel)
32. Zuǒyòu Lōuxī Àobù 左右搂膝拗步 (Brush Aside over the Knee in Reverse Forward Stance — Left and Right)
33. Shàngbù Zāichuí 上步栽捶 (Step Forward and Punch Downward)
34. Fānshēn Báishé Tǔxìn 翻身白蛇吐信 (Turn Around and White Snake Spits Poison)
35. Shàngbù Bānlánchuí 上步搬拦捶 (Step Forward, Deflect, Block and Punch)
36. Yòu Dēngjiǎo 右蹬脚 (Kick with the Right Heel)
37. Zuǒyòu Pīshēn Fúhǔ 左右披身伏虎 (Turn Around to Tame the Tiger Left and Right)
38. Huíshēn Yòu Dēngjiǎo 回身右蹬脚 (Turn Around and Kick with the Right Heel)
39. Shuāngfēng Guàn'ěr 双峰贯耳 (Strike the Opponent's Ears with Both Fists)
40. Zuǒ Dēngjiǎo 左蹬脚 (Kick with the Left Heel)

41. Zhuǎnshēn Yòu Dēngjiǎo 转身右蹬脚 (Turn Around and Kick with the Right Heel)
42. Jìnbù Bānlánchuí 进步搬拦捶 (Step In, Deflect, Block and Punch)
43. Rúfēng Sìbì 如封似闭 (Pull Back then Push, As if to Close)
44. Shízìshǒu 十字手 (Cross Hands)
45. Bàohǔ Guīshān 抱虎归山 (Hold the Tiger and Return to the Mountain)
46. Héng Dānbiān 横单鞭 (Horizontal Single Bian)
47. Zuǒyòu Yěmǎ Fēnzōng 左右野马分鬃 (Part the Wild Horse's Mane—Left and Right)
48. Jìnbù Lǎnquèwěi 进步揽雀尾 (Step In and Grasp the Peacock's Tail)
49. Dānbiān 单鞭 (Single Bian)
50. Yùnǚ Chuānsuō 玉女穿梭 (Jade Maiden Moves the Shuttle Left and Right)
51. Jìnbù Lǎnquèwěi 进步揽雀尾 (Step In and Grasp the Peacock's Tail)
52. Dānbiān 单鞭 (Single Bian)
53. Yúnshǒu 云手 (Move the Hands Like Clouds)
54. Dānbiān Xiàshì 单鞭下势 (Single Bian Downward)
55. Zuǒyòu Jīnjī Dúlì 左右金鸡独立 (Golden Rooster Stands on One Leg, Left and Right)
56. Zuǒyòu Dàoniǎnhóu 左右倒撵猴 (Drive the Monkeys Back Left and Right)
57. Xiéfēishì 斜飞势 (Diagonal Flying Posture)
58. Tíshǒu 提手 (Lift the Hands)
59. Báihè Liàngchì 白鹤亮翅 (White Crane Spreads Its Wings)
60. Lōuxī Àobù 搂膝拗步 (Brush Aside over the Knee in Reverse Forward Stance)
61. Hǎidǐzhēn 海底针 (Needle at the Bottom of the Sea)
62. Shàntōngbèi 扇通背 (Fan through the Back)
63. Piēshēnchuí 撇身捶 (Turn and Punch)
64. Jìnbù Bānlánchuí 进步搬拦捶 (Step In, Deflect, Block and Punch)
65. Shàngbù Lǎnquèwěi 上步揽雀尾 (Step Forward and Grasp the Peacock's Tail)
66. Dānbiān 单鞭 (Single Bian)
67. Yúnshǒu 云手 (Move the Hands Like Clouds)
68. Dānbiān 单鞭 (Single Bian)
69. Gāotànmǎ 高探马 (Gauge the Height of the Horse)
70. Zhuǎnshēn Shízìjiǎo 转身十字脚 (Turn Around and Cross the Feet)

71. Lōuxī Zhǐdāngchuí 搂膝指裆锤 (Brush Aside over the Knee and Punch Down toward the Crotch)
72. Shàngbù Lǎnquèwěi 上步揽雀尾 (Step Forward and Grasp the Peacock's Tail)
73. Dānbiān Xiàshì 单鞭下势 (Single Bian Downward)
74. Shàngbù Qīxīng 上步七星 (Step Forward and Seven Stars)*
75. Tuìbù Kuàhǔ 退步跨虎 (Step Back to Ride the Tiger)
76. Zhuǎnshēn Bǎilián 转身摆莲 (Turn Around and Lotus Swing)
77. Wāngōng Shèhǔ 弯弓射虎 (Draw the Bow and Shoot the Tiger)
78. Jìnbù Bānlánchuí 进步搬拦捶 (Step In, Deflect, Block and Punch)
79. Rúfēng Sìbì 如封似闭 (Pull Back then Push, As if to Close)
80. Shízìshǒu 十字手 (Cross Hands)
81. Hétàijí 合太极 (Return to Beginning Taiji Position)

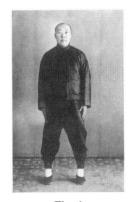
Fig. 1

Movements and Illustrations of Yang-style Taijiquan

1. Yùbèishì 预备势 (Ready Position)

Stand naturally straight, head and neck upright, feet parallel and shoulder-width apart. Let the hands hang naturally at the sides of the thighs. Look straight ahead. Imagine you are facing South. (Fig. 1)

Important Points

Stand straight, be calm, relaxed and natural with a peaceful mind and steady heart. Breathe naturally.

2. Tàijí Qǐshì 太极起势 (Begin Taiji Position)

2.1 Raise the Arms

Raise the arms slowly until the hands reach the level of the shoulders, shoulder-width apart, palms facing down. (Fig. 2)

2.2 Bend the Legs and Press Down with the Palms

Bend the legs slowly into a half squat. Press the palms

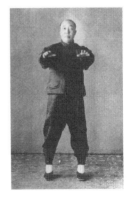
Fig. 2

---

* Shàngbù Qīxīng 上步七星 (Step Forward and Seven Stars): This name could refer to the shape the body takes in this position as being similar to the Big Dipper. It also could be a reference to the seven stars or "bright spots" of Taijiquan, the seven parts of the body that can be used as weapons: The head, the shoulders, the elbows, the hands, the hips, the knees and the feet.

of the open hands gently downward to the level of the abdomen. (Fig. 3)

Important Points

● Move gently, evenly and slowly as if swimming in water.

● Keep your body upright, comfortable and natural. Push up with the head and lower the shoulders. Relax the chest, keep the elbows down, keep the spine straight, relax the back, bend the knees, lower the hips.

● The level to which the knees bend can differ according to the individual. Do the best you can, naturally and appropriately. Don't push yourself too much. On the other hand, don't be too lax.

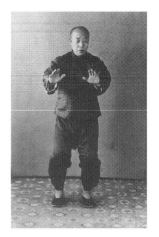

Fig. 3

Common Mistakes

● The torso leans too much forward or backward.

● The movements are too tense, the chest is thrust out, the buttocks stick out, the breath is held.

3. Lǎnquèwěi 揽雀尾 (Grasp the Peacock's Tail)

3.1 Ward Off in Left Bow Stance

3.1.1 Shift the body center to the right, move the toes of the right foot outward, turn the torso half to the right, the right arm should bend as if holding something in front of the right side of the chest. The left hand makes a circle to stop in front of the right side of the abdomen. The palms face each other as if holding a ball. Look at the right forearm. (Fig. 4)

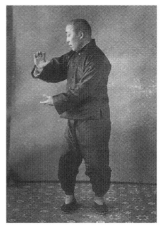

Fig. 4

3.1.2 Bring the left foot to the inside of the right ankle and step forward to the left gently with your heel touching the ground first, the whole foot stepping firmly on the ground. The center of the body moves forward, the right leg is naturally straightened, the right heel kicks down. Bend the left knee forward to form a left bow stance. Separate the hands, bend the left elbow half-way and extend the arm upward in front of the body with the hand at shoulder height, palm facing inside. Press the right hand down along the right side of the hip, palm down. Look at the left hand. (Fig. 5)

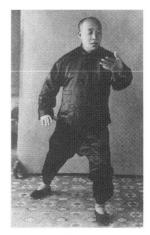

Fig. 5

3.2 Ward Off in Right Bow Stance

3.2.1 Turn the left hand downward, the right hand makes a circle and stops before the left side of the abdomen, the two palms facing each other as if holding a ball. Look at the left forearm. (Fig. 6)

3.2.2 Turn the torso to the right, bring the right foot to the inside of the left ankle and step forward to the right (West). Land the heel first, shift the body center forward, root the right foot, and straighten the left leg naturally. Bend the right knee to form a right bow stance. The hands separate in curves with the right arm bent in front of the body at shoulder height, right palm facing in. The left palm presses down alongside the left hip, palm down. Look at the right hand. (Fig. 7)

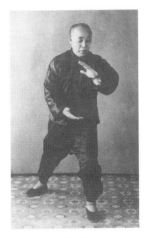

Fig. 6

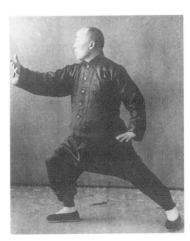

Fig. 7

Important Points

• The direction of the left bow stance should be the same as the beginning position, that is, South. The direction of the right bow stance should be West.

• Ward off (péng 掤), one of the major defensive techniques of Taijiquan, means to move forward to intercept the opponent in a counter-attack with the focus of power on the outside of the forearms.

• The movement of the feet in Taijiquan is "rise gently; fall gently" and "point, rise; point, fall" (Qīngqǐ qīngluò, diǎnqǐ diǎnluò. 轻起轻落，点起点落). That is, with the weight on one leg, raise the heel of the other foot first, then the whole foot steps forward. When touching the ground, gently lands the heel first, then the whole foot lands firmly as the body center shifts.

• Coordinate the arms and legs so that they work naturally together.

• Bow stance (gōngbù 弓步), one of the major stances in Taijiquan, requires the bending of the front leg so that the knee is above the front toes, the back leg thrust naturally straight but with the back knee a little flexed. Keep the waist and hips relaxed and steady. The width between the feet should be suitable.

Common Mistakes

● The timing of the legs and arms in motion is not synchronized: The hands are too slow and the feet too fast, or the hands are too fast and the feet too slow.

● When "holding the ball," the hands are limp, or when extending the arms, the hands are stiff.

● The feet land too heavily; the body center is unstable and the body sways.

3.3 Roll Back in Back Stance

3.3.1 Move the torso a little to the right. Turn the right hand and stretch it forward with the palm down. Move the left hand under the right forearm, with palm up. Look at the right hand. (Fig. 8)

3.3.2 Turn the torso to the left, shift the body center backward, bend the left leg and keep the right leg naturally straight. Press the hands down in a circular motion from the front to the left back until the left hand reaches shoulder height with palm down. The right hand reaches chest height with palm facing the inside. Look at the left hand and face Southeast. (Figs. 9, 10)

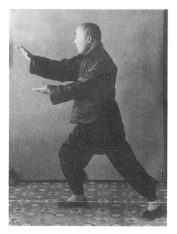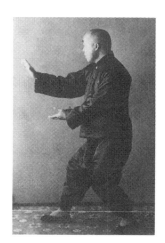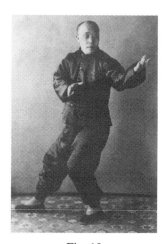

| Fig. 8 | Fig. 9 | Fig. 10 |

Important Points

● The hand technique called roll back (lǚ 捋) means to lead the opponent back by drawing the hands back, coordinated with bending the leg and sitting back.

● This technique should be synchronized with the shifting of the body center and turning of the waist.

● Keep the torso straight.

Common Mistakes

● The stroke back is not synchronized with the turning of the waist, making the shoulders and arms too tense.

● The head lowers, the waist bends.

3.4 Press Forward and Bow Stance

3.4.1 Turn the torso right toward the West. Stop the hands in front of the chest with the palms facing each other. Point the left fingers forward, touching the inside of the right wrist. Look straight ahead. (Fig. 11)

3.4.2 Shift the body center forward to form a right bow stance while pressing the back (left) hand forward against the front (right) hand with the palms facing each other, while bending the arms to make a circle at shoulder height. Look straight ahead. (Fig. 12)

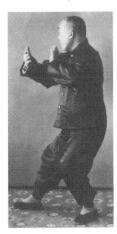

Fig. 11

Important Points

● The hand technique called pressing (jǐ 挤) involves moving forward into the opponent coordinated with the shifting of the legs into a bow stance.

● When fixing the form, extend the arms in curves with the torso straight and the head pushed up. Lower the shoulders and elbows and relax the lower back.

Common Mistakes

● The body leans forward, the head is lowered, the back is hunched.

● The body is not turned enough so that the side of the body pushes forward.

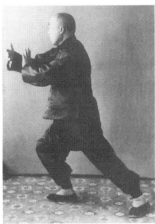

Fig. 12

3.5 Draw Back and Push Forward

3.5.1 Separate the hands to shoulder width and shift the center of the body back. Bend the left leg while straightening the right leg, lifting the right toes up. Pull the hands back to the chest, palms down. Look straight ahead. (Fig. 13)

3.5.2 Shift the body center forward to form a right bow stance again. Press the hands down in front of the chest to the ribs and then press forward until the arms are naturally straight at shoulder height, palms forward and fingertips

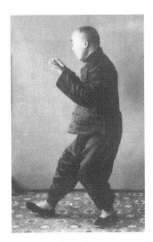

Fig. 13

upward. Look straight ahead. (Fig. 14)

Important Points

• The hand technique called pushing (àn 按) forward involves first leading the opponent in to thwart
an attack. Then take advantage of the opportunity to
push in a counter-attack.

• When drawing back the hands, do not touch them
to the chest. When pushing forward, bend the elbows
a little so that the arms are not completely straight. Pull
back the hands and push forward in a flowing and natural circular motion.

• The torso is always relaxed and straight. Coordinate the movements of the arms and legs with breathing.

Common Mistakes

• The hands are too stiff and straight when they are
pulled back and pushed forward.

• The timing is off in the movement of the hands and
the feet.

• The torso leans forward or backward.

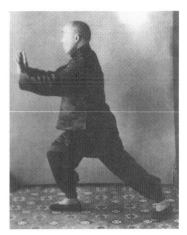

Fig. 14

4. Dānbiān 单鞭 (Single Bian)

4.1 Turn the Waist and Swing the Hand

Move the body center to the left. Turn the torso
left and bend the left leg. Keep the right leg straight,
turn the toes of the right foot inside while the hands
move horizontally from right to left. Swing the left
hand to the Southeast at shoulder height. Swing the
right hand in front of the left side of the chest, both
palms slanted downward. Look at the left hand. (Figs.
15, 16)

4.2 Hook the Hand and Draw In the Foot

Move the body center to the right, turning the
torso toward the right. Draw the left foot in to the
inside of the right foot, with the toes touching the
ground. Meanwhile, move the right hand right toward the Southeast while drawing the fingers of the
right hand together to form a hook at shoulder height
with the fingertips pointing downward. Press the left

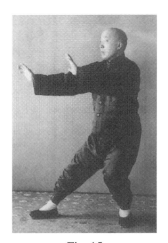

Fig. 15

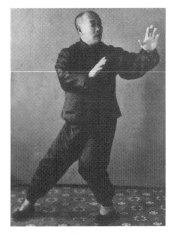

Fig. 16

hand downward to the right in a curve, past the abdomen and up to the right shoulder, palm facing in. Look at the hook hand. (Figs. 17, 18)

4.3 Bow Stance and Push with the Palm

Turn the torso to the right. Step the left foot forward to the North by East. Shift the body center forward, kicking the right leg straight. Bend the left leg to form a left bow stance. Turn the left hand and push forward past the chin at shoulder height, the elbow a little bent over the left knee. Raise the right hook hand to the left rear, to a position South by West, shoulder height. Look at the left hand. (Fig. 19)

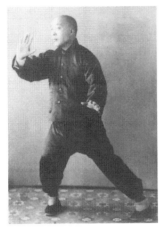 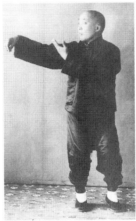 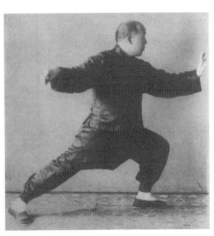

Fig. 17   Fig. 18   Fig. 19

Important Points

● The open-palm hand (zhǎng 掌) and the hook hand (gōushǒu 勾手) are basic Taijiquan hand techniques. When pushing the palm, naturally straighten and separate the five fingers and slightly CUP the palm, keep the wrist down and the fingers up. In the hook hand, hold the five fingertips together, bend the wrist and point the fingertips downward.

● Coordinate the left and right swing of the hands with the turning of the waist and the shifting of the body center.

● When forming a bow stance, kick the back leg straight with the turning of the waist while pushing back with the heel. The feet are at an angle of about 45 to 60 degrees. Keep the waist and hips relaxed and the torso straight.

Common Mistakes

● The shoulders are raised and the arms are straight, too tensed up and forced.

● The torso is turned too much, and the movements of the left leg and left arm are not coordinated.

5. Tíshǒu 提手 (Lift the Hands)

5.1 Turn the Waist and Swing the Hand

Turn the torso to the right with the body center shifting to the right leg while the left leg straightens and the left toes turn inside. Swing the left hand in front of the chest, palm facing the right. Look at the left hand. (Fig. 20)

5.2 Bring the Hands Together in Empty Stance

Shift the body center to the left leg, lift the right foot with the toes pointing up and the heel on the ground to form a right empty stance, facing Southwest; at the same time change the right hook hand to an open-palm hand, facing left, and raise it in front of the head, with the fingertips in line with the middle of the eyebrows. Raise the left hand in front of the abdomen, palm facing right. The left fingertips are at the same level as the right elbow, the two arms bend enough to make a curve. Look at the fingers of the right hand. (Fig. 21)

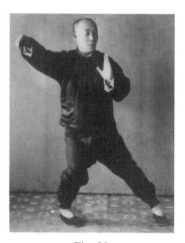
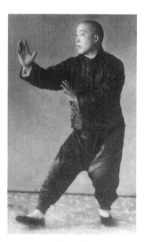

Fig. 20   Fig. 21

Important Points

● Empty stance (xūbù 虚步) is an important Taijiquan stance. Keep the body center mostly on the back leg. The front leg helps to support the body, with its knee slightly bent, and toe or heel on the ground. The two legs are distinct in the way they carry the body weight, one leg empty and the other solid. Keep the lower back relaxed with the hips steady, the spine upright, and the buttocks tucked in. Keep the torso relaxed, upright and steady.

● In the fixed empty stance, the right hand, the right foot and the eyes all face Southwest.

Common Mistakes

● The arms press toward each other too tightly, with too much force.

● The front leg is too straight in empty stance.

● The torso leans forward.

6. Báihè Liàngchì 白鹤亮翅 (White Crane Spreads Its Wings)

6.1 Turn the Foot In and Hold (Hands) in an Embrace

Turn the torso slightly to the left, push the hands down to the left and separate them in curves, then cross the hands and hold them as if holding something in front of the body; the left hand is in front of the right shoulder while the right hand is held in front of the left side of the abdomen. Meanwhile, shift the right foot slightly to the right, turn the right toes inside, then shift the body center to the right leg. Look straight to the right. (Figs. 22, 23)

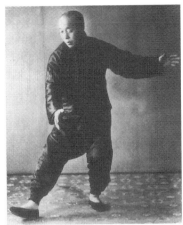

Fig. 22

6.2 Empty Stance with Palms Separated

Turn the torso to the left, shift the body center so it sits mostly on the right leg; turn the left foot slightly inside, the ball of the foot on the ground to make a left empty stance, facing East. Meanwhile, separate the hands — the right hand up and the left hand down — in curves, lift the right hand to the right side of the head, palm facing the temple, push the left hand down by the left side of the hip, a little in front of the hip with the fingertips pointing toward the front. Look straight ahead. (Fig. 24)

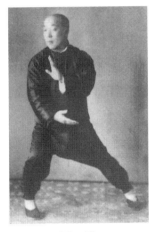

Fig. 23

Important Points

● After separating the hands, keep the arms in a half-circle; they should not be straight.

● Keep the posture upright, steady and relaxed.

Common Mistakes

● The chest is thrust out, the buttocks stick out, and the torso leans either forward or backward.

● There is a failure to make a clear distinction between empty and solid in the empty stance.

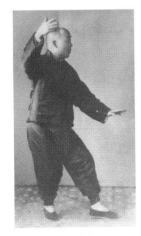

Fig. 24

7. Lōuxī Àobù 搂膝拗步 (Brush Aside Over the Knee in Reverse Forward Stance)

7.1 Turn the Waist and Swing the Hand

Turn the torso slightly to the left, then to the right. Lower the right hand down past the front of the body and raise it back to the right to shoulder height, palm up. Draw a curve with the left hand by raising it up past the head until it reaches the right side of the chest, palm down. Look at the right hand. (Figs. 25, 26)

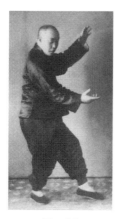

Fig. 25

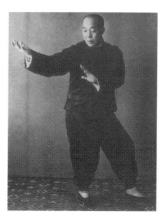

Fig. 26

7.2 Bow Stance and Push with the Palms

Turn the torso to the left. Step a half-step forward with left foot to the left, shift the body center forward, straighten the right leg, bend the left leg into a bow to make a left bow stance. Draw the right hand back past the shoulder and the side of the head and then push the right palm forward, shoulder height, the fingertips on the same line as the nose; drop the left hand over the left knee and brush aside to the left in a horizontal motion until the hand reaches the side of the left hip, palm down and fingertips pointing forward. Look at the right hand. (Figs. 27, 28)

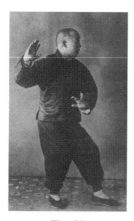

Fig. 27

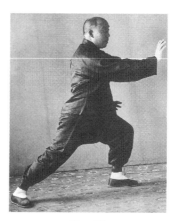

Fig. 28

Important Points

• The stepping technique here involves reverse forward step in bow stance (Àogōngbù 拗弓步). That is, the front leg of the bow stance is the opposite of the arm that is pushing forward. The feet in bow stance are fairly wide apart at about 8 to 12 inches or 20 to 30 centimeters.

• Pushing the palm forward means to make a forward attack. Brushing aside means to deflect an opponent's attack.

• Coordinate the movement of the hands as they cross with the turning of the waist. Also, coordinate and complete at the same time the pushing of the right palm, brushing aside with the left hand and bending the legs.

• Keep the torso relaxed and upright.

Common Mistakes

• The feet are on a straight line, or the feet cross so that the torso twists and tenses.

• The movements of the hands, feet and waist are not synchronized: The hands move but the waist does not turn. The feet complete their movement before the hands.

8. Shǒuhuī Pípā 手挥琵琶 (Play the Pipa)

8.1 Right Follow-Up Step

Move the right foot a half-step directly forward, landing the ball of the right foot behind the left foot on the right diagonal. (Fig. 29)

8.2 Bring Hands Together in Empty Stance

Shift the body center to the right leg, turn the torso to the right; move the left foot a half-step forward, landing the heel on the ground with the toes raised to make a left empty stance. Meanwhile, raise the left hand with the palm facing right, the fingertips in line with nose; also raise the right hand with palm facing left and lower the right hand to the inner side of the left upper arm, fingertips pointing toward the left elbow. Look at the fingers of the left hand. (Fig. 30)

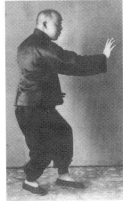

Fig. 29

Important Points

• The follow-up step (gēnbù 跟步), one of the basic foot techniques of Taijiquan, entails drawing the rear foot forward a half-step. Move the rear foot gently up and gently down; point, rise; point, fall. (Qīngqǐ qīngluò, diǎnqǐ diǎnluò. 轻起轻落，点起点落。) Make the shift of the body center gentle and steady.

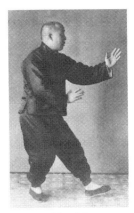

Fig. 30

- Keep the torso straight, relaxed and steady. Push the head up, straighten the spine, lower the shoulders and keep the elbows down. Arc in the chest and expand the back, relax the lower back and drop the hips.

Common Mistakes

- The torso leans forward or backward; the body center moves up and down.
- The arms are too tense, the legs make no distinction between empty and solid.

9. Zuǒyòu Lōuxī Àobù 左右搂膝拗步 (Brush Aside over the Knee in Reverse Forward Step — Left and Right)

9.1 Brush Aside over the Knee in Reverse Forward Stance — Left Side

9.1.1 Move the torso to the right. Lower the right hand in a curve to the left toward back and raise it at the back of the body to the right at shoulder height, palm up. At the same time, lower the left hand in a curve toward the right to the front of the right side of the chest, palm down. Look at the right hand. (Fig. 31)

9.1.2 Turn the torso to the left, step the left leg a half-step forward to the left, and shift the body center forward to make a left bow stance. Draw back the right hand past the shoulder and the side of the head and push forward at shoulder height. The fingertips are in line with the nose. Lower the left hand over the front of the left knee and brush aside horizontally to the left to stop at the side of the left hip, palm down and fingertips forward. Look at the right hand. (Fig. 32)

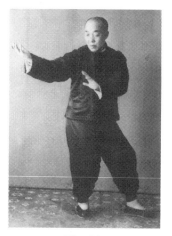

Fig. 31

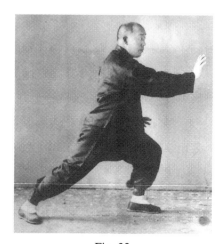

Fig. 32

Important Points and Common Mistakes are the same as 7. Lōuxī Àobù 搂膝拗步 (Brush Aside over the Knee in Reverse Forward Stance).

9.2 Brush Aside over the Knee in Reverse Forward Stance — Right Side

9.2.1 Shift the body center slightly back, turn the left toes out, turn the torso left.

Raise the left hand in a curve to the rear of the body on the diagonal, palm up. Lower the right hand in a curve to the left, palm down. Look at the left hand. (Fig. 33)

9.2.2 Step the right foot forward to the right; turn the torso to the right, shift the body center forward, straighten the left leg, and bend the right leg to make a right bow stance. Draw the left hand back past the shoulder and the side of the head and push forward at shoulder height, fingertips in line with the nose; lower the right hand over and in front of the right knee and brush aside in a level movement to the right until the hand reaches the side of the right hip, palm down, fingertips pointing forward. Look at the left hand. (Fig. 34)

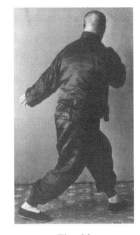
Fig. 33

Important Points

• Turn the body and swing the hand to the left towards the Northeast, extending as far as is comfortable without tensing.

• This is also a reverse forward stance. The width between the feet should be about 8 to 12 inches or about 20 to 30 centimeters to keep the body center stable.

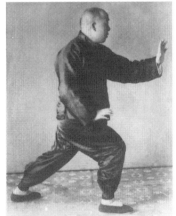
Fig. 34

Common Mistakes

• The left hand swings back too far or too much, the torso tenses and the body center becomes unstable.

• The stepping movement is not light and nimble, the foot is dragged, and the landing is too heavy.

9.3. Brush Aside over the Knee in Reverse Forward Stance — Left Side

9.3.1. Shift the body center slightly back, turn the right toes out, turn the torso to the right. Raise the right hand back on the diagonal in a curve, palm up. Lower the left hand in a curve to the right, palm down. Look at the right hand. (Fig. 35)

9.3.2. Step the left foot forward to the left, turn the torso to the left, move the body center forward to form a left bow stance. Draw the left hand past the shoulder and the side of the head and then push forward at shoulder height,

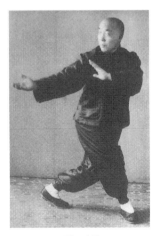
Fig. 35

fingertips in line with the nose. Lower the left hand and brush aside to the left in a level movement over and in front of the left knee until the hand reaches the side of the left hip. Look at the right hand. (Figs. 36, 37)

Important Points and Common Mistakes are the same as above.

10. Shǒuhuī Pípa 手挥琵琶 (Play the Pipa)

The same as 8. Shǒuhuī Pípā 手挥琵琶 (Play the Pipa). (Fig. 38)

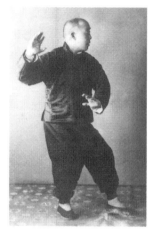 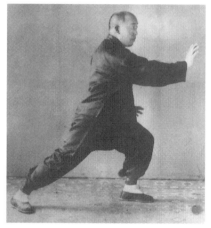 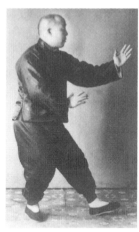

| Fig. 36 | Fig. 37 | Fig. 38 |

11. Jìnbù Bānlánchuí 进步搬拦捶 (Step In, Deflect, Block and Punch)

11.1 Hook Out Step and Make a Fist

11.1.1 Turn the torso to the left, turn the left toes out, shift the body center forward. Turn the left hand over and lower it to the side of the waist, palm down. Raise the right fist in front of the chest, the bottom of the fist down. Look straight ahead. (Fig. 39)

11.1.2 Step forward one step with the right foot, land on the heel, the toes turned out, then land the whole foot firmly on the ground. Turn the right fist and swing it with the arm in front of the body, up at shoulder height; push the left hand down at the side of the left hip, palm down. Look at the right fist. (Fig. 40)

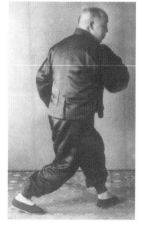 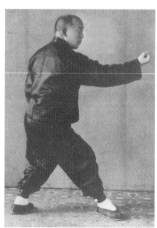

| Fig. 39 | Fig. 40 |

Important Points

Make a fist to deflect, push down and destroy the opponent's offensive by turning the back of the fist over. In this defensive move, focus the power on the back of the fist.

11.2 Step Forward and Block

Shift the body center forward, turn the torso to the right; step forward with the left foot, toes pointing straight ahead. Move the right hand upward and forward in a curve until it reaches the front of the body, palm slanted forward and fingertips slanted up at shoulder height. Draw the right fist back to the waist in a curve, palm up. Look at the left hand. (Fig. 41)

Important Points

In this defensive move, focus the power in the middle of the palm as you use your blocking hand to thwart an opponent's offensive. Both "Make a Fist" and "Block" here are meant for defense.

11.3 Attack with the Fist in Bow Stance

Shift the body center forward, turn the torso to the left, kick the right leg straight, bend the left leg to make a left bow stance. Punch forward with the right fist from the waist to the front at shoulder height, the thumb-side of the fist (the acupuncture point of Hǔkǒu 虎口) is up. Draw the left hand back with fingertips pointing upward lightly touching the inside of the right forearm. Look at the right fist. (Fig. 42)

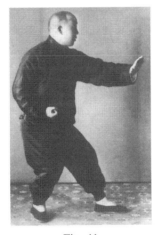 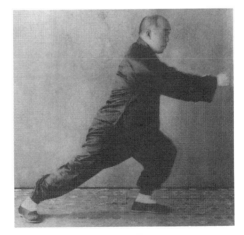

Fig. 41   Fig. 42

Important Points

• From its inclusion in the name of the art, Tàijíquán, it is obvious that quán (拳)

or fist is one of major hand techniques of Taijiquan. Fold the fingers into the palm with the thumb pressing against the bent index and middle fingers between the first and second knuckles. Do not make the fist too tight.

● Use this technique in a forward offensive with the fist against an opponent. Focus the power in the front of the fist.

● Stepping in (jìnbù 进步) is a two-step sequence. In the first step, the foot lands on the heel in a hook-out step (bǎibù 摆步). In the second step, the foot lands with the toes pointing forward which is called a step forward (shàngbù 上步). Stepping in should be light, nimble, balanced, gentle and continuous.

● Bend the arm somewhat in each of the movements of making a fist, blocking with the palm and punching with the fist. Relax the shoulders, lower the elbows. Seek straightness in the curve (qǔzhōng qiúzhí 曲中求直).

Common Mistakes

● The feet move too quickly during the stepping in. They are lifted too high and land too heavily. The torso becomes unsteady, twisting and swaying. The moving foot does not come close enough to the supporting foot.

● When punching, the arm is stretched too straight, the fist is too tight and the front of the fist is not flat.

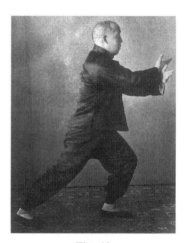

Fig. 43

12. Rúfēng Sìbì 如封似闭 (Pull Back then Push, As if to Close)

12.1 Sit Back and Draw In the Hands

Move the left hand forward from below the right wrist, the right fist opens, cross the hands with palms up. (Fig. 43) Then shift the body center backward, bend the right leg and sit back, straighten the left leg with the toes pointing up; separate the hands and draw them in to the front of the chest, palms slant backward and upward. Look straight ahead. (Fig. 44)

12.2 Push in Bow Stance

Turn the hands inward and make the palms slant slightly downward, then shift the body center to make a left bow stance; at the same time push both hands forward shoulder-width apart to shoulder height, palms forward and

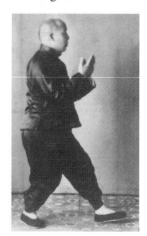

Fig. 44

fingertips upward. Look straight ahead. (Fig. 45)

Important Points

• Complete the pushing movement and the bow stance at the same time. Coordinate the movements of the arms and legs.

• Always keep the body upright. Push the head up and straighten the spine. Relax the shoulders, keep the elbows down, relax the chest and expand the back. Bend the knees and relax the hips. Breathe naturally.

• In the fixed posture, keep the wrists down, the fingers relaxed. Push the head up, and keep the shoulders down. In a long and deep exhale, the breath (qì 气) sinks to the Dantian (dāntián 丹田).

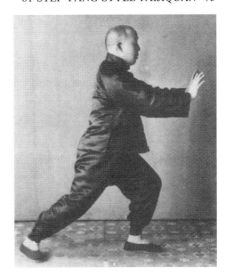

Fig. 45

• When drawing in the hands, bend and sink the elbows. Keep the forearms turned in; they should not turn up.

Common Mistakes

• When sitting back, the torso leans backward. In bow stance, the torso leans forward.

• When drawing in the hands, the breath is exhaled. When pushing forward, the breath is inhaled. The breathing and hand techniques are not in harmony.

13. Shízìshǒu 十字手 (Cross Hands)

13.1 Turn the Waist and Separate the Hands

Shift the body center to the right and turn the torso to the right; turn the left toes in and the right toes out to make a right side-bow stance. Move the right hand with the body from left to right horizontally. Raise both hands at either side of the body with the palms facing forward. Look at the right hand. (Fig. 46)

13.2 Draw In the Feet and Hold in Embrace

Shift the body center to the left leg, draw the right foot in a half-step toward

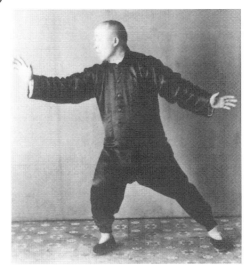

Fig. 46

the left, place the feet parallel, shoulder-width apart. The body center rises as the legs straighten naturally. The weight falls evenly on both feet to make a standing feet-apart stance. Lower the hands in curves together at the same time, cross the wrists in front of the abdomen, raise the hands and hold them in front of the chest, with the right hand outside, the left hand inside. The arms form a circle, the palms facing inside. Look straight ahead. (Figs. 47, 48)

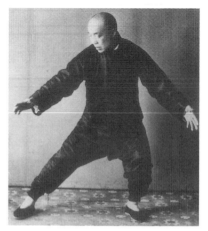

Fig. 47

Important Points

- Make one continuous, smooth, flowing and coordinated movement in doing Cross Hands. Do not stop half way and do not accelerate the speed during the process.

- Keep the torso straight.

Common Mistakes

- The arms are too straight when the hands separate; the arms are too tense and pressed in the position of holding something in front of the body.

- The torso hunches, the waist bends.

- The movement stops midway which interrupts the flow of power.

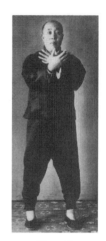

14. Bǎohǔ Guīshān 抱虎归山 (**Hold the Tiger and Return to the Mountain**)

Fig. 48

14.1 Turn Around and Push with an Open-Palm Hand

14.1.1 Turn the right toes inside and turn the torso to the right; bend both knees, shift the body center to the right leg. Lower the left hand in an arc backward to the left, raising it to the Southeast at shoulder height, palm up. Turn over and lower the right hand to the left side of the chest, palm down. Look straight ahead to the right. (Fig. 49)

14.1.2 Step to the Northwest with the right foot, shift the body center forward to make a right bow stance. Draw in the left hand past the shoulder and the side of the head and push forward at shoulder height. The right hand brushes aside horizontally over

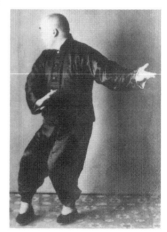

Fig. 49

the front of the right knee until it reaches the right side of the hip. Look at the left hand. (Fig. 50)

Important Points

The same as 7. Lōuxī Àobù 搂膝拗步 (Brush Aside over the Knee in Reverse Forward Stance) but in the opposite direction, facing West by North.

14.2 Roll Back in Back Stance

14.2.1 Move the right hand up to the right and in a curve to the front of the body at shoulder height, palm down. Turn the left hand up and close to the right forearm. Look at the right hand. (Fig. 51)

14.2.2 The same as 3. Lǎnquèwěi 揽雀尾 (Grasp the Peacock's Tail). (Fig. 52)

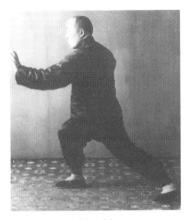
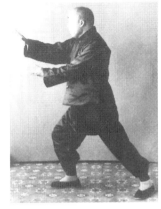
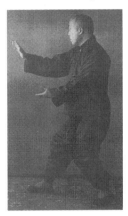

Fig. 50   Fig. 51   Fig. 52

14.3 Press (Jǐ 挤) and Bow Stance

The same as 3. Lǎnquèwěi 揽雀尾 (Grasp the Peacock's Tail). (Fig. 53)

14.4 Draw Back and Push Forward (Àn 按)

The same as 3. Lǎnquèwěi 揽雀尾 (Grasp the Peacock's Tail). (Figs. 54, 55)

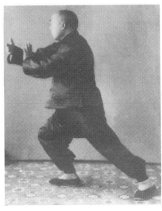
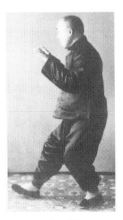
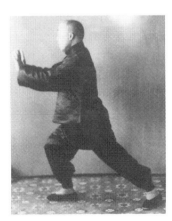

Fig. 53   Fig. 54   Fig. 55

Important Points

- The direction of this stance is West by North, about 30 degrees.

- This is a long movement. In modern times, most works on Taijiquan divide it into two movements: Bàohǔ Guīshān 抱虎归山 (Hold the Tiger and Return to the Mountain), and Xié Lǎnquèwěi 斜揽雀尾 (Grasp the Peacock's Tail on the Diagonal).

Common Mistakes

- The direction of Turn Around and Push with the Open-Palm Hand and the direction of bow stance are not aligned.

- Refer to 3. Lǎnquèwěi 揽雀尾 (Grasp the Peacock's Tail) and 7. Lōuxī Àobù 搂膝拗步 (Brush Aside over the Knee in Reverse Forward Stance).

15. Zhǒudǐ Kànchuí 肘底看捶 (Fist Under the Elbow)

15.1 Turn around and Swing the Hand

15.1.1 Shift the body center backward, bend the left leg and sit back; turn the right toes inside and turn the torso to the left. The hands move from right to left, swinging horizontally with the turn of the body (the right hand slightly lower). Swing the left hand to the left side of the body; swing the right hand to the left side of the chest, palms down. Look at the left hand. (Fig. 56)

15.1.2 Shift the body center to the right, bend the right leg and sit back; turn the torso to the right. Move the right hand in a curve to the right past the head; move the left hand to the right in a curve past the abdomen. Look at the right hand. (Fig. 57)

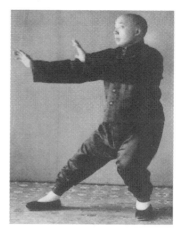

Fig. 56

15.2 Hook-Out Step and Bring the Arm Across ([lit.] Forming a Horizontal Palm)

Raise the left foot to the inside of the right foot, then return the foot to the original place with the toes turned out in a hook-out step. Turn the torso with the foot movement to the left. Raise the right hand forward to the left in a curve past the head to form a "horizontal palm" (héngzhǎng 横掌) in front of the body at shoulder height, palm facing out, the fingertips facing right. Lower the right hand to the right side of the waist, palm

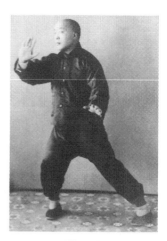

Fig. 57

down. Look at the left hand. (Fig. 58)

15.3 Follow In with the Foot and Make a Fist

15.3.1 Draw the right foot in a half-step forward, landing it behind although not directly behind the left foot, with about a foot's distance between the two feet. Turn the torso continuously to the left and shift the body center to the right leg. Move the right hand in a curve to the right and then forward to the front of the head and make a fist, the bottom of the fist facing left. Lower the left hand to the left in a curve to the left side of the waist, palm facing right. Look at the right fist. (Fig. 59)

15.4 Empty Stance and Chop

Step the left foot forward a half step, landing on the heel with the toes pointing up to form a left empty stance. Meanwhile, turn the torso to the left; thread the left hand past the chest from the inside of the right arm forward to chop with the side of the hand in front of the body, palm facing right, fingertips slanted upward on line with the nose. Lower the right fist and stop it below, although not exactly below, the left elbow, the thumb-side of the fist facing upward, the palm the fist facing left. Look at the left hand. (Fig. 60)

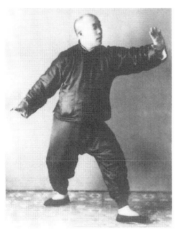
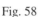
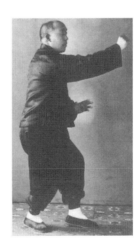
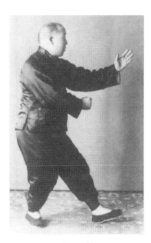

Fig. 58   Fig. 59   Fig. 60

Important Points

● The chop (pī 劈) focuses power on the edge of the hand to slash the opponent.

● The offensive/defensive meaning of this technique is: Turn around and push the opponent aside with the left horizontal hand, then grab the opponent with your right hand and chop the opponent with the left hand.

● The fixed position faces East. Keep the body upright, comfortable, steady, composed. The whole process should be continuous with the hands, feet and waist in good coordination.

Common Mistakes

● The hook-out step strays too far away from the starting point, thus making a stepping around in a circle.

● In the fixed position, the elbows press too tightly against the body, the armpits close and the upper arms are too tense.

16. Zuǒyòu Dàoniǎnhóu 左右倒撵猴 (Drive the Monkeys Back Left and Right) Or Dàojuǎngōng 倒卷肱 (Step Back and Curl the Arms)

16.1 Drive the Monkeys Back — Right Side

16.1.1 Open the right fist into an open-palm hand. Lower it back past the abdomen in a curve, then raise it, bend the elbow, and lift it to shoulder height, hand with palm forward. At the same time, turn the left hand upward and raise it up to shoulder height in front of the body. Lift the left foot lightly. Look straight ahead. (Figs. 61, 62)

16.1.2 Step back one step with the left foot, landing on the ball of the foot, then shift the body center back until the entire left foot settles firmly on the ground; bend the left leg and sit back, lift the right heel lightly, turning the right toes to point straight to make a right empty stance. Meanwhile, turn the torso to the left, push the right palm forward from above shoulder, the fingertips pointing up in line with the nose. Draw the left palm to the left side of the hip, palm up. Look at the right hand. (Fig. 63)

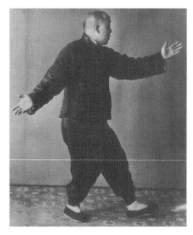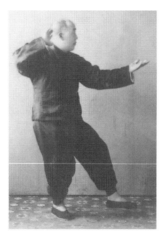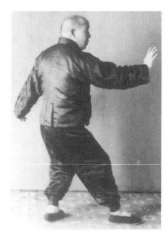

| Fig. 61 | Fig. 62 | Fig. 63 |

16.2 Drive the Monkeys Back — Left Side

16.2.1 Move the left hand up and back in a curve, bend the elbow and lift it to shoulder height, palm facing forward; turn the right hand over with the movement of the elbow and raise it up in front of the body to shoulder height. Lift the right foot lightly. Look straight ahead. (Fig. 64)

16.2.2 Step one step back with the right foot, landing on the ball of the foot first, then shift the body center backward until the entire right foot settles firmly on the ground. Bend the right leg and sit back, lift the left heel lightly, turning the left toes to point straight to make a left empty stance. Meanwhile, turn the torso to the right, push the left palm forward from above the shoulder, the fingertips pointing up in line with the nose. Draw the right palm to the right side of the hip, palm up. Look at the left hand. (Fig. 65)

16.3 Drive the Monkeys Back — Right Side

16.3.1 Move the right hand up and back in a curve, bend and draw the right hand over the right shoulder; turn the left hand so the palm is up and raise it up in front of the body. Lift the left foot lightly. Look straight ahead. (Fig. 66)

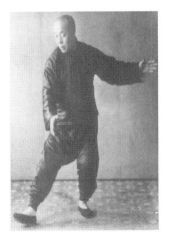
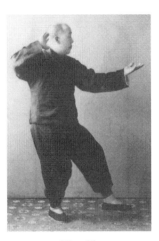

Fig. 64   Fig. 65   Fig. 66

16.3.2 Step the left foot back one step, shift the body center and sit back to form a right empty stance. Meanwhile, turn the torso to the left and press the right palm forward, fingertips in line with the nose. Draw the left hand to the left side of the hip, palm up. Look at the right hand. (Fig. 67)

Important Points

• The offensive and defensive meaning of this movement is to counter-attack by pushing in retreat.

• Retreating step (tuìbù 退步) is an important step in Taijiquan. It requires a light, nimble, calm, and steady movement. Point, rise; point, fall; first land on

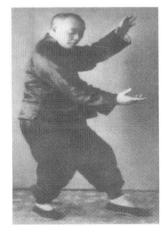

Fig. 67

the ball of the foot then shift the body center backward until the whole foot is solid, bending the knee in a squat. When the front leg moves into in empty stance, the toes turn straight and the knee is naturally bent. The front leg should not be straight. The width between feet is about 4 inches or 10 centimeters, the feet do not cross each other. The torso does not twist and the body center does not move up and down.

• When pushing the palm forward, keep both the elbows and shoulders down, bending the elbows appropriately. When drawing the hand backward past the side of the body, raise it in a curve at the back of the body.

Common Mistakes

• The feet land too heavily in retreat, the body center shifts too fast, the body center goes up and down, the torso sways and twists.

• When swinging the hand back, the angle is too big; the chest is thrust out, the shoulders raised, and the head turned to look back.

17. Xiéfēishì 斜飞势 (Diagonal Flying Posture)

17.1 Shift the Gaze and Hold the Ball

Turn the torso to the left; raise the left hand up to the left in a curve and hold it in front of the right chest, palm down. Lower the left hand to the left in an arc and hold it in front of the abdomen, palm up, as if holding a ball. Look at the left hand. (Fig. 68)

17.2 Turn Around and Separate the Hands

Draw the right foot back on the diagonal of the left foot, landing on the ball of the foot, turn the body back to the right on the left heel and the ball of the right foot; then step forward with the right foot to the Southwest and shift the body center forward to make a right bow stance. Separate the hands in curves, right hand up and left hand down, lift the right hand in front of the right shoulder, palm slanted upward, the fingertips in line with the nose. Press the left hand down by the side of the left hip, palm down. Look at the right hand. (Fig. 69)

Important Points

• This is a turning and leaning movement, meant to press the opponent with the arm or the body. Thrust the right arm under the armpit of the opponent and squeeze and weigh down the opponent with the force from the turning and charging of the body.

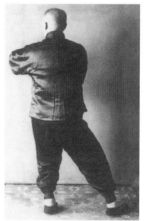

Fig. 68

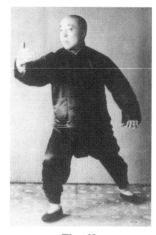

Fig. 69

- When turning back to the right, the right toes can land or not as you will, so just turn on the left foot. In any case, when turning always make a smooth flowing motion with the center of the body stable.

Common Mistakes

- The body is not turned enough or the movement stops midway which interrupts the flow of power.

- The center of the body is not steady when stepping forward with the right leg.

- The power of the right arm is not focused and pressed on the right spot so the arm is extended upward.

18. Tíshǒu 提手 (**Lift the Hands**)

18.1 Follow-In Step and Draw In the Hands

Draw in the left foot a half-step, landing about 8 inches or 20 centimeters behind the right foot on the diagonal. Turn the right hand slightly inside, palm facing left. Draw the left hand to the waist, palm facing the right. Look straight to the Southwest. (Fig. 70)

18.2 Bring Hands Together in Empty Stance

Move the right foot half a step to Southwest and land on the heel, with the toes turning upward to make a right empty stance. Close the hands (vertically) with fingertips up in front of the body. Point the right fingertips slanted upward in line with the nose, bending the elbow a little; lower the left hand below the right elbow, fingertips in line with the right elbow; half bend the left arm. Look at the right palm. (Fig. 71)

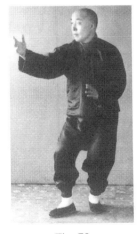 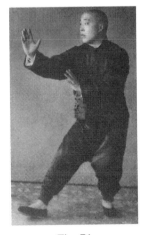

Fig. 70   Fig. 71

Important Points and Common Mistakes are the same as 5. Tíshǒu 提手 (Lift the Hands).

19. Báihè Liàngchì 白鹤亮翅 (White Crane Spreads Its Wings)

The same as 6. Báihè Liàngchì 白鹤亮翅 (White Crane Spreads Its Wings). (Fig. 72)

20. Lōuxī Àobù 搂膝拗步 (Brush Aside over the Knee in Reverse Forward Stance)

The same as 7. Lōuxī Àobù 搂膝拗步 (Brush Aside over the Knee in Reverse Forward Stance). (Fig.73)

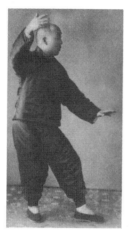

Fig. 72

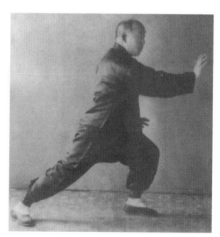

Fig. 73

21. Hǎidǐzhēn 海底针 (Needle at the Bottom of the Sea)

21.1 Right Follow-Up Step

Move the right foot a half-step forward and land about 8 inches or 20 centimeters behind the left foot on the diagonal. Look straight ahead. (Fig. 74)

21.2 Empty Stance and Spear the Hand

Move the left foot half a step forward, landing on the ball of the foot to make a left empty stance. Turn the torso to the right then to the left while leaning slightly forward. Lower the right hand past the side of the waist and lift it to the front of the right shoulder, then spear the right hand forward and downward, palm facing left, fingers slanted down but higher than the crotch. Swing the left hand to the right first horizontally and then in an arc, then it brushes aside to the left horizontally before it stops at the side of the left hip, palm down. Look down and forward. (Fig. 75)

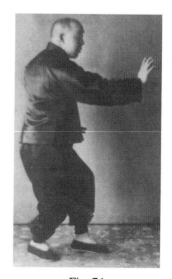

Fig. 74

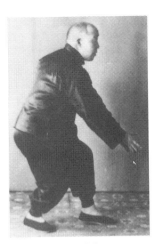

Fig. 75

Important Points

• The technique of spearing the hand (chāzhǎng 插掌) entails using the fingers to spear an opponent. Here, direct the attack at the opponent's crotch.

• Draw and raise the right hand and then spear it down and forward. Swing the hand in a vertical circle. Draw the left hand from right to left in a horizontal circle. Both hands must act in coordination with the turn of the body.

• In the fixed position, naturally stretch the torso straight, leaned forward within 45 degrees.

Common Mistakes

• When spearing, power is not focused on the fingers so that the technique becomes instead a "chopping" or "slicing" (pīzhǎng 劈掌).

• When leaning forward, the head lowers, the back hunches and the waist bends.

22. Shàntōngbèi 扇通背 (Fan Through the Back)

Keep the torso erect and turn a little to the right; move the left foot forward half a step and shift the body center forward to form a left bow stance. Lift the right hand past the front of the body and stop over the side of the head, palm slanted up and fingertips pointing to the left. Push the left hand forward in front of the chest at shoulder height, with the fingertips pointing up at the nose level. Look at the left hand. (Fig. 76)

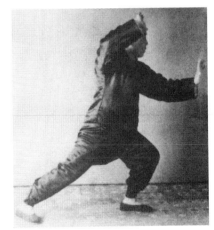

Fig. 76

Important Points

• Keep the torso upright and natural. Arc in the chest and expand the back, while pushing up the head and lowering the shoulders.

• Bend the left arm a little and hold the right arm in a curve. The hands are separated, one in front and the other drawn back.

Common Mistakes

• The torso turns too much to the right so that the left bow stance becomes a side-bow stance.

• The right hand is lower than the head because the right arm bends too much.

23. Piēshēnchuí 撇身捶 (Turn and Punch)

23.1 Turn Around Holding the Fists

23.1.1 Shift the body center to the right, turn the left toes inside and turn the torso to the right. Raise the left hand over the side of the head, palm facing outside; lower the right hand in front of the chest, palm down. Look straight ahead. (Fig. 77)

23.1.2 Shift the body center to the left leg and continue to turn the torso to the right. Keep holding the left hand over the side of the head. Hold the right fist by the left rib. Turn the head and look to the right. (Fig. 78)

23.2 Punch in Bow Stance

Lift and draw the right foot to the inside of the left ankle and step to the Northwest with the turn of body; shift the body center forward and bend the right leg to make a right bow stance. Raise the right fist, turn it over past the front of the head and strike to the Northwest at head level, with the palm of the fist slanted upward. Lower the left palm along the inside of the right arm until it reaches the side of the waist, palm down. Eyes follow the right fist. (Fig. 79)

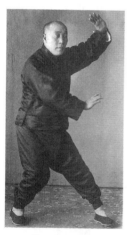 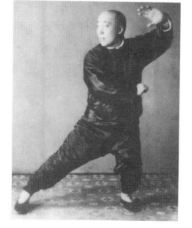 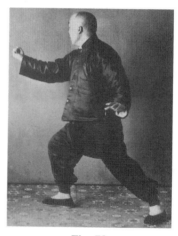

Fig. 77   Fig. 78   Fig. 79

23.3 Bow Stance and Push with the Palm

Turn the torso slightly to the right; push the left palm forward from the side of the waist at shoulder height, fingertips pointing upward. Meanwhile draw the right fist to the right side of the waist, with the palm of the fist facing up. Look at the left palm. (Fig. 80)

23.4 Strike with the Fist in Bow Stance

Turn the torso slightly to the left; turn/rotate the right fist in to make a vertical fist and punch forward at shoulder height, with thumb-side of the fist facing upward; draw back the left palm a little, the fingertips touching lightly the inside of the right forearm. Look at the right fist. (Fig. 81)

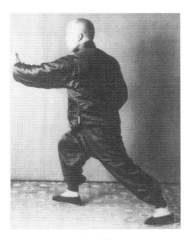

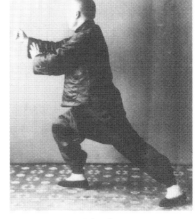

Fig. 80   Fig. 81

Important Points

● Make the strike with the back of the fist by rotating the forearm and striking the opponent with the back of the fist from up to down, with the power focused on the back of the fist. Make the punch with the fist by straightening the bent arm and attacking the opponent with the fist, with the power focused on the face of the fist.

● This movement involves three offensive hand techniques: striking with the back of the fist, pushing with the palm and punching with the fist, all facing Northwest in the same direction as the bow stance. Coordinate the arm and leg actions and keep the torso straight.

● When striking with the back of the fist, the right arm is in line with the right leg. Make the width of the feet in bow stance about 4 to 8 inches or 10 to 20 centimeters to keep the body steady and relaxed.

Common Mistakes

● In bow stance, the feet stand on the same line so that the body is unsteady.

● The torso turns too much so the hands are not in line with the feet.

24. Jìnbù Bānlánchuí 进步搬拦捶 (Step In, Deflect, Block and Punch)

24.1 Hook Out Step and Make a Fist

24.1.1 Shift the body center back (by sitting back), turn the torso to the left, draw back the right foot half a step, landing on the ball of the foot. Swing the left palm down to the left in an arc until it reaches the side of the left hip, palm down. Turn/rotate the right fist in and lower it in front of the abdomen, palm down and thumb-side of the fist facing inward. Look straight to the West. (Fig. 82)

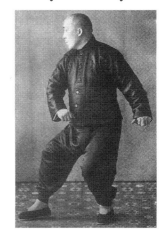

Fig. 82

24.1.2 Step to the West with the right foot, landing on the heel with toes turning outward. Draw a vertical curve with the left hand at the side of the body upward, to the right and downward and press it down at the side of the left hip, palm down. Stretch the right hand to make a fist past the inside of the left arm to the front of the body at shoulder height, palm up. Look at the right fist. (Fig. 83)

24.2 Step Forward and Block

Shift the body center forward and turn the torso to the right. Step forward with the left foot, landing on the heel with the toes forward, then let the whole foot stand firmly. Raise the left hand forward in a curve and stop in front of the body at shoulder height, palm facing right with fingertips slanted upward. At the same time turn and draw the right fist to the waist, palm up. Look at the left palm. (Fig. 84)

24.3 Strike with the Fist in Bow Stance

Shift the body center forward and turn the torso to the left, bend the left leg and kick straight the right leg to make a left bow stance. Turn the right fist inside and punch forward vertically at shoulder height with the thumb-side of the fist facing up. Draw back the left palm a little, the fingertips touching lightly on the inside of the right forearm. Look at the right fist. (Fig. 85)

Important Points and Common Mistakes are the same as 11. Jìnbù Bānlánchuí 进步搬拦捶 (Step In, Deflect, Block and Punch), except that the direction of this movement is West.

25. Shàngbù Lǎnquèwěi 上步揽雀尾 (Step Forward and Grasp the Peacock's Tail)

25.1 Ward Off in Right Bow Stance

25.1.1 Shift the body center slightly backward, turn the left toes outside and turn the torso to the left. Lower the left hand to the left and then upward in an arc, and hold it in front of the body, palm down. Hold the right hand in a fist, and swing it downward

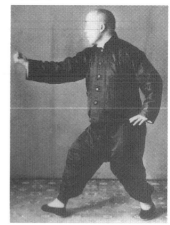

Fig. 83

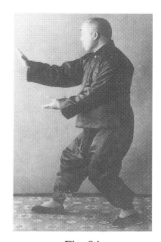

Fig. 84

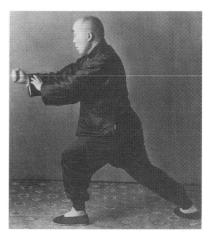

Fig. 85

in a curve to the right and then to the left before holding it in front of the abdomen, palm upward with the hands facing each other as if holding a ball. Look at the left hand. (Fig. 86)

25.1.2 Step forward with the right foot and shift the body center forward to make a right bow stance. Then separate the hands in curves, hold the right hand extended in front of the body at shoulder height, palm facing inward, and press the left hand at the side of the left hip, palm down. Look at the right hand. (Fig. 87)

25.2 Roll Back in Back Stance, Press and Bow Stance, Draw Back and Push Forward are the same as their counterparts in 3. Lǎnquèwěi 揽雀尾 (Grasp the Peacock's Tail). (Figs. 88 - 92)

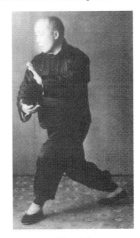

Fig. 86

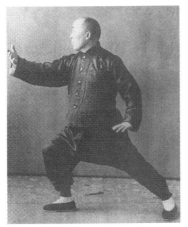

Fig. 87

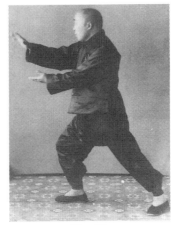

Fig. 88

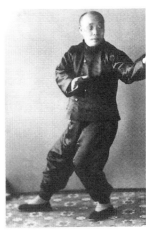

Fig. 89

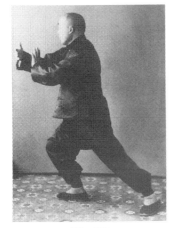

Fig. 90

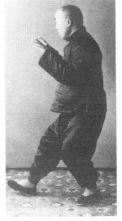

Fig. 91

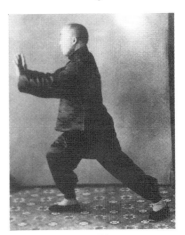

Fig. 92

26. Dānbiān 单鞭 (Single Bian)

The same as 4. Dānbiān 单鞭 (Single Bian). (Figs. 93 - 96)

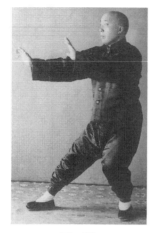

Fig. 93

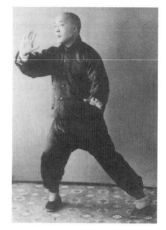

Fig. 94

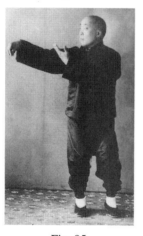

Fig. 95

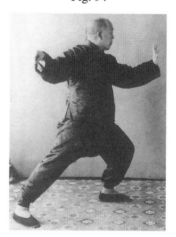

Fig. 96

27. Yúnshǒu 云手 (Move the Hands Like Clouds)

27.1 Move the Hands Like Clouds (First Time)

27.1.1 Shift the body center to the right leg as the torso turns to the right, and turn the left toes inside. Lower the left hand past the abdomen to the left in a curve until it reaches the front of the right shoulder. Change the right hook hand to an open-palm hand and raise it at the side of the body, both palms slanted down. Look at the left hand. (Fig. 97)

27.1.2. Shift the body center to the left as the torso turns to the left. Turn the left hand over to the inside, past the front of the head and move it in a curve to the left; lower the right hand past the abdomen and move it to the left in an arc, palm facing left.

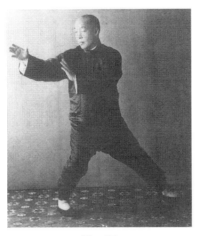

Fig. 97

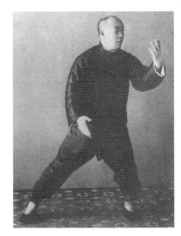

Fig. 98

Eyes follow the left hand. (Fig. 98)

27.1.3 Shift the body center again to the left as the torso turns to the left. Draw the right foot half a step to the left, landing on the ball of the foot, followed by the whole foot firmly on the ground, about 20-30 centimeters or 8-12 inches from the left foot. The feet are parallel (Facing South). Continue circling both hands to the left in curves, move the left hand to the left front of the body, facing East, palm turning outward; and move the right hand to the inside of the left elbow, palm facing inward. Eyes follow the left hand. (Fig. 99)

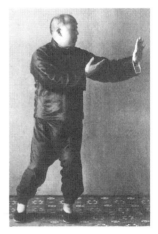

Fig. 99

27.2 Move the Hands Like Clouds (Second Time)

27.2.1 Shift the body center to the right as the torso turns to the right. Move the right hand to the right past the head in an arc, palm facing inward; lower the left hand to the right in an arc to the front of the abdomen, palm facing right. Eyes follow the right hand. (Fig. 100)

27.2.2 Shift the body center to the right again as the torso turns to the right. Move the left foot half a step to the left, landing on the inside (right side) on the left ball of the foot before the whole foot is firmly on the ground, the toes facing South. Move the hands to the right continuously in curves — the right hand to the right front of the body, pointing to the West, palm turning outside; the left hand to the inside

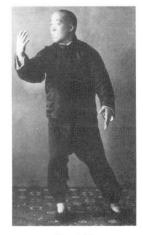

Fig. 100

of the right elbow, palm facing inward. Eyes follow the right hand. (Fig. 101)

27.2.3 Shift the body center to the left as the torso turns to the left. Move the left hand to the left past the head in a curve, palm facing inward; lower the right hand to the left in a curve to the front of the abdomen, palm facing left. Eyes follow the left hand. (Fig. 102)

27.2.4 Continue to shift the body center to the left as the torso turns to the left. Move the right foot to the left half a step, landing on the ball of the foot before the whole foot is firmly on the ground. Keep the feet about 8-12 inches or 20-30 centimeters apart, parallel to the South. Move the left hand to the left front of the body, facing East, palm turned outward; move the right hand to the inside of the left elbow, palm facing inward. Eyes follow the left hand. (Fig. 103)

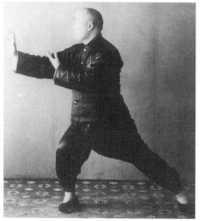 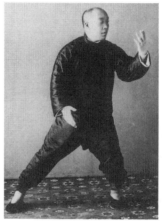 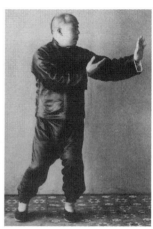

Fig. 101   Fig. 102   Fig. 103

27.3 Move the Hands like Clouds (Third Time)

The movements are the same as above in Move the Hands like Clouds (Second Time). (Fig. 104-107)

Important Points

● To deflect an opponent's left and right attacks, move the hands in vertical circles that cross each other in front of the body.

● Move the feet sideways to the left. Both the left foot stepping out and the right foot following in should rise gently, fall gently, i.e. "point, rise; point, fall." Keep the body center steady and move at an even speed.

● Move the head, waist, hands and legs in synchronization, with nothing out of step.

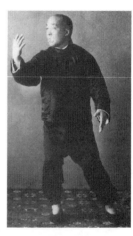

Fig. 104

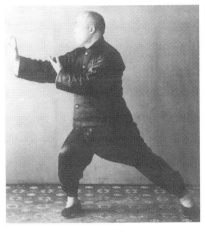

Fig. 105

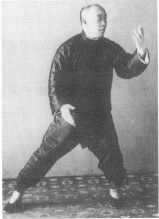

Fig. 106

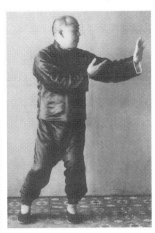

Fig. 107

● Keep the torso straight, and don't let the body center move up and down.

● This movement can also be repeated five times, depending on the size of the place and the distance between the beginning position and the closing position.

Common Mistakes

● When stepping sideways, the feet are put together next to each other side-by-side or in the shape of the Chinese character for the numeral eight, which is: 八.

● The waist does not turn with the hand movements.

● The buttocks and hips sway; the arms and legs are not coordinated.

● The eyes do not follow the hands.

● The torso leans forward or sways left and right.

28. Dānbiān 单鞭 (Single Bian)

28.1 Turn Around and Hook the Hand

Shift the body center to the right as the torso turns to the right, lifting the left heel. While moving the right hand to the right in a curve past the head to the right front of the body (Southwest), turn the palm inside and draw the fingers together to form a hook turning in toward the outside, with the wrist bent and the fingertips pointing downward. The left hand presses down to the left in a curve, passes the abdomen to the inside of the right elbow, palm facing in. Look at the hook hand. (Fig. 108)

28.2 Bow Stance and Push with the Palm

Turn the torso to the left, step forward with the left foot to the East by North and shift the body center for-

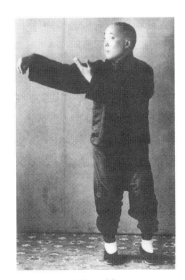

Fig. 108

ward to make a left bow stance. Turn the left palm over in front of the chin and push forward, shoulder height, with the elbow and the left knee on the same line. Hook the right hand and raise it behind the body on the diagonal to the left, facing South by West at shoulder height. Look at the left hand. (Fig. 109)

Important Points and Common Mistakes are the same as 4. Dānbiān 单鞭 (Single Bian)

29. Gāotànmǎ 高探马 **(Gauge the Height of the Horse)**

29.1 Follow-Up Step and Turn Over the Hands

Move the rear right foot half a step forward, landing on the ground about one foot's length behind the left foot to the right. Shift the body center backward and turn the torso slightly to the right. Turn the left hand so the palm faces upward, then change the right hook hand into an open-palm hand with the palm facing upward. Look at the left hand. (Fig. 110)

29.2 Empty Stance and Push the Palm

Move forward half a step with the left foot, landing on the ball of the foot to make a left empty stance. Turn the torso slightly to the left, draw back the right hand and push it forward at head level past the side of the head, the fingertips pointing upward. Withdraw the left hand to the front of the abdomen, palm upward. Look at the right hand. (Fig. 111)

Important Points

● Coordinate pushing the palm with turning the waist, moving of the shoulder and landing on the ball of the left foot.

● Keep the torso upright, steady, and relaxed.

Common Mistakes

● The height of pushing the palm and the position where the left palm is drawn back are confused with those in the movement of "Drive the Monkeys Back."

● The left arm presses against the ribs too tightly, so the armpit closes.

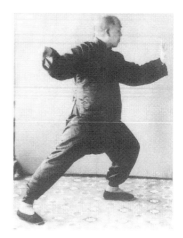

Fig. 109

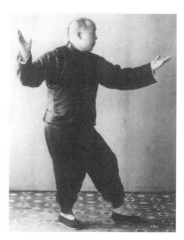

Fig. 110

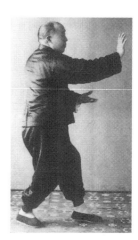

Fig. 111

• The timing of the hands and feet is off with the feet moving faster than the hands.

30. Zuǒyòu Fēnjiǎo 左右分脚 (Separate Feet Right and Left)

30.1 Lift the Right Foot

30.1.1 Turn the torso to the left. Move the left foot half a step forward to the left (Northeast) so the body center is shifted forward, bending the left leg like a bow. Meanwhile move/thread the left hand over the back of the right hand and cross the hands back to back. Then separate the hands to either side of the body in curves, palms facing outside. Look at the right hand. (Fig. 112)

30.1.2 Turn the torso to the right and draw the right foot to the inside of the left foot, landing on the ball of the foot. Lower both hands in curves and cross them in front of the abdomen, then lift them to the front of the chest, crossing the wrists with the right hand outside (or the left hand closer to the chest), both palms turning from inside to outside. Look straight to the Southeast. (Fig. 113)

30.1.3 Stand on the left leg, bend the right knee and lift it, slowly kick up to the right front with the top of the foot level and toes forward, keeping the right leg higher than level in the Eastern direction but 30 degrees to the South. Separate the arms simultaneously to the sides of the body, right arm directly over the right leg. Extend the left arm back on the diagonal to the left in the Northern direction. Both palms face outside at shoulder height. Look at the right palm. (Fig.114)

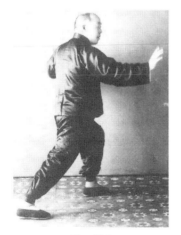
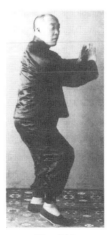
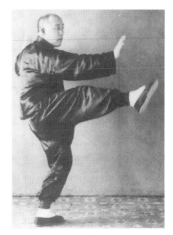

| Fig. 112 | Fig. 113 | Fig. 114 |

30.2 Lift the Left Foot

30.2.1 Lower the right leg by bending the knee, step forward to the right with the right foot, bend the right leg like a bow and turn the torso to the right. Move the left hand over the back of the right hand, cross the hands back to back, then separate the hands to either side of the body in curves, palms facing out. Look at the left hand. (Fig. 115)

30.2.2 Draw in the left foot to the inside of the right foot, landing on the ball of the foot. Press both hands down in curves, cross them in front of the abdomen as if holding something, and raise them to the front of the chest. The wrists cross each other, right hand on the outside, and both palms facing out. Look at the Northeast. (Fig. 116)

30.2.3 Stand on the right leg only, bend and lift the left leg, slowly kick up to the left front with the top of the left foot level and toes forward, keeping the left leg above level in the Eastern direction 30 degrees to the North. Separate the arms simultaneously to either side of the body in curves, left arm directly over the left leg; extend the right arm back on the diagonal to the right in the Southern direction; both palms face out at shoulder height. Look at the left palm. (Fig.117)

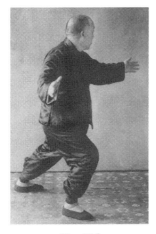
Fig. 115

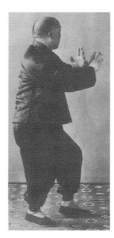
Fig. 116

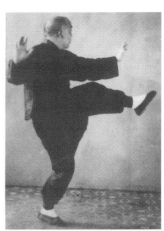
Fig. 117

Important Points

• Separating the feet (fēnjiǎo 分脚), a basic kicking techniques of Taijiquan, involves kicking an opponent with power focused on the toes.

• When separating the feet, bend the supporting leg a little and keep it steady. Keep the torso naturally upright and do not lean forward or backward. Bend the arms slightly and raise them up, one in front and other back at one side. Keep both wrists down and fingertips up. Breath naturally.

• As the hands swing to separate and join together, two overlapping vertical circles are formed. The movement should be continuous, gentle and even.

Common Mistakes

• The standing leg is not steady or bends too much.

- The torso leans forward or backward.
- One of the arms is higher than the other when they are separated.
- The arm stretched forward is not in line with the kicking leg and foot.
- The head is lowered and waist bent, the body too tensed up and the breathing forced.

31. Zhuǎnshēn Zuǒ Dēngjiǎo 转身左蹬脚 (Turn and Kick with the Left Heel)

31.1 Turn the Body and Hold in an Embrace

Bend and raise the left knee in front of the body, standing on the right leg; turn the toes of the right foot in on the heel and turn the body back to the left. Lower both hands in curves and to a position of holding something in front of the abdomen before raising them to the front of the chest; cross the wrists with the right hand on the outside, and turn both palms from inside to outside. Turn the head to the West. (Fig. 118)

31.2 Separate the Hands and Heel Kick

Slowly straighten the left leg, kick the left foot forward and upward, toes pointing up, in the Western direction, the left leg higher than level. The arms separate in curves to either side of the body, the left arm in line with the left leg, while the right arm stretches up backward to the right in the Northeastern direction; both palms face out at shoulder height. Look at the left hand. (Fig. 119)

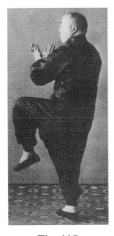
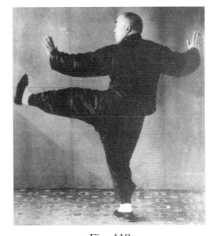

Fig. 118   Fig. 119

Important Points

- Focus the power of Heel Kick on the heel.
- The other points are the same as 30. Zuǒyòu Fēnjiǎo 左右分脚 (Separate Feet Right and Left).

Common Mistakes

The same as 30. Zuǒyòu Fēnjiǎo 左右分脚 (Separate Feet Right and Left).

32. Zuǒyòu Lōuxī Àobù 左右搂膝拗步 (Brush Aside over the Knee in Reverse Forward Stance — Left and Right)

32.1 Brush Aside over the Knee in Reverse Forward Stance — Left Side

Bend and lower the left knee, step forward with the left foot, shift the body center forward, and bend the left knee to make a left bow stance. Meanwhile, turn the torso to the right then to the left; turn the right hand over and draw it back past the side of the head and push forward at shoulder height; press down the left hand to the right in a curve past the right shoulder and the right side of the abdomen, then brush aside over the left knee horizontally to the left before stopping the left hand at the side of the left hip. Look at the right hand. (Fig. 120)

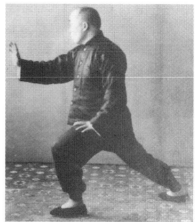
Fig. 120

32.2 Brush Aside over the Knee in Reverse Forward Stance—Right Side

32.2.1 Shift the body center backward a little; turn the left toes outward and torso to the left. Swing the right hand to the left until it reaches the front of the left shoulder, palm facing left; raise the left hand to the left in a curve and swing backward on the diagonal, palm facing up. Look at the left hand. (Fig. 121)

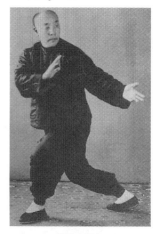
Fig. 121

32.2.2 Step forward with the right foot, shift the body center forward, and bend the right leg to make a right bow stance. At the same time, turn the torso to the right; draw back the left hand and push forward past the shoulder; lower the right hand in a curve, brush over the front of the right knee to the right horizontally and stop at the side of the right hip. Look at the left hand. (Fig. 122)

Important Points and Common Mistakes are the same as 9. Zuǒyòu Lōuxī Àobù 左右搂膝拗步 (Brush Aside over the Knee in Reverse Forward Stance — Left and Right).

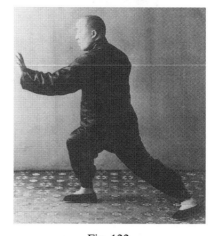
Fig. 122

33. Shàngbù Zāichuí 上步栽捶 (Step Forward and Punch Downward)

33.1 Turn Around and Make a Fist

Shift the body center backward a little, turn the right toes outward and the torso to the right. Move the left palm to the front of the right shoulder, palm facing right; turn over the right hand and raise it backward to the right in a curve to make a fist, the bottom of the fist facing up. Look at the right fist. (Fig. 123)

33.2 Bow Stance and Punch Downward

Step forward with the left foot, shift the body center forward, and bend the left leg to make a left bow stance. Meanwhile turn the torso to the left and lean slightly forward; draw back the right fist and then punch forward and downward past the side of the head, the thumb-side of the fist is toward the left and the face of the fist is slanted forward and downward at abdomen level; sweep the left palm down in a curve to the side of the left hip, palm facing downward. Look at the right fist. (Fig. 124)

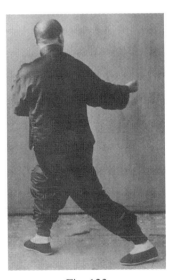
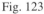
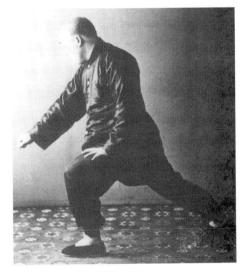

Fig. 123   Fig. 124

Important Points

● Punching downward involves attacking the opponent with the fist. The wrist is straight and the power focused on the face of the fist.

● To make such a forward and downward punch, lean the torso slightly forward to help with the attack, but keep the torso straight for correct posture even when bending down.

Common Mistakes

● The waist is bent and back hunched so that the torso is twisted and not straight.

● The wrist bends when punching downward.

34. Fānshēn Báishé Tǔxìn 翻身白蛇吐信 (**Turn Around and White Snake Spits Poison**)

34.1 Turn Around and Raise the Fist

Bend the right leg and sit back to shift the body center backward, turn the left foot in and the torso to the right. Raise the right fist in front of the head, with the thumb side of the fist inward and the palm downward; turn the left hand over and raise it to the side of the body. Look at the right fist. (Fig. 125)

34.2 Turn Around and Strike with the Back of the Palm

Shift the body center to the left, straighten the right leg, and turn the torso continuously to the right to face East. Change the right fist into an open-palm hand, turn over and strike with the forearm toward the East, shoulder height, palm facing up; draw back the right hand to the side of the head over the shoulder, palm facing forward. Look ahead to the East. (Fig. 126)

34.3 Resting Stance and Push the Palm

Raise the right foot to move to the left a little, toes turning outside; turn the torso half to the right, leaning slightly forward; cross the legs to sit down with the back knee against the front knee, sitting a little more on the back leg, the left heel lifted and with the ball of the left foot touching the ground to make a resting stance. Push the left palm forward, the palm slanted downward slightly below shoulder height; draw back the right hand to the right side of the waist, palm facing up. Look at the left hand. (Fig.127)

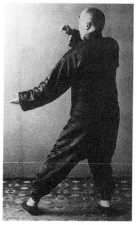
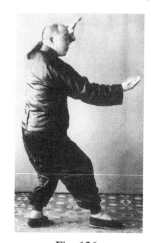
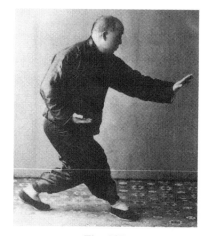

Fig. 125   Fig. 126   Fig. 127

Important Points

● Resting stance (xiēbù 歇步), also called Squatting High on Crossed Knees, is a major stance in the martial arts rarely seen in Taijiquan. It is done by half squatting on crossed knees that are pressed together with the front foot pointing horizontally outward and planted firmly on the ground, and the back foot pointing vertically ahead, touching the ground with the ball of the foot; the torso leans forward on the diagonal, body center over both legs or slightly more on the back leg.

• When turning around, shift the body center completely with a clear distinction between the empty leg and the solid leg. Turn the left foot inward and straighten the right foot, then move to the right to turn the foot out. The movement should flow continuously and smoothly, coordinated with the turn of the body to the right.

• Push the palm to the East. Lower the body center a little; the leaning forward of the torso should be no more than 30 degrees.

Common Mistakes

• The feet are not agile enough when turning around, and the legs make no distinction between empty and solid.

• There is too much space between the feet in the Resting Stance. The torso is not turned enough to the right and the legs are not crossed together and pressed tightly.

35. Shàngbù Bānlánchuí 上步搬拦捶 (Step Forward, Deflect, Block and Punch)

Step forward with the left foot, shift the body center forward, bend the left leg to make a left bow stance. Meanwhile turn the torso to the left, make a fist with the right palm and punch forward, shoulder high, with the thumb-side of the fist facing up; draw back the left palm a little, with the four fingers touching lightly on the inside of the right forearm. Look at the right fist. (Fig. 128)

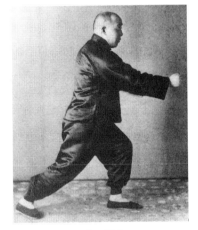

Fig. 128

Important Points

• The footwork of this movement is to step forward. Punching is the only hand technique involved. In some places it is done like "Bow Stance and Push Forward" in Báishé Tǔxìn 白蛇吐信 (White Snake Spits the Poison), but here we still follow the order of Step Forward, Deflect, Block and then Punch.

• The torso should be relaxed and upright. After punching, the shoulders and elbows are down and relaxed, with a deep breath sinking to the lower abdomen (qìchén Dāntián 气沉丹田).

• To best sink the breath to the lower abdomen, coordinate punching with a deep exhaled breath to keep the lower abdomen tense and solid, the body center steady and the body full of energy and strength.

Common Mistakes

The feet bump up against each other in stepping forward and the body center is unsteady.

36. Yòu Dēngjiǎo 右蹬脚 (Kick with the Right Heel)

36.1 Turn the Waist and Hold in an Embrace

Turn the left toes outward and the torso to the left. Raise both hands and separate them to either side in curves, press down in a curve to a position of holding something with wrists crossed in front of the abdomen, palms facing in, the left hand closer to the body. Look straight ahead. (Fig. 129)

36.2 Draw In the Feet and Hold in Embrace

Shift the body center forward, turn the torso slightly to the right; draw in the right foot to the inside of the left foot, landing on the ball of the foot. Have the hands in a position of holding something in front of the chest, palms turning outward. Look ahead to the right. (Fig. 130)

36.3 Kick and Separate the Hands

Stand on the left leg, bend and raise the right knee, kick slowly with the right foot up to the left in front of the body in the direction of the East 30 degrees to the South, toes pointing upward and the right leg higher than level. Meanwhile separate the hands in curves past the head, raise them one in front of the body and the other at back on the diagonal, both shoulder height. Keep the right arm and the right leg in the same line; stretch the left arm back on the diagonal, facing North. Look at the right hand. (Fig. 131)

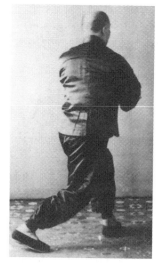 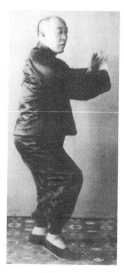 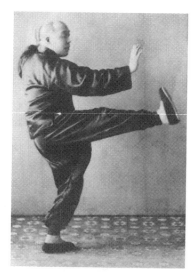

Fig. 129   Fig. 130   Fig. 131

Important Points

The same as in 31. Zhuǎnshēn Zuǒ Dēngjiǎo 转身左蹬脚 (Turn and Kick with the Left Heel), only in the opposite direction.

Common Mistakes

Refer to 30. Zuǒyòu Fēnjiǎo 左右分脚 (Separate Feet Right and Left).

37. Zuǒyòu Pīshēn Fúhǔ 左右披身伏虎 (Turn Around to Tame the Tiger Left and Right)

37.1 Tame the Tiger on the Left

37.1.1 Bend and lower the right knee, pull back and land the right foot on the diagonal to the left, cross the legs, land the right foot on the ball of the foot; move the left hand forward past the side of the head to the inside of the right forearm, palm facing right and fingertips slanted upward; turn/rotate the right hand outward, palm facing left and fingertips slanted upward. Look at the right hand. (Fig. 132)

37.1.2 Lift the left foot and step back on the diagonal to the left past the inside of the right ankle, shift the body center forward, bend the left leg to make a left bow stance, facing North. Meanwhile turn the torso to the left; lower both hands to the right in curves to make fists at the left side of the body; then raise the left fist in an arc to the right to punch at the left side of the head, the palm of the fist facing out and the thumb-side of the fist slanted down to the right; swing the right fist to the front of the left chest in line with the left fist, the palm of the fist facing down and the thumb-side of the fist facing in. Turn the head to look ahead to the right. (Fig. 133)

37.2 Tame the Tiger on the Right

37.2.1 Shift the body center back a little, turn the left toes in and the torso to the right; shift the body center to the left and lift the right foot. Stretch both fists to the left, raise them at the left side of the body, and move them with the body. Turn the head to look South. (Fig. 134)

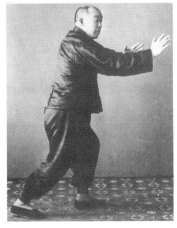

Fig. 132

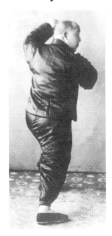

Fig. 133

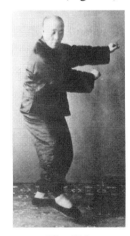

Fig. 134

37.2.2 Step forward to the right with the right foot, shift the body center forward, bend the right leg to make a right bow stance, facing South. Turn the torso right, lower both fists to the right side of the body in curves; swing the right fist in a penetrating strike to the left at the right side of the head, the palm of the fist facing out and the thumb-side of the fist slanted down to the left; swing the left fist to the front of the right chest in line with the right fist, the palm of the fist facing down and the thumb-side of the fist facing in. Turn the head to look ahead to the left. (Fig. 135)

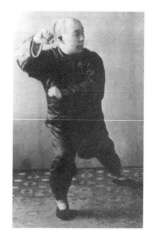

Fig. 135

Important Points

● Penetrating Strike (guàndǎ 贯打) is an important fist technique of Taijiquan. Attack by swinging the fist forward in a half-circle curve past the side of the body, turning in the arm and at the same time bending the arm in an arc, the thumb-side of the fist slanted down, with power focused on the front of the fist.

● The bow stances in this movement face North and South. The left bow stance is completed by pulling the right foot back, and stepping forward with the left foot to the North; the right bow stance is completed by turning in the foot and the body, stepping forward with the right foot to the South. The movement should be done continuously, the body center steady with hands and feet in coordination.

● Cross-step (chabù 插步) is footwork often found in the martial arts. Lift one foot past the back of the supporting foot, in the opposite direction.

● In the fixed posture, relax the shoulders, push up with the head, arc the chest in and expand the back; relax the lower back and the hips while leaning the torso slightly forward.

Common Mistakes

● When stepping sideward, the crossed feet are too far apart so the torso sways and the body center is unsteady.

● The waist and hips are turned too much in the bow stances, thus forming side-bow stances.

● In the fixed posture, the shoulders and hips are tense so the posture is not naturally relaxed.

38. Huíshēn Yòu Dēngjiǎo 回身右蹬脚 (**Turn Around and Kick with the Right Heel**)

38.1 Turn Around and Separate the Hands

Shift the body center backward, turn the right toes in and the left toes out, turn the torso backward to the left. Hold both hands in fists, separate them from the front of the head to either side of the body in curves, palms facing out. Look straight ahead. (Fig. 136)

38.2 Draw In the Feet and Hold in Embrace

Turn the torso to the right, draw the right foot in to the inside of the left foot, landing the ball of the right foot. Lower the hands in curves toward the inside and hold the hands crossed in front of the abdomen, then raise them up in front of the chest, palms turning over outward, wrists crossed with the right hand on the outside. Look ahead to the right. (Fig. 137)

38.3 Heel Kick and Separate the Hands

Bend and lift the right knee, kick up slowly forward to the right, toes pointing upward and the right leg higher than level, facing East and 30 degrees South. Separate the hands to the sides of the body in curves at shoulder height, palms facing out; keep the right arm in line with the right leg, raise the left arm backward on the diagonal in the direction of the North. Look at the right hand. (Fig. 138)

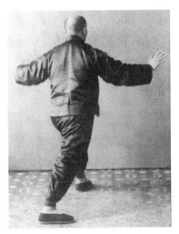 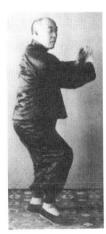 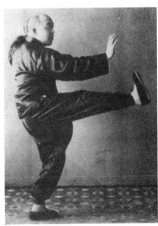

Fig. 136   Fig. 137   Fig. 138

Important Points and Common Mistakes are the same as those in 31. Zhuǎnshēn Zuǒ Dēngjiǎo 转身左蹬脚 (Turn and Kick with the Left Heel).

39. Shuāngfēng Guàn'ěr 双峰贯耳 (Strike the Opponent's Ears with Both Fists)

39.1 Draw In the Foot and Bring the Hands Together

Bend the right knee and lift the right foot in front of the body, pointing the toes downward. Move the left hand past the side of the head to the front of the body, bring it parallel with the right hand directly above the right knee, and turn palms upward as if holding a ball. Look straight ahead. (Fig. 139)

39.2 Bow Stance and Strike with Both Fists

Land the right foot lightly in front, shift the body center forward, bend the right knee to make a right bow stance. Draw back the hands to the waist to make fists, then swing the fists to both sides of the body in curves and round-house punch forward in front of the head at the height of the ear with the fists stopping a head-width's distance apart, the thumb-side slanted down; bend the arms slightly in a curve. Look straight ahead. (Fig. 140)

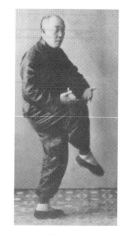

Fig. 139

Important Points

• The direction of this movement is the same as 38. Huíshēn Yòu Dēngjiǎo 回身右蹬脚 (Turn Around and Kick with the Right Heel), i.e. East and 30 degrees to the South.

• The distance between the feet should be 8-12 inches or 10-20 centimeters to keep the body steady, upright and relaxed.

Common Mistakes

• The head is lowered, shoulders and elbows raised, and the torso is tense and turned.

• In the fixed posture, the arms are straight and the thumbs face each other so that the power is not focused on the front of the fists.

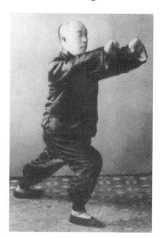

Fig. 140

40. Zuǒ Dēngjiǎo 左蹬脚 (Kick with the Left Heel)

40.1 Turn the Waist and Hold Hands in Embrace

Turn the right toes out and the torso to the right; change the fists into open-palm hands and bring them to the sides of the body in curves, then press them down and hold them crossed in front of the abdomen; cross the wrists with the right below the left, palms facing up. Look ahead to the left. (Fig. 141)

40.2. Heel Kick and Separate the Hands

Stand on the right leg with the knee slightly bent. Bend and lift the left leg, slowly kicking the left foot forward to

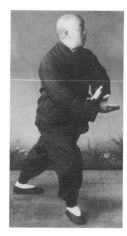

Fig. 141

the left toward the East, toes pointing up and the left leg higher than level. Cross and raise the hands past the front of the chest, turn the palms over and separate them in curves to either side of the body; raise the left arm right above the left leg, hold up the right arm back to the right toward the Southwest; keep both hand at shoulder height, palms facing out. Look at the left hand. (Fig. 142)

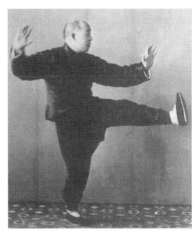

Fig. 142

Important Points and Common Mistakes are the same as in 31. Zhuǎnshēn Zuǒ Dēngjiǎo 转身左蹬脚 (Turn and Kick with the Left Heel).

41. Zhuǎnshēn Yòu Dēngjiǎo 转身右蹬脚 (Turn Around and Kick with the Right Heel)

41.1 Turn Around and Hold Hands in Embrace

Bend the left leg and turn it in, turn the body back to the right pivoting on the ball of the right foot, landing the left foot on the outside behind the right foot; then shift the body center to the left leg, lift the right heel, and turn the torso continuously to the right, facing East. Lower the hands in curves with the turn of the body, hold them crossed in front of the abdomen then up to the chest, with the right wrist crossing the left on the outside, palms turning outward. Look ahead to the right. (Fig. 143)

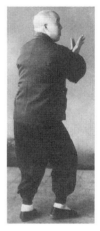

Fig. 143

41.2 Heel Kick and Separate the Hands

Standing firmly on the left leg, bend and lift the right leg, kick the heel upward and forward slowly toward East, toes pointing upward and the right leg higher than level. Separate the hands in curves to either side of the body, keep the right arm directly above the right leg, raise the left arm backward to the left toward North by West, both hands at shoulder height, palms facing outward. Look at the right hand. (Fig. 144)

Important Point

• To make a smooth turn, coordinate lowering and drawing in the left leg and holding the hands down together with the turning of the body. Meanwhile, keep the body upright and body center steady.

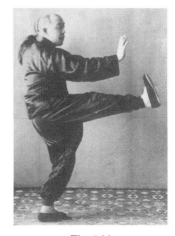

Fig. 144

- The same as 31. Zhuǎnshēn Yòu Dēngjiǎo 转身左蹬脚 (Turn and Kick with the Left Heel).

Common Mistakes

- The body turn is clumsy so the torso sways.
- The landing of the left foot is not coordinated with the turning of the body and turning in of the leg, and so it does not land in the right place.

42. Jìnbù Bānlánchuí 进步搬拦捶 (Step In, Deflect, Block and Punch)

42.1 Land the Foot and Draw In the Fist

Turn the torso to the left; draw in and land the right foot in front of the left foot; draw in and hold the left hand in a front of the chest, palm down, half bending the left arm in a curve; make a fist with the right hand and lower it in front of the left abdomen, the thumb-side of the fist facing in and the palm of the fist down. Look at the left hand. (Fig. 145)

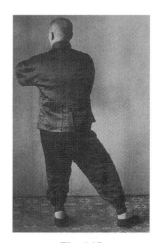

Fig. 145

42.2 Hook Out Step and Make a Fist

42.3 Step Forward and Block

42.4 Strike with the Fist in Bow Stance

42.2, 42.3, and 42.4 are all the same as in 11. Jìnbù Bānlánchuí 进步搬拦捶 (Step In, Deflect, Block and Punch). (Figs. 146, 147, 148)

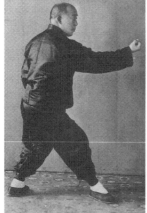
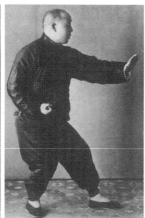
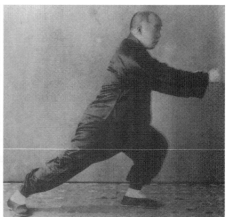

Fig. 146   Fig. 147   Fig. 148

43. Rúfēng Sìbì 如封似闭 (Pull Back then Push, As if to Close)

The same as 12. Rúfēng Sìbì 如封似闭 (Pull Back then Push, As if to Close). (Figs. 149, 150)

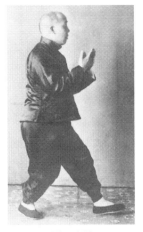

Fig. 149

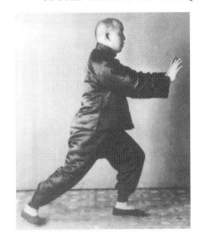

Fig. 150

44. Shízìshǒu 十字手 (Cross Hands)

The same as 13. Shízìshǒu 十字手 (Cross Hands). (Figs. 151, 152)

45. Bàohǔ Guīshān 抱虎归山 (Hold the Tiger and Return to the Mountain)

The same as 14. Bàohǔ Guīshān 抱虎归山 (Hold the Tiger and Return to the Mountain). (Figs. 153, 154, 155)

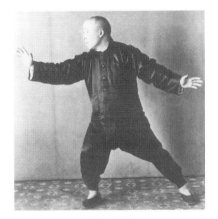

Fig. 151

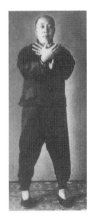

Fig. 152

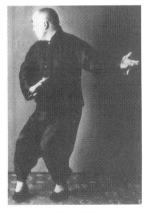

Fig. 153

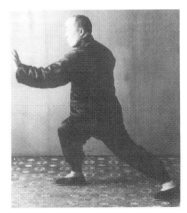

Fig. 154

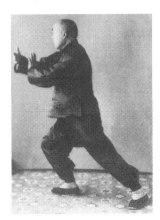

Fig. 155

46. Héng Dānbiān 横单鞭 (Horizontal Single Bian)

The same as 4. Dānbiān 单鞭 (Single Bian). The only difference is that the final fixed posture here faces South. (Fig. 156)

47. Zuòyòu Yěmǎ Fēnzōng 左右野马分鬃 (Part the Wild Horse's Mane — Left and Right)

47.1 Part the Wild Horse's Mane — Right Side

47.1.1 Turn the torso to the left; change the right hook hand to an open-palm hand and arc it down to the left to the front of the left abdomen, palm upward; bend the right elbow and hold the right hand in front of the chest, palm downward; hold the hands as if holding a ball. Look at the left hand. (Fig. 157)

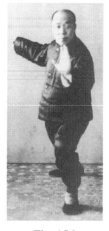

Fig. 156

47.1.2 Turn the torso to the right; draw in and lift the right foot, past the inside of the left ankle and step forward to the right (30 degrees West by North), shift the body center forward, and bend the right leg to make a right bow stance. Draw the hands apart in arcs, move the right hand to the front of the body at head level, palm slanted upward; move the left hand to the side of the left hip, palm downward. Look at the right hand. (Fig. 158)

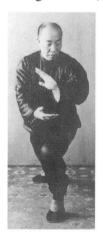

Fig. 157

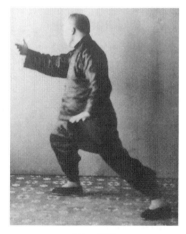

Fig. 158

47.2 Part the Wild Horse's Mane — Left Side

47.2.1 Turn the torso to the right; hold the hands in front of the right chest as if holding a ball, right hand higher. Look at the right hand. (Fig. 159)

47.2.2 Step forward with the left leg past the inside of the right ankle to the left (30 degrees West by South) to make a left bow stance. Draw the hands apart, move the left hand to the front of the body at head level, palm slanted upward; move the right hand to the side of the right hip, palm downward. Look at the left hand. (Fig. 160)

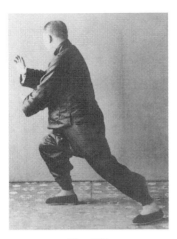

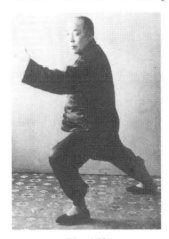

Fig. 159

Fig. 160

47.3 Part the Wild Horse's Mane — Right Side

47.3.1 Turn the torso to the left; hold the hands in front of the left chest as if holding a ball, left hand higher. Look at the left hand. (Fig. 161)

47.3.2 Step forward with the right foot past the inside of the left ankle to the right (30 degrees West by North) to make a right bow stance. Draw the hands apart, move the right hand to the front of the body at head level, palm slanted upward; move the left hand to the side of the left hip, palm downward. Look at the right hand. (Fig. 162)

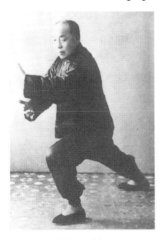

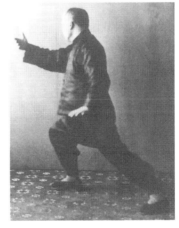

Fig. 161

Fig. 162

Important Points

● The hand technique of Parting the Wild Horse's Mane involves pushing aside an attack and knocking the opponent over. That is, catch and press down the opponent's hand, then thrust the other hand under his/her armpit to throw the opponent by using the force of the turning of the waist.

• This movement is repeated three (or five) times. The direction of pushing aside and throwing over in bow stance is about 30 degrees on the diagonal.

• Keep the torso upright; coordinate the separating of the hands, turning of the waist and bow stance. Bend the elbows slightly after separating the hands to keep the shoulders relaxed, elbows down, chest in, hips naturally down, with a deep breath sinking to the lower abdomen (qìchén Dāntián 气沉丹田).

Common Mistakes

• The arms are too tight while "holding the ball," and they are too straight when separated.

• The movements of the arms and legs are not synchronized. The feet are faster than the hands so when the bow stance is done, the hands are still parting.

• There is not enough space between the feet in bow stance, so the torso is tense and body center unsteady.

• When drawing in the foot to step forward, the foot does not pass the inside of the supporting foot.

48. Jìnbù Lǎnquèwěi 进步揽雀尾 (Step In and Grasp the Peacock's Tail)

48.1 Ward Off (Péng 掤) in Left Bow Stance

48.1.1 Turn the torso to the right; hold the hands in front of the right chest as if holding a ball, with the right hand on top. Look at the right hand. (Fig. 163)

48.1.2 Turn the torso to the left; step forward to the left with the left foot past the inside of the right ankle, shift the body center forward to make a left bow stance; separate the hands with the left held extended in front of the body, palm facing inward at shoulder height, and the right hand pressing down at the side of the right hip. Look at the left hand. (Fig. 164)

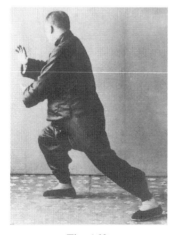

Fig. 163

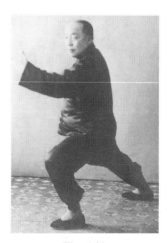

Fig. 164

48.2 Ward Off in Right Bow Stance

48.2.1 Turn the torso to the left; hold the hands in front of the left chest as if holding a ball, with the left hand on top. Look at the left hand. (Fig. 165)

48.2.2 Turn the torso to the right; step forward toward the East with the right foot passing the inside of the left ankle, shift the body center forward to make a right bow stance; separate the hands with the right hand extended in front of the body, palm facing inward at shoulder height, and the left hand pressing down at the side of the left hip. Look at the right hand. (Fig. 166)

48.2.3 Roll Back in Back Stance, 48.2.4. Press Forward and Bow Stance and 48.2.5. Draw Back and Push Forward are all the same as in 3. Lǎnquèwěi 揽雀尾 (Grasp the Peacock's Tail). (Figs. 167, 168, 169)

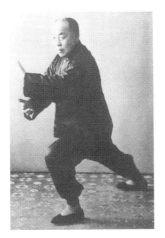

Fig. 165

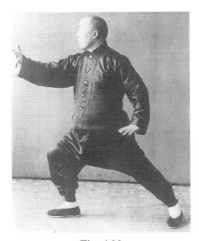

Fig. 166

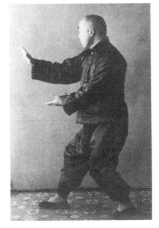

Fig. 167

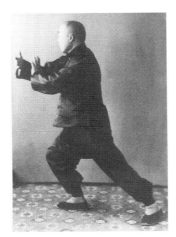

Fig. 168

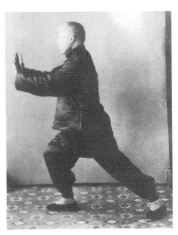

Fig. 169

Important Points and Common Mistakes are the same as for 3. Lǎnquèwěi 揽雀尾 (Grasp the Peacock's Tail), except that the direction for the Left Bow Stance is 30 degrees West by South.

49. Dānbiān 单鞭 (Single Bian)

The same as 4. Dānbiān 单鞭 (Single Bian). (Fig. 170)

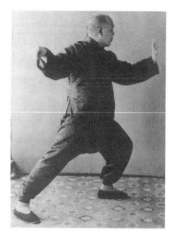

Fig. 170

50. Yùnǚ Chuānsuō 玉女穿梭 (Jade Maiden Moves the Shuttle Left and Right)

50.1 Jade Maiden Moves the Shuttle to the Left

50.1.1 Shift the body center backward, turn the left toes in and turn the torso back toward the right; lift the right foot and land it horizontally, toes pointing outward; arc the left arm down to the right until the hand is in front of the right abdomen, palm facing up; change the right hook hand into an open-palm hand in front of the right chest, palm down; have the two hands as if holding a ball. Look ahead to the left. (Fig. 171)

50.1.2 Step forward to the left (Southwest) with the left foot, turn the torso to the left, shift the body center forward, and bend the left knee to make a left bow stance; raise the left palm past the front of the body and hold it high at the side of the head, palm slanted upward with the thumb-side of the palm pointing to the left temple, arm bent slightly in a curve; draw back the right hand past the right chest and push forward in front of the body, palm facing forward and fingertips in line with the nose. Look at the right hand. (Figs. 172, 173)

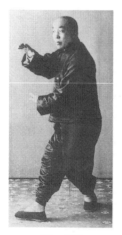

Fig. 171

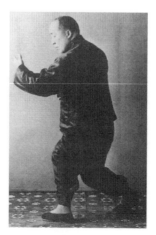

Fig. 172

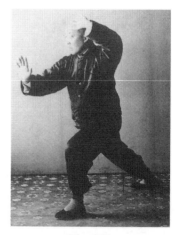

Fig. 173

50.2 Jade Maiden Moves the Shuttle to the Right

50.2.1 Shift the body center backward a little, turn the left toes in and the torso to the right. Place the hands in front of the left chest as if holding a ball, the left hand over the right. Look at the left hand. (Fig. 174)

50.2.2 Pull the right foot back on the diagonal to the left foot, landing the ball of the foot, turn the left foot and the body continuously to the right; then step forward to the right (Southeast) with the right foot, shifting the body center forward to make a

right bow stance. Raise the right palm past the front of the body and hold it high at the side of the head, the palm slanted upward with the thumb-side of the palm pointing to the right temple, the right arm bent slightly in a curve; draw back the left hand past the left chest and push it forward in front of the body, fingertips in line with the nose. Look at the left hand. (Fig. 175)

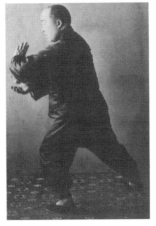 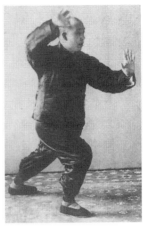

Fig. 174   Fig. 175

50.3 Jade Maiden Moves the Shuttle to the Left

50.3.1 Turn the torso to the right; hold the hands in front of the right chest with the right over the left. Look at the right hand. (Fig. 176)

50.3.2 Turn the torso to the left; draw in the left foot and step forward past the inside of the right ankle to the left (Northeast), shift the body center forward, bend the left leg to make a left bow stance. At the same time, push the right hand past the chest to the front of the body, raising the left hand high past the front of the body to the side of the head. Look at the right hand. (Fig. 177)

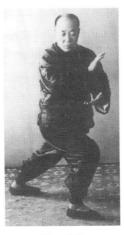 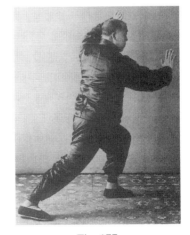

Fig. 176   Fig. 177

50.4 Jade Maiden Moves the Shuttle to the Right

50.4.1 Shift the body center backward a little, turn the left toes in and the torso to the right. Place the hands in front of the left chest as if holding a ball, the left hand over the right. Look at the left hand. (Fig. 178)

50.4.2 Draw in the right foot backward on the diagonal to the left foot, landing the ball of the foot, turn the left foot and the body continuously to the right; then step forward to the right (Northwest) with the right foot, shift the body center forward, bend the right knee to make a right bow stance. At the same time push the left hand past the left chest to the front of the body; raise the right hand past the front of the body and hold it high at the side of the head. Look at the left hand. (Fig. 179)

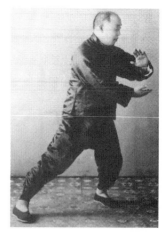

Fig. 178

Important Points

• Keep the line of the hands and the stance parallel in pushing with the palms in this movement, making four oblique angles. This is a defensive hand technique, meant to block overhead attacks from an opponent.

• The movement involves pushing the palms in bow stance with reverse step forward. Keep a width of about 12 inches or 30 centimeters between the feet to assure that the body is relaxed, straight, and steady.

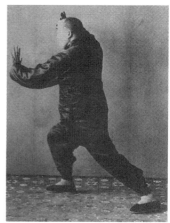

Fig. 179

• In Jade Maiden Weaves the Shuttle to the Right, turn the body in a steady and smooth movement. The right foot need not touch the ground when drawn in, but can step forward directly to the right with the left foot and the turning of the body.

Common Mistakes

• In the fixed posture, the feet in bow stance are not parallel, so the torso is not straight; the palms are not pushed in the same direction as the bow stance.

• The turning of the body stops midway or the speed is accelerated.

• When holding up the palms over the head, the shoulders are raised, the head is not upright and the elbows are raised.

51. Jìnbù Lǎnquèwěi 进步揽雀尾 (Step In and Grasp the Peacock's Tail)

The same as 48. Jìnbù Lǎnquèwěi 进步揽雀尾 (Step In and Grasp the Peacock's Tail). (Fig. 180)

52. Dānbiān 单鞭 (Single Bian)

The same as 4. Dānbiān 单鞭 (Single Bian). (Fig. 181)

53. Yúnshǒu 云手 (Move the Hands Like Clouds)

The same as 27. Yúnshǒu 云手 (Move the Hands Like Clouds). (Fig. 182)

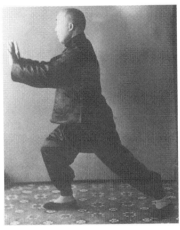
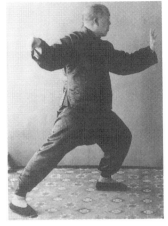
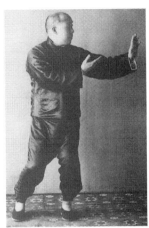

| Fig. 180 | Fig. 181 | Fig. 182 |

54. Dānbiān Xiàshì 单鞭下势 (Single Bian Downward)

54.1 Bow Stance and Push with the Palm

The same with 28. Dānbiān 单鞭 (Single Bian). (Fig. 183)

54.2 Crouch Stance and Thread with the Palm

54.2.1 Shift the body center backward, turn the torso to the right; turn the left foot in and straighten the left leg; turn the right foot out and bend the right leg. Swing the left hand past the front of the head in a curve to the front of the right shoulder, palm facing right; raise the right hook hand to the right front of the body, pointing to the Southwest, shoulder high. Look at the right hook hand. (Fig. 184)

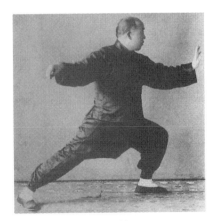

Fig. 183

54.2.2 Bend the right knee and crouch completely on the right leg, stretching the left leg straight to the left to make a crouching stance. Turn the torso to the left; lower the left palm past the front of the abdomen and thread it along the inside of the left leg to the left, palm facing out and fingertips pointing to the left; raise the right hook hand at the right side of the body, shoulder high, fingertips downward. Look at the left hand. (Fig. 185)

Important Points

● The Crouching Stance (pūbù 仆步) is an important stance of Taijiquan. It is performed with one leg completely crouching and the other, stretching straight out to the side; the feet are parallel or turning slightly outward, touch the ground with the whole foot. The torso is straight or leans forward a little.

● In threading the palm, the hand stretches along the body, arm or thigh. Its attacking point is along the fingertips.

● Beginners should proceed step-by-step when doing the crouching stance and kick. The situation varies from person to person; be sure not to tense and hold the breath or force yourself too much.

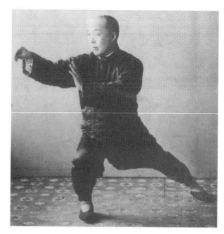

Fig. 184

Common Mistakes

● The head is lowered and the buttocks stick out when crouching. By raising up the heel or the outer side of the foot, the foot does not touch the ground completely.

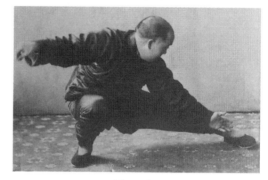

Fig. 185

● The hook hand is placed behind the back, with fingertips pointing upward.

55. Zuǒyòu Jīnjī Dúlì 左右金鸡独立 (Golden Rooster Stands on One Leg, Left and Right)

55.1 Stand on the Left Leg and Spear Up the Hand

55.1.1 Shift the body center forward, turn the left toes out and the right toes in, turn the torso to the left, and bend the left knee forward. Raise the left palm to the front of the body, palm facing right and fingertips pointing upward; change the right hook hand to an open-palm hand and lower it at the side of the body, palm facing inside. Look at the left palm. (Fig. 186)

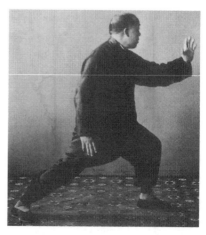

Fig. 186

55.1.2 Stand on the left leg, bend the right knee and lift it forward, toes slanted downward. Turn the torso to the left; raise the right palm up to the front of the head, palm facing left and fingertips pointing upward, with the arm bent slightly in a curve and the elbow in line with the right knee; press the left hand down at the side of the left hip, palm facing down. Look at the right fingertips. (Fig. 187)

55.2 Stand on the Right Leg and Spear Up the Hand

Bend the left knee and squat down, land the right foot backward on the diagonal of the left foot; shift the body center to the right, stand steadily on the slightly bent left leg; bend the right knee and lift it upward and forward, toes slanted down. Turn the torso to the right; raise the left hand to the front of the head, arm half bent in a curve, the elbow directly above the left knee; press down with the right hand at the side of the right hip. Look at the left hand. (Fig. 188)

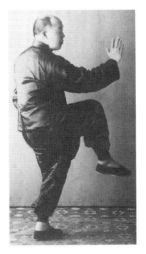 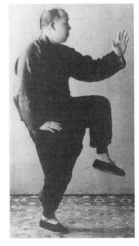

Fig. 187   Fig. 188

Important Points

• One-leg stance (dúlìbù 独立步) is an important stance of Taijiquan. Stand on one leg, knee slightly bent, while bending and lifting the other leg, thigh above level. Keep the torso steady and straight.

• Spearing up the hand (tiǎozhǎng 挑掌) focuses power on the thumb-side of the open-hand as it lifts up to deflect an opponent's attack.

• Keep the torso upright and relaxed naturally, lower the shoulders and push up with the head, arc in the chest and expand the back.

Common Mistakes

• The supporting leg is too bent, and the other leg is not lifted high enough. The body is not balanced steadily on one leg.

• The waist is bent and the back is hunched.

• The palm swings up too close to the body, and the arm bends too much.

56. Zuǒyòu Dàoniǎnhóu 左右倒撵猴 (Drive the Monkeys Back Left and Right)

The same as 16. Zuǒyòu Dàoniǎnhóu 左右倒撵猴 (Drive the Monkeys Back

Left and Right), except that the first "Drive the Monkeys Back — Right Side" begins with the one-leg stance. (Figs. 189, 190)

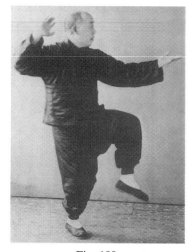
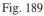
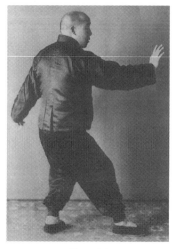

| Fig. 189 | Fig. 190 |

57. Xiéfēishì 斜飞势 (Diagonal Flying Posture)

The same as 17. Xiéfēishì 斜飞势 (Diagonal Flying Posture). (Fig. 191)

58. Tíshǒu 提手 (Lift the Hands)

The same as 18. Tíshǒu 提手 (Lift the Hands). (Fig. 192)

59. Báihè Liàngchì 白鹤亮翅 (White Crane Spreads Its Wings)

The same as 6. Báihè Liàngchì 白鹤亮翅 (White Crane Spreads Its Wings). (Fig. 193)

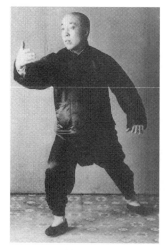
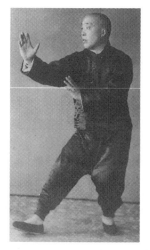
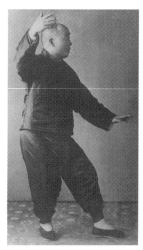

| Fig. 191 | Fig. 192 | Fig. 193 |

60. Lōuxī Àobù 搂膝拗步 (**Brush Aside over the Knee in Reverse Forward Stance**)

The same as 7. Lōuxī Àobù 搂膝拗步 (Brush Aside over the Knee in Reverse Forward Stance). (Fig. 194)

61. Hǎidǐzhēn 海底针 (**Needle at the Bottom of the Sea**)

The same as 21. Hǎidǐzhēn 海底针 (Needle at the Bottom of the Sea). (Fig. 195)

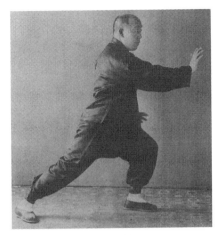
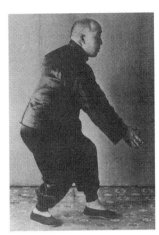

Fig. 194   Fig. 195

62. Shàntōngbèi 扇通背 (**Fan Through the Back**)

The same as 22. Shàntōngbèi 扇通背 (Fan Through the Back). (Fig. 196)

63. Piēshēnchuí 撇身捶 (**Turn and Punch**)

The same as 23. Piēshēnchuí 撇身捶 (Turn and Punch). (Fig. 197)

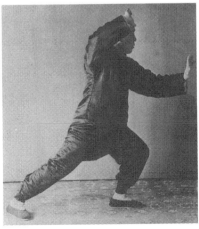
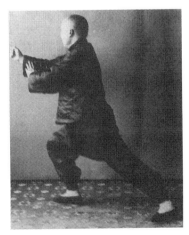

Fig. 196   Fig. 197

64. Jìnbù Bānlánchuí 进步搬拦捶 (Step In, Deflect, Block and Punch)

The same as 24. Jìnbù Bānlánchuí 进步搬拦捶 (Step In, Deflect, Block and Punch). (Fig. 198)

65. Shàngbù Lǎnquèwěi 上步揽雀尾 (Step Forward and Grasp the Peacock's Tail)

The same as 25. Shàngbù Lǎnquèwěi 上步揽雀尾 (Step Forward and Grasp the Peacock's Tail). (Fig. 199)

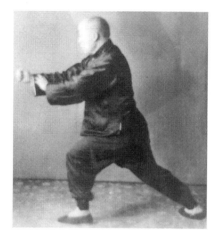 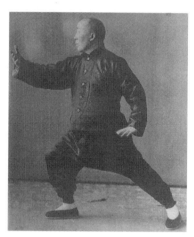

Fig. 198 Fig. 199

66. Dānbiān 单鞭 (Single Bian)

The same as 4. Dānbiān 单鞭 (Single Bian). (Fig. 200)

67. Yúnshǒu 云手 (Move the Hands Like Clouds)

The same as 27. Yúnshǒu 云手 (Move the Hands Like Clouds). (Fig. 201)

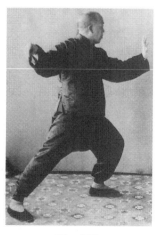 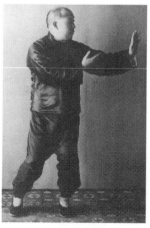

Fig. 200 Fig. 201

68. Dānbiān 单鞭 (Single Bian)

The same as 28. Dānbiān 单鞭 (Single Bian). (Fig. 202)

69. Gāotànmǎ 高探马 (Gauge the Height of the Horse)

The same as 29. Gāotànmǎ 高探马 (Gauge the Height of the Horse). (Fig. 203)

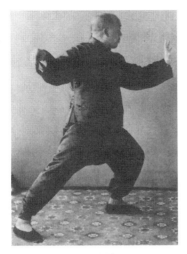

Fig. 202

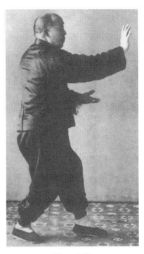

Fig. 203

70. Zhuǎnshēn Shízìjiǎo 转身十字脚 (Turn Around and Cross Feet)

70.1 Bow Stance and Thread the Palm

Move half a step forward with the left foot, shift the body center forward, bend the left leg to make a left bow stance. Turn the torso to the right; thread the left hand over the back of the right hand, raise it as high as the head, palm slanted upward; draw in the right hand to the front of the chest, rest it below the left elbow, palm facing downward. Look at the left palm. (Fig. 204)

70.2 Turn Around and Sweep the Leg

70.2.1 Sit back, turn the left toes in and the torso backward to the right; then shift the body center to the left leg, continue to turn the torso back to the right, straighten the right foot. Raise the left hand up over the side of the head, palm facing out (West); draw in the right hand to the left side of the

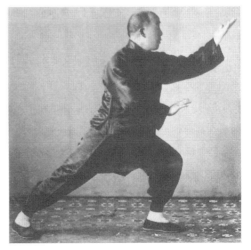

Fig. 204

waist, palm down. Turn the eyes to look ahead to the right. (Fig. 205)

70.2.2 Stand on the left leg, turn the torso to the right; lift the right leg to the left, sweep it past the front of the body upward and outward to the right in a fan-shaped arc, with the top of the foot level and higher than the waist. When the right foot sweeps in front of the body, stretch the left hand to pat the top of the right foot; move the right hand with the turn of the waist to the right side of the body at shoulder height, palm facing right and fingertips upward. Look at the left hand. (Fig. 206)

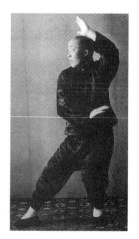

Fig. 205

Important Points

• Sweeping out the leg (wàibǎituǐ 外摆腿) is an important kicking technique in Taijiquan. Turn the waist and move the hips, swinging the leg from the opposite side back to its same side in a fan-shaped arc to kick the opponent with the outside of the foot. When sweeping the right leg, pat the top of the right foot with the left hand with accuracy to make a loud sound. This technique is also called Single-Foot Lotus Swing.

• In the fixed posture, the body turns to face the West. When turning the body to a different direction, coordinate the body center shift with the turning of the feet.

• When patting the top of the foot, the body takes on the form of a cross with the left arm stretched forward and the other to the right. Keep the torso upright and steady, leaning slightly forward.

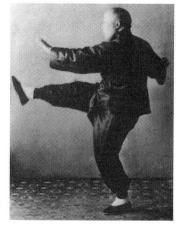

Fig. 206

Common Mistakes

• The kicking leg is swung upward instead of in a fan-shaped arc.
• The patting hand misses the foot; the patting point is lower than the waist.
• The outstretched arms do not cross.
• The torso is bent, the head lowered and the back hunched.

71. Lōuxī Zhǐdāngchuí 搂膝指裆锤 (Brush Aside over the Knee and Punch Down Toward the Crotch)

71.1 Land the Foot and Draw In the Fists

Land the right foot in the right front, turn the toes out, shift the body center forward, bend the right leg, and lift the left heel. Circling the left palm to the right before it stops in front of the right abdomen, palm facing down and fingertips pointing to the right; make a fist with the right hand and hold it at the waist, the palm of the fist facing up. Look ahead downward. (Fig. 207)

71.2 Strike with the Fist in Bow Stance

Shift the body center forward, step forward with the left foot, bend the knee to make a left bow stance. Turn the torso to the left; strike forward with a vertical right fist from the waist at a height of the lower abdomen, the thumb-side of the fist facing up; the left palm sweeps horizontally to the left over the front of the left knee until it stops at the side of the left hip. Look at the right fist. (Fig. 208)

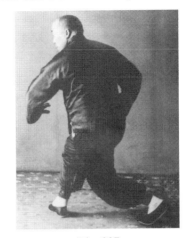

Fig. 207

Important Points

● The strike is made at the height of the lower abdomen, with the torso leaning slightly forward.

● The right foot should land gently, with the heel touching the ground first.

Common Mistakes

● Landing too heavily.

● Lowering the head and bending the waist.

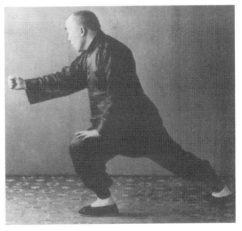

Fig. 208

72. Shàngbù Lǎnquè wěi 上步揽雀尾 (Step Forward and Grasp the Peacock's Tail)

The same as 25. Shàngbù Lǎnquèwěi 上步 揽雀尾 (Step Forward and Grasp the Peacock's Tail). (Figs. 209, 210)

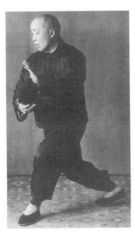

Fig. 209

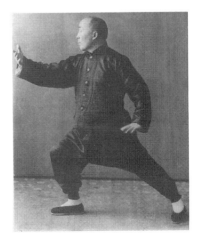

Fig. 210

73. Dānbiān Xiàshì 单鞭下势 (Single Bian Downward)

The same as 54. Dānbiān Xiàshì 单鞭下势 (Single Bian Downward). (Figs. 211, 212)

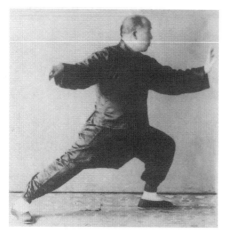

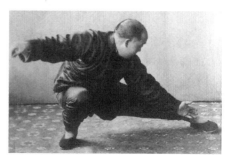

Fig. 212

Fig. 211

74. Shàngbù Qīxīng 上步七星 (Step Forward and Seven Stars)

Shift the body center forward; bend the left leg, turn the left foot out and the right foot in, and turn the torso to the left; step forward with the right foot, landing on the ball of the foot to make an empty stance. Raise the left hand up and make a fist; lower the right hook hand down to make a fist, then move it to the front of the right chest and cross the right wrist with the left wrist; the left fist is inside with the bottom of the fist facing backward; the right fist is outside with the palm of the fist facing forward; half bend the arms in curves. Look straight ahead. (Fig. 213)

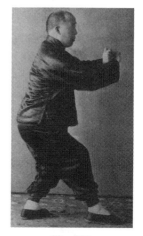

Important Points

Keep the body upright, the lower back relaxed and hips down; push the head up, straighten the spine, and relax the shoulders;

Fig. 213

keep the elbows down, the chest in and the back expanded; bend the knees and tuck in the buttocks, holding the arms in a circle. The direction of this movement is East.

Common Mistakes

The body is leaned either forward or backward; the lower back is pressed forward with the buttocks sticking out; the shoulders are raised as are the elbows; the chest is thrust out and the back tightened; the arms are bent too much with the armpits pressed to the body; the head is lowered and waist bent; the breath is held.

75. Tuìbù Kuàhǔ 退步跨虎 (Step Back to Ride the Tiger)

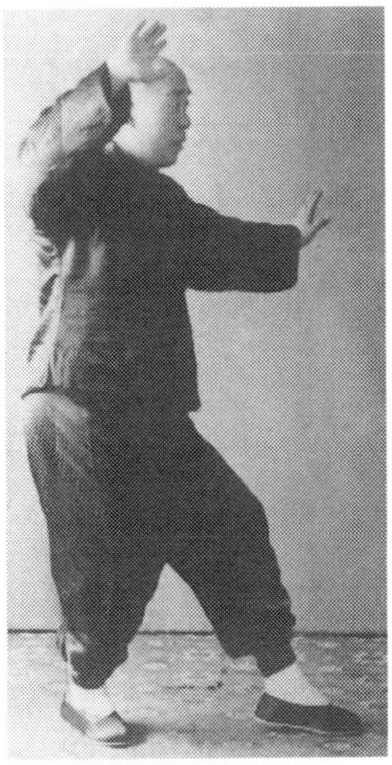

Step backward with the right foot, turning the toes out a little, then shift the body center backward and bend the right leg to sit back; draw in the left foot a little, landing the ball of the foot to make a left empty stance. Turn the torso to the right a little, then turn to the front (East); change the fists into open-palm hands, separate and lower them to either side in curves. Hold the right hand over the head at the right side, palm slanted up to the right, the thumb-side in line with the right forehead; hold the left hand at the side of the body, waist high, palm slanted down to the left. Look straight ahead. (Fig. 214)

Important Points

• Hold the arms half bent in curves to separate and block the opponent's attack.

Fig. 214

• The Important Points for 74. Shàngbù Qīxīng 上步七星 (Step Forward and Seven Stars) also apply here.

Common Mistakes

Same as 74. Shàngbù Qīxīng 上步七星 (Step Forward and Seven Stars).

76. Zhuǎnshēn Bǎilián 转身摆莲 (Turn Around and Lotus Swing)

76.1 Turn Around and Stride

Switch the left heel and then the right toes out, turn the body backward to the right; bend and lift the left leg with the turn of the body and stride to the right turning 270 degrees to land toward the North, shifting the body center forward to make a left bow stance. Move the hands with the body backward to the right, change them to fists when the left foot makes the stride; raise the left fist high at the side of the head, palm of the fist facing out and the thumb-side of the fist slanted down to the right; draw in the right fist to the front of the left chest, palm of the fist facing down and the thumb-side in. Turn the head to look ahead to the right. (Fig. 215)

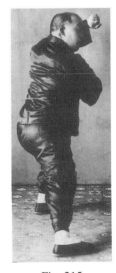

76.2 Sweep the Leg and Pat the Foot

Shift the body center to the right, turn the left foot in and the torso to the right; stand steadily on the left supporting leg, lift the

Fig. 215

right foot and sweep it to the left, upward and to the right in a fan-shaped arc higher than level, extending the top of the foot. Change the fists into open-palm hands and sweep them to the right; when the right leg sweeps out in a fan-shaped arc, the palms sweep from right to left, and pat the top of the right foot in front of the body with two striking sounds. Look straight ahead. (Fig. 216)

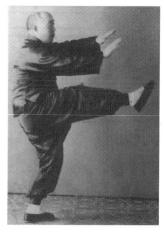

Important Points

• Keep the body balanced and steady when turning backward to the right to stride, raise the left leg while turning in the knee and moving the hips, pivoting on the ball of the right foot. The movement should be continuous and the torso straight.

• When sweeping the leg and patting the foot, the lower back and hips should be relaxed, the hips drawn in

Fig. 216

first and then moved out; keep the sweeping leg agile and relaxed so as to widen the span of sweeping; the height of sweeping may differ from person to person, but the foot must be patted in front of the head or chest, accurately and loudly. Keep the torso relaxed and straight, leaning slightly forward.

Common Mistakes

• The turning of the body and the stride are too heavy and slow; the movement is not continuous and nimble.

• The sweeping leg is not raised high enough; and the patting hands miss the sweeping foot.

• The head is low, waist bent, and breath is held.

77. Wāngōng Shèhǔ 弯弓射虎 (Draw the Bow and Shoot the Tiger)

77.1 Sweep the Arm and Make a Fist

Bend and draw in the right leg after it sweeps outward, turn the torso to the right, step forward with the right leg and land to the right, shifting the body center forward to make a right bow stance. Press down the hands from the left to the right in curves past the front of the abdomen, make fists at the right side of the body, the right fist at shoulder level and the left fist in front of the right chest, palms of both fists facing down. Turn the head to look at the right fist. (Fig. 217)

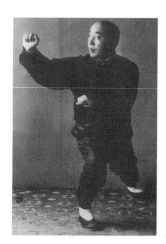

77.2 Strike with Fist in Bow Stance

Keep the right leg bending in right bow stance. Turn the torso to the left; bend the right arm and punch forward to the left, with the right fist by the side of the head, the

Fig. 217

palm of the fist outward and the thumb-side slanted down to the left; punch the left fist forward to the left from the front of the chest, shoulder height, the thumb-side of the fist slanted down to the right. Look at the left fist. (Fig. 218)

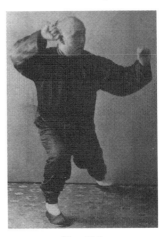

Important Points

● Be light, nimble and steady when landing the right foot, coordinate the swinging of the arm to the right with the turning of the waist.

● Punch with the fists and the bow stance should be coordinated with the left turning of the torso.

● The bow stance faces South by East, while the punches are directed to East by North.

Fig. 218

Common Mistakes

● The bow stance is made before the punch, that is, the feet move faster than the hands.

● Punching with the right fist becomes an overhead block.

● The landing of the right foot is too heavy.

● The body is over-turned so that the bow stance becomes side-bow stance.

78. Jìnbù Bānlánchuí 进步搬拦捶 (Step In, Deflect, Block and Punch)

78.1 Turn Around and Draw In the Fist

Shift the body center to the left, turn the right toes in and the left toes out, and turn the torso to the left to make a left bow stance. Curve the right arm down to the right and rest the right fist in front of the left abdomen; change the left fist into an open-palm hand, facing upward, lower it past the front of the chest, then raise it to the left in a curve until holding it in front of the left shoulder, palm downward. Look ahead to the right. (Fig. 219)

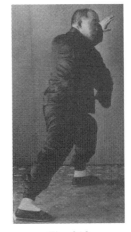

Fig. 219

78.2 Hook Out Step and Make a Fist, 78.3. Step Forward and Block and 78.4. Strike with Fist in Bow Stance are all the same as in 11. Jìnbù Bānlánchuí 进步搬拦捶 (Step In, Deflect, Block and Punch). (Figs. 220, 221, 222)

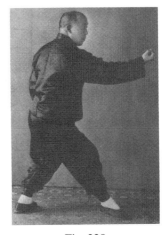

Fig. 220

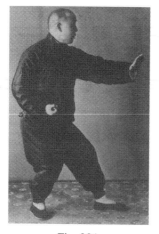

Fig. 221

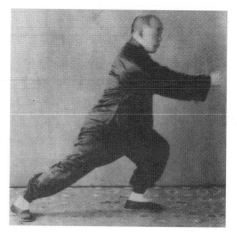

Fig. 222

79. Rúfēng Sìbì 如封似闭 (Pull Back then Push, As if to Close)

The same as 12. Rúfēng Sìbì 如封似闭 (Pull Back then Push, As if to Close). (Figs. 223, 224)

80. Shízìshǒu 十字手 (Cross Hands)

The same as 13. Shízìshǒu 十字手 (Cross Hands). (Figs. 225, 226)

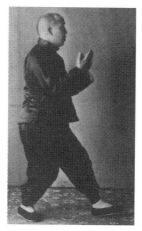

Fig. 223

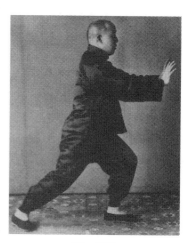

Fig. 224

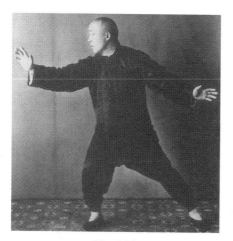

Fig. 225

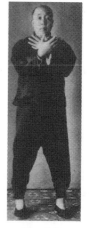

Fig. 226

81. Hétàijí 合太极 (Return to Beginning Taiji Position)

Turn the hands over, stretch forward and separate the arms, raise them to the front of the body at shoulder height and width, palms down. Then lower the elbows and shoulders, press down the hands slowly in front of the hips, palms downward and fingertips forward. Look straight ahead. (Fig. 227)

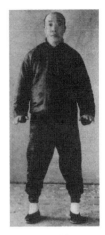

Fig. 227

Important Points

● Be gentle and slow in the movement; keep the body upright, steady and at ease; relax naturally, with peace of mind and even breath.

● To adapt to the rules of martial arts competition in modern times, Ready Position in Taijiquan mostly begins with standing straight, feet parallel and shoulder-width apart. After concluding Taiji, draw the feet together and return to the posture of standing upright.

Common Mistakes

● The concluding movement is done in a rushed, perfunctory and inattentive manner.

● There is a loss of concentration, with irregular breathing.

CHAPTER VI

24-STEP TAIJIQUAN

Èrshísì Shì Tàijíquán   二十四式太极拳

Introduction

After the State Physical Culture and Sports Commission in 1954 established a Martial Arts Research Institute to "explore, classify, research and promote" the martial arts in China, the decision was made to standardize and simplify instructional materials to make martial arts more accessible to the public, starting with Taijiquan. In this regard, the State Physical Culture and Sports Commission invited Taijiquan experts like Wu Tunan (1883-1989), Chen Fake (1887-1957), Gao Ruizhou, Tian Zhenfeng, Li Tianji (1914-1996), Tang Hao (1897-1959) and others to discuss and make a proposal on simplifying Taijiquan. This group made a draft proposal based on representative movements of all the major Taijiquan styles. However, this first proposal was not implemented after it was deemed too complicated for beginners, and therefore inappropriate as a way to promote Taijiquan.

In 1955, Mao Bohao, Li Tianji, Tang Hao, Wu Gaoming and others of the Martial Arts Department of the State Physical Culture and Sports Commission restudied the problem and found a solution: By selecting the main parts of the popular Yang-style Taijiquan, they created an easy-to-learn-and-to-practice sequence of movements, concise and clear, that preserved the traditional features of Taijiquan, emphasized the health benefits of Taijiquan and encouraged wide public participation. Because this sequence had 24 basic steps, it was given the name 24-Step Taijiquan.

The 24-Step Taijiquan was first published in China as *Simplified Taijiquan*, a martial arts textbook written and illustrated by Li Tianji. In 1956, the Martial Arts Department of the State Physical Culture and Sports Commission revised the book and after several editions distributed the work to physical education departments on all levels throughout China.

24-Step Taijiquan has the following features:

1. All the movements were selected from Yang-style Taijiquan. The movements are soft and smooth, with straight and balanced postures. They are suitable for both the young and old, therefore widely accessible to everyone.

2. It takes between 4 to 6 minutes to complete. This compares to some 16 to 24 minutes it takes to complete the traditional Yang form on which the 24-Step Taijiquan is based. The shorter time interval makes the 24-Step Taijiquan suitable for practice during morning exercises as well as work breaks.

3. While retaining the main techniques of traditional Taijiquan, 24-Step Taijiquan eliminates much of the repetition. In the traditional routines of Taijiquan, over half of the movements are repeated.

4. The order of movements in 24-Step Taijiquan does not follow the order of the traditional form. The principle behind the arrangement of the order of 24-Step Taijiquan: From simple to complicated, from easy to difficult. At the beginning, the order calls for forward movements, then back and sideward movements. Later in the sequence come movements with complicated transitions such as kicking, lowering the body down, and standing on one leg.

5. The 24-Step Taijiquan offers a complete and balanced exercise. In key movements, corresponding left or right forms were added to avoid the phenomenon of having one Push Down and Stand on the Left Leg and one Grasp the Peacock's Tail on the Right. This gives practitioners the benefits of an all-round workout.

The 24-Step Taijiquan has preserved martial arts heritage and promoted its teaching. Some worried when it was first created that a simplified Taijiquan would betray tradition by discarding the essence of Taijiquan. These critics gradually have changed their views with the realization that traditional martial arts can maintain their vitality only through adapting to changes in society and people's needs. This has been the reality of Taijiquan throughout history. After 24-Step Taijiquan was introduced in 1956, it immediately became popular throughout China. Now, it has become the beginning step for Taijiquan enthusiasts in every country, playing a positive role in promoting Taijiquan not only in China but also throughout the world.

Names of the Movements of 24-Step Taijiquan

Pinyin Chinese (English)

1. Qǐshì 起势 (Beginning Position)

2. Zuǒyòu Yěmǎ Fēnzōng 左右野马分鬃 (Part the Wild Horse's Mane — Left and Right)

3. Báihè Liàngchì 白鹤亮翅 (White Crane Spreads Its Wings)

4. Zuǒyòu Lōuxī Àobù 左右搂膝拗步 (Brush Aside over the Knee in Reverse Forward Stance — Left and Right)

5. Shǒuhuī Pípā 手挥琵琶 (Play the Pipa*)

6. Zuǒyòu Dàojuǎngōng 左右倒卷肱 (Step Back and Curl the Arms — Left and Right)

7. Zuǒ Lǎnquèwěi 左揽雀尾 (Grasp the Peacock's Tail on the Left)

8. Yòu Lǎnquèwěi 右揽雀尾 (Grasp the Peacock's Tail on the Right)

9. Dānbiān 单鞭 (Single Bian**)

10. Yúnshǒu 云手 (Move the Hands like Clouds)

11. Dānbiān 单鞭 (Single Bian)

12. Gāotànmǎ 高探马 (Gauge the Height of the Horse)

13. Yòu Dēngjiǎo 右蹬脚 (Kick with the Right Heel)

14. Shuāngfēng Guàn'ěr 双峰贯耳 (Strike the Opponent's Ears with Both Fists)

15. Zhuǎnshēn Zuǒ Dēngjiǎo 转身左蹬脚 (Turn and Kick with the Left Heel)

16. Zuǒ Xiàshì Dúlì 左下势独立 (Push Down and Stand on the Left Leg)

17. Yòu Xiàshì Dúlì 右下势独立 (Push Down and Stand on the Right Leg)

18. Zuǒyòu Chuānsuō 左右穿梭 (Move the Shuttle Left and Right)

19. Hǎidǐzhēn 海底针 (Needle at the Bottom of the Sea)

20. Shǎntōngbì 闪通臂 (Send a Flash Through the Arms)

21. Zhuǎnshēn Bānlánchuí 转身搬拦捶 (Turn the Body, Deflect, Block and Punch)

22. Rúfēng Sìbì 如封似闭 (Pull Back then Push, As if to Close)

23. Shízìshǒu 十字手 (Cross Hands)

24. Shōushì 收势 (Closing Position)

Movements and Illustrations of 24-Step Taijiquan

Yùbèishì 预备势 (Ready Position)

Stand naturally straight, calm and relaxed. The arms hang naturally at the sides. Keep the head and neck straight, chin slightly drawn in. Close the mouth and bring the

---

* Shǒuhuī Pípā 手挥琵琶 (Play the Pipa): A pipa is a pear-shaped Chinese four-stringed musical instrument made of wood, plucked, and usually held perpendicular with the body of the instrument on the performer's knee.

** Dānbiān 单鞭 (Danbian): "Dān" means single. "Biān" here refers to an ancient weapon, an iron rod that is either rectangular in shape or edged as in bamboo, or other patterns. Bian were often used in pairs, hence Danbian means Single Bian.

teeth together. Touch the tip of the tongue to the roof of the mouth. Concentrate and breathe naturally, eyes to the front. (Fig. 1 Assume that the direction faced is South.)

1. Qǐshì 起势 (Beginning Position)

1.1 Step to the Left and Stand with the Feet Shoulder-Width Apart

Step to the left to form a stance with the feet shoulder-width apart, pointing parallel forward. (Fig. 2)

1.2 Raise the Arms

Raise the arms slowly until the hands reach shoulder height, shoulder-width apart. Extend the arms forward naturally with the elbows slightly bent and the palms facing down, fingers forward. (Fig. 3)

1.3 Bend the legs slowly into a half squat. Keep the body center balanced on both feet to form a horse stance. At the same time, press the palms of the open hands gently down to abdomen level, the torso upright. Look straight ahead. (Fig. 4)

Important Points

● Horse stance (mǎbù 马步) is one of the basic stances of Taijiquan. Keep the torso upright; lift the head and straighten the spine, drop the shoulders and relax the chest. Bend the knees and tuck in the buttocks. Keep the body center balanced between both feet.

● When stepping into horse stance, follow the footwork principle of "rise gently; fall gently; point, rise, point, fall" (Qīngqǐ qīngluò, diǎnqǐ diǎnluò. 轻起轻落，点起点落). First shift the body center to the right leg, then raise the left heel gently and move the left foot half a step to the left without raising it above the right ankle height. Touch the toes of the left foot on the ground first, and point the left toes straight ahead. Then set the whole foot.

● Raise the arms and lower the open-palm hands according to the principle of "slow and steady." Lift the arms and let them down as if they were moving through

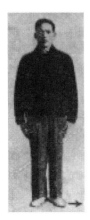 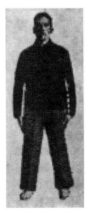 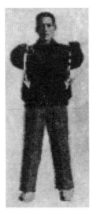 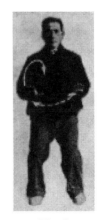

| Fig. 1 | Fig. 2 | Fig. 3 | Fig. 4 |

water — controlled but not stiff; relaxed but not slack.

● Before raising the arms, turn the hands at the outer sides of the thighs so the palms face back. Then slowly raise the arms.

● Coordinate the lowering of the palms with the bending of the legs. When the hands reach the abdomen level, the palms stretched out and fingers are relaxed.

● The level to which the knees are bent can differ according to the individual. Most Taijiquan routines are executed at the level of a half squat. The level to which the knees are bent at the beginning should be maintained throughout the routine. The level should not be raised or lowered. Therefore, to assure a steady posture throughout, practitioners in the beginning position should squat neither too low nor too high.

Common Mistakes

● When stepping to the left, the body wavers.

● When raising the arms and lowering the hands, the elbows move outward or are raised up; the shoulders are shrugged.

● When bending into a squat, the torso leans forward or backward.

● When raising the arms and lowering the palms, the wrists are too lax.

● The knees are bent and the hands lowered at different speeds, without synchronization.

2. Zuǒyòu Yěmǎ Fēnzōng 左右野马分鬃 (Part the Wild Horse's Mane — Left and Right)

Zuǒ Yěmǎ Fēnzōng 左野马分鬃 (Part the Wild Horse's Mane — Left Side)

2.1 Hold a Ball and Draw In the Foot

Turn the torso slightly to the right; draw the right arm in a curve to the right of the chest, with the right hand not higher than shoulder height and the right elbow slightly lower than the right hand, the right palm down. Keep the left arm in a curve in front of the abdomen, the left palm up; the two hands face each other in a position as if to hold a ball in front of the right ribs. Draw in the left foot to the inside of the right foot, toes on the ground. Look at the right hand. (Fig. 5)

2.2 Turn the Body and Step Forward

Turn the torso to the left; move the left foot one step to the left front, with the heel landing gently on the ground. The body center still stays on the right leg. (Fig. 6)

2.3 Bow Stance (Gōngbù 弓步) and Separate the Hands

Continue to turn the torso to the left; shift the body center forward, plant the left foot firmly, and bend the left knee forward into a bow, with the right leg naturally straight and the right heel pushed down and outward, to form a left bow stance. At the same time, pull the hands apart — up to the front and down to the back until the left hand in front reaches the eye level in front of the body, with the left palm slanted up; and the right hand in back reaches the side of the right hip, with the right palm pressing down, fingertips forward. Both arms are slightly bent. Look at the left hand. (Fig. 7)

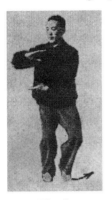
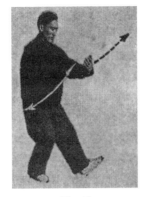
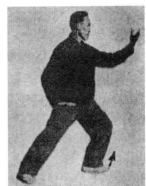

Fig. 5   Fig. 6   Fig. 7

Yòu Yěmǎ Fēnzōng 右野马分鬃 (Part the Wild Horse's Mane — Right Side)

2.4 Turn the Body and Lift the Ball of the Foot Up and Outward

Shift the body center slightly back, and raise the left ball of the foot up and slightly outward; turn the torso slightly to the left; be ready to turn the hands and "hold a ball." Look at the left hand. (Fig. 8)

2.5 Hold a Ball and Draw In the Foot

Continue to turn the torso to the left. Turn the left hand until the palm faces down, circling the left hand in front of the left chest; turn the right hand and swing it forward and curve it in front of the abdomen, the palm up; the palms face each other in a position in front of the left ribs as if to hold a ball. Shift the body center to the left leg, plant the left foot firmly, and draw in the right foot to the inside of the left foot, toes on the ground. Look at the left hand. (Fig. 9)

2.6. Turn the Body and Step Forward

Turn the torso slightly to the right; move the right foot one step forward to the right, with the heel landing gently on the ground. (Fig 10)

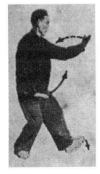
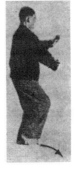
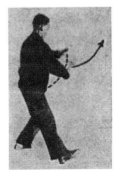

Fig. 8   Fig. 9   Fig. 10

2.7 Bow Stance and Separate the Hands

Continue to turn the torso to the right; shift the body center forward, plant the right foot firmly. Bend the right knee forward into a bow; at the same time the left leg is naturally straight, draw the left heel outward, forming a right bow stance; separate the hands until the right hand reaches the eye level in front of the body, right palm slanting up, while the left hand is pressing down at the outside of the left hip, palm down and fingertips forward. Both arms are slightly bent. Look at the right hand. (Fig. 11)

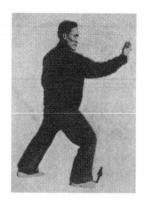

Fig. 11

Zuǒ Yěmǎ Fēnzōng 左野马分鬃 (Part the Wild Horse's Mane — Left Side)

2.8 Turn the Body and Lift the Ball of the Foot Up and Outward

Shift the body center slightly back, and raise the right toes and ball of the foot up and outward; turn the torso slightly to the right; be ready to turn the hands and "hold a ball." (Fig. 12)

2.9 Hold a Ball and Draw In the Foot

Continue to turn the torso to the right; turn the right hand until the palm faces down, with the arm circled in front of the right chest; turn the left hand and swing it forward in a circle in front of the abdomen; the palms face each other in a position in front of the right ribs as if to hold a ball. Shift the body center forward and plant the right foot firmly, and draw in the left foot to the inside of the right foot, with toes landing on the ground. Look at the right hand. (Fig. 13)

2.10 Turn the Body and Step Forward

Turn the torso to the left; move the left foot a step forward to the left, with the left heel landing on the ground gently. Keep the body center on the right leg. (Fig. 14)

2.11 Bow Stance and Separate the Hands

Continue to turn the torso to the left; shift the body center forward, plant the left

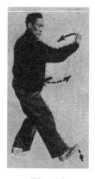

Fig. 12

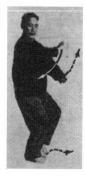

Fig. 13

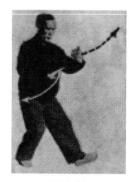

Fig. 14

foot firmly. Bend the left knee forward into a bow; the right leg is naturally straight, draw the right heel outward, forming a left bow stance; at the same time separate the hands until the left hand reaches the eye level in front of the body, palm slanted up, while the right hand is pressed down at the side of the right hip, palm down and fingers forward. Both arms are slightly bent. Look at the left hand. (Fig. 15)

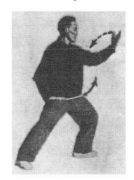

Fig. 15

Application

Yěmǎ Fēnzōng (Part the Wild Horse's Mane) applies to pulling an opponent off balance and then moving in on him/her. For example, when an opponent attacks with his/her right hand, I catch the opponent's right wrist with my right hand and pull the opponent down. At the same time, I step forward with my left foot behind the opponent and thrust my left forearm under the opponent's right armpit to throw the opponent by using the force of the turning of my waist.

Important Points

Zuǒ Yěmǎ Fēnzōng 左野马分鬃 (Part the Wild Horse's Mane — Left Side)

• Turning the body and holding a ball are done as one; that is, they happen simultaneously, and holding a ball must be coordinated through the turning of the body. "To hold a ball" is a vivid metaphor. Keep the arms curved as if to hold a balloon without touching the body — the arms relaxed but not limp. Keep the right arm in a curve at shoulder height, relax the shoulders with the elbows a little lower than the shoulders and the wrists a little lower than the hands, fingers slightly bent and apart. The distance between the forearms and the chest is about 8 to 12 inches or 20 to 30 centimeters. When drawing the left arm into a curve, rotate the forearm at the same time. Keep the left arm curved when it reaches its final position.

• When "drawing in the left foot to the inside of the right foot, toes landing on the ground," most of the body center is on the right leg, and the left leg just helps support the body. Here "toes landing on the ground" means the ball of the foot lands on the ground. Beginners should do it this way. However, after becoming proficient in the movement, do not land the toes on the ground when drawing in the left foot to the inside of the right foot. This applies also to Yòu Yěmǎ Fēnzōng (Part the Wild Horse's Mane — Right Side).

Assuming that the student is facing South at the beginning, the first bow stance in "Zuǒ Yěmǎ Fēnzōng" or "Part the Wild Horse's Mane — Left" ends up facing due East. To accomplish this, turn the torso to the Southeast before making the step forward to the left, then continue to turn the torso with the step until facing due East. Make the two turnings of the body in a continuous movement.

- When stepping forward with the left foot, land the left heel on the ground first. The footwork of Taijiquan requires that one leg be bent to support the body and stabilize the body center while the other leg steps out gently with agility. Do not abruptly drop the foot and do not shift the body center too early.

- The bow stance (gōngbù 弓步) of Taijiquan requires that the rear leg be naturally straight, not as tight as the leg in Long Fist Boxing. If it were, the waist and hips would not be as relaxed as they should be for Taijiquan. However, do not relax the waist and hips so much that the knee bends too much, which makes the whole body look soft and weak. In addition, after the right leg naturally straightens, root the right foot firmly on the ground. Do not let the outside of the foot or the heel come up. When fixing the bow stance, have two-thirds of the body center on the front leg and one-third on the back leg.

- When separating the hands, slant the left palm up. Focus power on the outside of the forearm. Push the forearm to the left upper left corner on the diagonal. At this time, keep the left shoulder low and relaxed, the elbow slightly bent. At the same time, move the right hand down to the right until it reaches the right side of the hip. The right palm is down, fingertips forward, the elbow slightly curved. When the right hand reaches its lowest point, extend the right palm and relax the fingers. Seat the wrist and lower the shoulder slightly. When the hands are separated to their farthest distance, the palms should be spread open and fingers relaxed, demonstrating an air of moving from agility to stability.

- The expression of the eyes is an important component of Taijiquan. In the beginning of this movement, look straight ahead, then shift the attention to the right hand, then shift the attention to the left hand. When fixing the form, look at the left hand. That is to say, the eyes sometimes focus with attention, and sometimes they soften and relax. Let the eyes continually and appropriately adjust.

- At the moment when finishing this movement, have the idea of sending power to the limbs and to the top of the head. At the same time, exhale. In this way, the end of the form will be more stable and the change between solid and empty will be more distinct. But don't overdo it. Especially, the arms should not be stretched tight nor should the legs be so bent that the body is deliberately lowered.

Yòu Yěmǎ Fēnzōng 右野马分鬃 (Part the Wild Horse's Mane — Right)

- When turning the body and raising the ball of the left foot, shift the body center slightly back, steadily, with a turning of the body to the left. In the execution of turning the body, keep the torso upright.

- When the hands start to turn into an arc until they "hold a ball," first relax the hands from solid to empty, then turn the left hand palm inward while the right hand moves outward in a curve. At the same time, draw in the rear foot.

- When drawing in the foot by shifting the body center forward, use the power of the thigh to raise the rear foot gently, then slowly bend the back knee to place the rear foot to the inside of the front foot.

• The footwork of successive forward stepping is an essential point to study in this movement. Practice both bow stance and successive forward stepping by themselves to address any problem that might arise from paying too much attention to the hands in the movement without considering the feet.

• Other important points are the same as those for Zuǒ Yěmǎ Fēnzōng (Part the Wild Horse's Mane — Left).

Common Mistakes

• In executing the first Zuǒ Yěmǎ Fēnzōng (Part the Wild Horse's Mane — Left) the body is not turned enough so that the left foot falls too far to the right, twisting the legs in the left bow stance. This throws off the next two bow steps, as well, creating stances that are too narrow in their width.

• In making a bow step, the toes of the front foot are turned outward.

• When fixing the bow stance, the rear heel is not pushed outward and rooted, creating the mistakes of thrusting out the chest, leaning the body, leaving the hip joints open instead of closed.

• The fingers are too stiff or too soft. When turning the hand, a "wrist flower" or extraneous turning of the wrist is made.

• During the movement, the torso leans, the head lowers, the waist bends, and the body center is not steady.

3. Báihè Liàngchì 白鹤亮翅 (White Crane Spreads Its Wings)

3.1 Follow-Up Step and Hold a Ball

Turn the torso slightly to the left; move the right foot half a step forward, with the ball of the right foot landing on the ground gently one-foot length away from the left heel; at the same time, turn the hands until they face each other, and bend the arms and "hold a ball" before the chest, the left hand above and palm down, the right hand below and palm up. Look at the left hand. (Fig. 16)

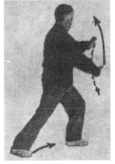

Fig. 16

3.2 Sit Back and Turn the Body

Shift the body center back, plant the right foot firmly on the ground; at the same time the torso sits back and turns to the right; cross the hands and separate them, with the right hand raised up and the left hand lowered. Look at the right hand. (Fig. 17)

3.3 Empty Stance and Separate Hands

Turn the torso to the front; move the left foot slightly forward,

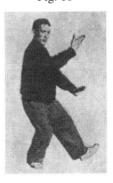

Fig. 17

with the sole of the foot landing on the ground, to form a left empty stance; at the same time, the right hand is raised up to the front of the right forehead, the palm facing inward. Lower the left hand to the side of the left thigh, pressing the left palm down. Look straight ahead. (Fig.18)

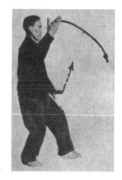

Fig. 18

Application

Báihè Liàngchì (White Crane Spreads Its Wings) has two applications. When an opponent attacks with both hands, I move both hands up then down to separate the opponent's hands. Also, when the opponent initiates a right-hand attack, I grab the opponent's right wrist with my left hand, thrust, my right arm under his/her left armpit and then throw him/her through the power generated by my turning waist.

Important Points

• Empty stance and follow-up step are used in this movement. Empty stance requires relaxing the torso while keeping it upright and making a clear distinction in the legs between empty and solid. Keep the body center stable. When executing the follow-up step, shift the body center first, then raise the right foot gently and move it half a step forward. Land the right foot one foot's length away from the left foot, then slowly shift the body center back, gradually planting the whole right foot. The stance of the right leg changes from empty to solid, supporting most of the body center. Finally, move the left foot forward slowly, forming a left empty stance with the ball of the left foot touching the ground. The whole process requires gentle and agile footwork, steady shifting of the body center and a clear expression in the feet of the change between empty and solid.

• When executing the above movements, pay attention to the turning of the waist to assure coordination in a complete movement that involves the whole body. That is to say, when stepping forward with the right foot, turn the waist slightly to the left. When sitting back, turn the waist slightly to the right. Finally, when fixing the stance, turn the body directly to the front (due East).

Coordinate the eye movements with the movements of the hands. When executing the follow-up step and holding a ball, look at the left hand; when sitting back and turning the body, shift the focus to the right hand; finally, when turning the torso to the front, look straight ahead.

• As the two hands separate, keep the head held high and the spine erect, with the waist and hips relaxed. Concentrate. Show an air of composure and stability in the fixed posture.

Common Mistakes

• When fixing the empty stance, the torso leans back, with the hips and the abdomen thrust forward. Or the torso leans forward, with the chest and buttocks thrust back. The left knee is straightened, the right knee is drawn inward. The width between the feet is too long or too short. There is no clear distinction between empty and solid in the two feet, so the body center is balanced on both feet.

● The hands are not extended enough; the elbows are too bent, causing tension in the armpits and a break in the line of the extended arms.

4. Zuǒyòu Lōuxī Àobù 左右搂膝拗步 (Brush Aside over the Knee in Reverse Forward Stance — Left and Right)

Zuǒ Lōuxī Àobù 左搂膝拗步 (Brush Aside over the Knee and Reverse Forward Stance — Left Side)

4.1 Turn the Body and Swing the Arms

Turn the torso slightly to the left; swing the right hand to the front of the body, palm up. Look at the right hand. (Fig. 19)

4.2 Swing the Arms and Draw In the Foot

Turn the torso to the right; swing the arms to the right overlapping, left over right. The right hand drops down from the front of the head in a semi-circle past the right hip side and up to the upper rear right until it reaches head level, palm up. Meanwhile, the left hand swings in an arc up from the left side past the front of the head to the right where it then lowers to the front of the right chest, palm down; draw the left foot to the inside of the right foot, with toes landing on the ground. Turn the head with the body. Look at the right hand. (Fig. 20)

4.3 Step Forward and Bend the Elbow

Turn the torso slightly to the left; move the left foot one step forward to the left, with the heel landing on the ground gently; bend the right elbow, bring the right hand to the side of the head above the shoulder, with the "tiger's mouth" (Hǔkǒu 虎口) or the web between the thumb and index finger facing the ear and the palm slanted forward, drop the left hand to the front of the abdomen. Look at the right hand. (Fig. 21)

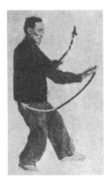
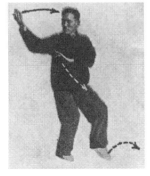
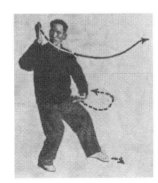

Fig. 19   Fig. 20   Fig. 21

4.4 Bow Stance and Brush Aside and Push

Continue to turn the torso to the left; shift the body center forward, plant the left foot firmly. Bend the left leg, the right leg is naturally straight to form a left bow stance; the left hand brushes aside over the front of the left knee and presses down to the outside of the left thigh, palm down, fingers forward. Push the right hand forward, fingertips level with the nose, palm forward, fingers up. The right arm is naturally straight, the right elbow slightly bent. Look at the right hand. (Fig. 22)

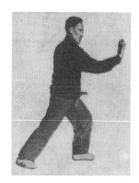

Fig. 22

Yòu Lōuxī Àobù 右搂膝拗步 (Brush Aside over the Knee and Reverse Forward Stance — Right Side)

4.5 Turn the Body and Draw the Ball of the Foot Outward

Shift the body center to the back slightly, raise the ball of the left foot up and outward, turn the torso to the left; turn the arms outward and begin to swing them to the left. Look at the right hand. (Fig. 23)

4.6 Swing the Arms and Draw In the Foot

Continue to turn the torso to the left; shift the body center forward, plant the left foot firmly on the ground, and draw in the right foot to the inside of the left foot, with the toes landing on the ground; swing the right hand in an arc past the front of the head until it reaches the front of the left shoulder, palm down; raise the left hand in an arc to the upper left until it reaches the head level, palm up. The left arm is naturally straight, the elbow is slightly bent. Turn the head and look at the left hand. (Fig. 24)

4.7 Step Forward and Bend the Elbow

Turn the torso slightly to the right; move the right foot a step forward to the right, with the heel landing on the ground gently; bend the left elbow, pull back the left hand to the side of the head above the shoulder, with the "tiger's mouth" facing the ear, palm slanted forward; at the same time, drop the right hand to the abdomen, palm down, the elbow slightly bent. Begin to turn the head to look forward. (Fig. 25)

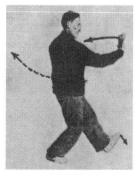
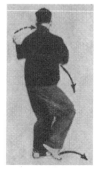
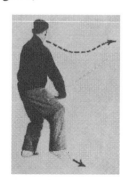

Fig. 23   Fig. 24   Fig. 25

4.8 Bow Stance and Brush Aside and Push

Continue to turn the torso to the right; shift the body center forward, plant the right foot firmly, bend the right leg, the left leg naturally straight to form a right bow stance; brush aside with the right hand past the right knee to the right and down by the outside of the right leg, palm down, fingers forward. Push the left hand forward, fingertips level with the nose, palm forward, fingers up. The left arm is naturally straight, the elbow slightly bent. Look at the left hand. (Fig. 26)

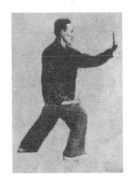

Fig. 26

Zuǒ Lōuxī Àobù 左搂膝拗步 (Brush Aside over the Knee and Reverse Forward Stance — Left Side)

4.9 Turn the Body and Draw the Ball of the Foot Outward

Shift the body center to the back slightly, raise the ball of the right foot outward, turn the torso to the right; turn the arms outward and begin to swing them to the right. Look at the left hand. (Fig. 27)

4.10 Swing the Arms and Draw In the Foot

Continue to turn the torso to the right; shift the body center forward, plant the right foot firmly, draw in the left foot to the inside of the right foot, with toes on the ground; swing the left hand in an arc past the front of the head until it reaches the front of the right shoulder, palm down; raise the right hand in an arc to the upper right until it reaches head level, palm up. The right arm is naturally straight; the elbow is slightly bent. Turn the head and look at the right hand. (Fig. 28)

4.11 Step Forward and Bend the Elbow

Turn the torso slightly to the left; move the left foot a step forward to the left with the heel landing on the ground gently; bend the right elbow, pull the right hand to the side of the head above the shoulder, with the "tiger's mouth" (the web between the index finger and thumb) facing the ear, palm slanted forward; at the same time, drop the left hand to the front of the abdomen, palm down and the elbow slightly bent. Begin to turn the head to look forward. (Fig. 29)

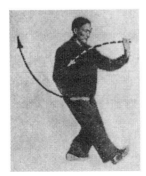

Fig. 27

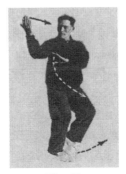

Fig. 28

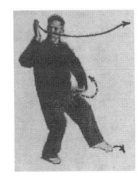

Fig. 29

4.12 Bow Stance and Brush Aside and Push

Continue to turn the torso to the left; shift the body center forward, plant the left foot firmly, bend the left leg, the right leg is naturally straight to form a left bow stance; brush aside with the left hand past the left knee to the left and press it down at the outer side of the left leg, palm down, fingers forward. Push the right hand forward, fingertips level with the nose, palm forward, fingers up. The right arm is naturally straight, the elbow slightly bent. Look at the right hand. (Fig. 30)

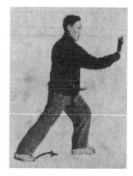

Fig. 30

Application

This movement can be used to intercept an attack, using one hand to deflect and the other hand to counter-attack the opponent.

Important Points

• Both Lōuxī Àobù (Brush Aside over the Knee and Reverse Forward Stance) and Yěmǎ Fēnzōng (Part the Wild Horse's Mane) involve three successive forward steps into bow stance. The difference is: Lōuxī Àobù employs a reverse bow stance in which the opposite arm and leg are forward. To keep the body center steady and to assure that the torso does not lean, place the feet about 12 inches or 30 centimeters apart in the width of the stance. Do not have the feet on the same line; do not cross them.

• When stepping forward, beginners who have trouble keeping their balance can touch their toes to the ground as they draw in the rear foot to the inside of the supporting foot. Once they become proficient in this body shifting, students should skip the landing of the toes and step forward continuously and steadily with the rear foot passing the inside of the supporting foot without the toes landing on the ground.

• When executing Lōuxī Àobù, coordinate the movements of pushing forward, brushing aside and bending the leg.

Common Mistakes

• When pushing, the front hand stretches out too straight or too far. When the hand brushes aside over the knee to deflect an attack, the elbow is bent and drawn back, causing tension in the shoulders and arms and a leaning forward of the torso.

• When swinging the arms, the waist doesn't move. This creates a stiff, puppet-like movement.

• Not enough distance between the feet in the width of the bow stance. The torso is tense and leans with the body center unsteady.

• The movements of pushing forward, brushing palms and bending legs are not coordinated.

5. Shǒuhuī Pípā 手挥琵琶 (Play the Pipa)

5.1 Follow-Up Step and Extend the Arm

Move the right foot half a step forward, with the ball of the foot landing at the back of the left foot, about one foot's length away from the left foot. Extend the right arm forward slightly, relax the wrist. (Fig. 31)

5.2 Sit Back and Lead Back the Hand

Shift the body center to the back, plant the right foot firmly. Turn the torso to the right; swing the left hand to the upper left in an arc to the front of the body, with the arm naturally straight, palm slanted down; bend and lead back the right arm to the front of the chest, palm slanted down. Look at the left hand. (Fig. 32)

5.3 Empty Stance and Bring the Hands Together

Turn the torso to the left, move the left foot slightly forward with the heel on the ground, to form a left empty stance; turn the arms outward, bend the elbows, with the left hand in the front of the right one, the hands brought together on the vertical in front of the body; the left hand is level with the nose, left palm facing toward the right; the right hand is level with the left elbow, right palm facing left, as if to play a lute. Look at the left hand. (Fig. 33)

Application

When an opponent attacks with the right hand, I use my right hand to grab hold of the opponent's right wrist and pull it back. At the same time, I put my left hand on the opponent's elbow and twist or lock the elbow joint with both hands by using Qin Na [techniques used to control joints] to dislocate his or her right arm.

Important Points

● Play the Pipa requires good coordination of the body, hands and feet to avoid stiff movements. For example, when sitting back and drawing back the hand, move and draw back the arms using the power of the turning of the body and the shifting back of the body center. When closing the hands in empty stance, control the movements of both the upper and lower body through the turning of the body to the left.

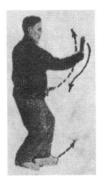 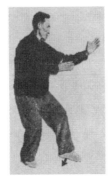 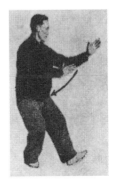

Fig. 31   Fig. 32   Fig. 33

- When fixing the form, have the arms both curved and extended. At the same time, lift the head and straighten the spine, relax the waist and exhale, bend the legs and lower the hips. Exude steadiness, uprightness and vitality.

Common Mistakes

- The movements of the body and the hands are not coordinated. There are usually two problems: One is that the body turns too much, and the movements are too lax. This can cause the torso to lean to the side with movements of the waist and limbs that are not coordinated. The other problem occurs when the body turns too little. This is usually characterized by hand techniques that are unsteady and stiff.

- When fixing the form, the arms are bent too much. The arms are tense and clamp to the ribs. The movements are not smooth.

- The empty stance is incorrect. The body leans forward and the buttocks are thrust out, or the body leans back and the abdomen is thrust forward.

6. Zuǒyòu Dàojuǎngōng 左右倒卷肱 (Step Back and Curl the Arms — Left and Right)

Yòu Dàojuǎngōng 右倒卷肱 (Step Back and Curl the Arms — Right Side)

6.1 Turn the Body and Pull Back the Hands

Turn the torso slightly to the right; rotate both hands up, move the right hand down past the waist then up and back in a circular (curling) motion with the turning of the body until the right hand reaches head level, with the right arm slightly bent. Turn the left arm in front of the body; the head turns with the body, first looking at the right hand and then the left. (Fig. 34)

6.2 Step Back and Curl the Arms

Turn the torso slightly to the left; raise the left foot and move it one step back, with the ball of the foot landing on the ground gently; bend the right elbow and curl the right hand to the right ear above the shoulder, palm slanted down; begin to draw the left hand back. Look at the left hand. (Fig. 35)

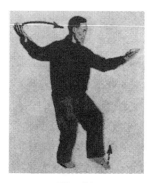

Fig. 34

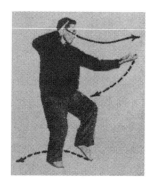

Fig. 35

6.3 Empty Stance and Push Palm

Continue to turn the torso to the left; shift the body center back, plant the left foot firmly, pivot on the ball of the right foot to turn the right foot straight, with the heel off the ground. Bend the right knee slightly to form a right empty stance; push the right hand to the front of the body, the wrist at shoulder height, palm forward; draw the left hand down to the back in an arc, drawing it back to the left side of the waist, palm up. Look at the right hand. (Fig. 36)

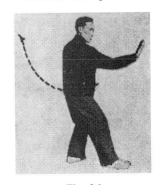

Fig. 36

Zuǒ Dàojuǎngōng 左倒卷肱(Step Back and Curl the Arms — Left Side)

6.4 Turn the Body and Pull Back the Hands

Turn the torso slightly to the left; move the left hand to the left upper back in an arc until it reaches the head level, palm up and the left arm slightly bent. Turn the right arm in the front of the body; the head turns with the body, first looking at the left hand and then the right. (Fig. 37)

6.5 Step Back and Curl the Arms

Turn the torso to the right; raise the right foot and move it one step back, with the ball of the foot landing on the ground gently; bend the left elbow to curl the left hand to the left ear above the shoulder, palm slanted down; begin to draw the right hand back. Look at the right hand. (Fig. 38)

6.6 Empty Stance and Push Palm

Continue to turn the torso to the right; shift the body center back, plant the right foot firmly, pivot the ball of the left foot until the foot is straight, with the heel off the ground. Bend the left knee slightly to form a left empty stance; push the left hand to the front of the body, the wrist at shoulder height, palm forward; move the right hand back and down in an arc to the right side of the waist, palm up. Look at the left hand. (Fig. 39)

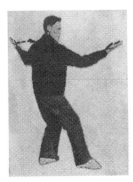
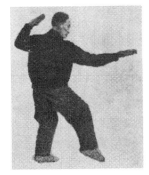
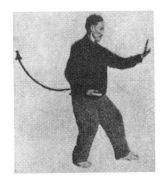

Fig. 37   Fig. 38   Fig. 39

Yòu Dàojuǎngōng 右倒卷肱(Step Back and Curl the Arms — Right Side)

6.7 Turn the Body and Pull Back the Hands

Turn the torso slightly to the right; move the right hand from below up in a circular motion to the upper rear with the turning of the body until the right hand reaches head level, the right arm slightly bent and palm up. Turn the left hand to the front of the body; the head turns with the body, first looking at the right hand and then the left. (Fig. 40)

6.8 Step Back and Curl the Arms

Turn the torso slightly to the left; raise the left foot and move it one step back, with the ball of the foot landing on the ground gently; bend the right arm, bring the right hand to the right side of the ear over the shoulder, palm slanted down; begin to draw the left hand back. Look at the left hand. (Fig. 41)

6.9 Empty Stance and Push Palm

Continue to turn the torso to the left; shift the body center back, plant the left foot firmly, pivot the ball of the right foot to turn the right foot straight, with the heel off the ground; bend the right knee slightly to form a right empty stance. Push the right hand to the front of the body, the wrist at shoulder height, palm forward; move the left hand back and down in an arc to the left side of the waist, palm up. Look at the right hand. (Fig. 42)

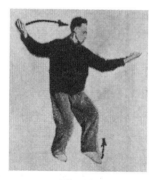 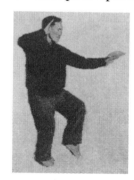 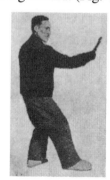

Fig. 40   Fig. 41   Fig. 42

Zuǒ Dàojuǎngōng 左倒卷肱 (Step Back and Curl the Arms — Left Side)

6.10 Turn the Body and Pull Back the Hands

Turn the torso slightly to the left; move the left hand to the left upper back in an arc until it reaches to head level, palm up, the left arm slightly bent. Turn the right hand to the front of the body; the head turns with the body, first looking at the left hand and then the right. (Fig. 43)

6.11 Step Back and Curl the Arms

Turn the torso slightly to the right; raise the right foot and move it one step back, with the ball of the foot landing on the ground gently; bend the left elbow and curl the left hand to the side of the ear over the left shoulder, palm slanted down; begin to draw the right hand back. Look at the right hand. (Fig. 44)

6.12 Empty Stance and Push Palm

Continue to turn the torso to the right; shift the body center back, plant the right foot firmly, pivot on the ball of the left foot to turn the left foot pointing straight ahead, with the heel off the ground; bend the left knee slightly to form a left empty stance. Push the left hand to the front of the body, the wrist at shoulder height, palm forward; pull the right hand down and back in an arc to the right side of the waist. Look at the left hand. (Fig. 45)

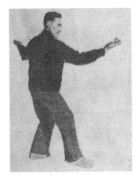 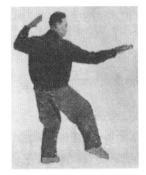 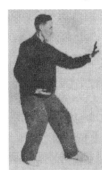

Fig. 43   Fig. 44   Fig. 45

Application

The meaning of this form applies to fighting back when retreating. Take Yòu Dàojuǎn Gōng (Step Back and Curl the Arms — Right Side) as an example: When the opponent attacks with the right hand, use your right hand to grab the opponent's right hand and pull it back. At the same time, step back and use your left hand to strike the opponent's chest.

Important Points

● The footwork of this form involves consecutive back steps based on empty stance. During this process, attention should be paid to these key principles: "Keep the body center stable" (zhòngxīn píngwěn 重心平稳), "point, rise; point, fall" (diǎnqǐ diǎnluò 点起点落) and "rise gently, fall gently" (qīngqǐ qīngluò 轻起轻落).

— "Keep the body center stable" means the body center must not be raised when a leg is being raised; the body center must not be lowered when the foot is landing. The body must not go up and down when stepping back.

— "Point, rise; point, fall" and "rise gently, fall gently" means to aim for movements that are soft, gentle, agile and slow that change in their body center distribution on the ground from a single point to a wider area. When raising the foot, raise the heel first; when landing the foot, land the ball of the foot first (when stepping forward, land the heel first). When raising the foot, avoid any sudden kick or sudden drawing back; when lowering the foot, avoid any sudden landing like a "stamping."

- When executing juǎngōng (curl the arms), pay attention to bending the elbows to curl the arms; avoid bending the fingers and rotating the wrists. Curl the Arms should not be turned into Rotate the Wrists. When pushing the palm to the highest point, keep the idea of seating the wrists, stretching out the palms, relaxing the fingers, and showing the change of power from empty to solid.

- Pull the hand back in an arc. Do not pull it back in a straight line to the front of the chest. In addition, the pushing forward and the pulling back of the hands should be coordinated. The hands cross each other in front of the body. The hands should not be too far apart when they cross.

- Allow the eyes to follow the turning of the body: Look first to the side hand, then to the front hand.

Common Mistakes

- Students can't tell when to fix the form, therefore the movements are not coordinated. Fix the form when completing the third group movements of "Step Back and Curl the Arms," that is "Empty Stance and Push Palm." (Figs. 36, 39, 42) At this time, the eyes are on the front hand, and the torso is straight and relaxed. Some students turn to look back after pushing the palm. The movements of the hands are not coordinated with the eyes.

- When stepping back, the foot lands too far inside the other foot, throwing the feet off-line and causing the torso to lean and the feet to twist together.

- When stepping back, the body center is not under control. The body is seated back too early so that the foot lands too heavily. The foot moves faster than the hand, leading to uncoordinated movements between the upper and lower body.

7. Zuǒ Lǎnquèwěi 左揽雀尾 (Grasp the Peacock's Tail on the Left)

7.1 Turn the Body and Pull the Hand Back

Turn the torso slightly to the right back; move the right hand past the side of the waist back to the upper right in an arc, the right arm slightly bent, the hand at shoulder height, and the palm slanted up; relax the left hand in front of the body, palm down; turn the head with the body. Look straight ahead to the right. (Fig. 46)

7.2 Hold a Ball and Draw In the Foot

Bend the right arm in front of the right chest, turn the right palm down; move the left hand in an arc down before the abdomen, palm up. The hands face each other as if to hold a ball. Draw the left foot in to the inside of the right foot, the left toes on the ground. Look at the right hand. (Fig. 47)

7.3 Turn the Body and Step Forward

Turn the torso slightly to the left, move the left foot a step forward to the left, with the heel landing on the ground gently. Look straight ahead. (Fig. 48)

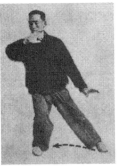
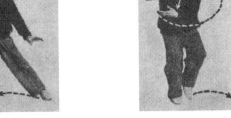
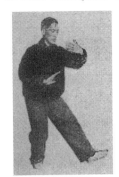

Fig. 46   Fig. 47   Fig. 48

7.4 Bow Stance and Ward Off (Péng 掤)

Continue to turn the torso to the left; shift the body center forward, plant the left foot firmly, bend the left knee forward into a bow, and straighten the right leg naturally to form a left bow stance; part the hands, bend the left arm and extend the left arm up, the wrist at shoulder height, palm down and fingers forward. Press the right hand down in an arc to the right side of the hip, palm down and fingers forward. Look at the left hand. (Fig. 49)

7.5 Turn the Body and Swing the Arm

Turn the torso slightly to the left; stretch the left hand out to the left front, palm down; at the same time, turn the right arm outward and move the right hand past the front of the abdomen up and forward to the inside of the left forearm, palm up. Look at the left hand. (Fig. 50)

7.6 Turn the Body and Roll Back (Lǚ 捋)

Turn the torso to the right; at the same time, both hands stroke back in an arc past the front of the abdomen to the right back. The right hand is raised at the back to the side of the body, at head level, palm outward; the left arm is bent horizontally before the chest, palm inward; shift the body center back, seat the body back, bend the right knee, and straighten the left leg naturally. Look at the right hand. (Fig. 51)

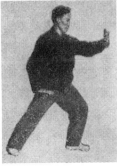
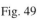
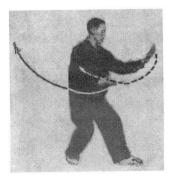
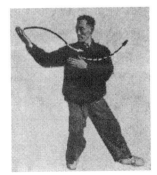

Fig. 49   Fig. 50   Fig. 51

7.7 Turn the Body and Touch the Wrist

Turn the torso to the left to face the front; bend the right elbow, pull the right hand back in front of the chest, and touch it to the inside of the left wrist, palm forward; the left forearm is still bent before the chest, palm inward, fingertips to the right. Look straight ahead. (Fig. 52)

7.8 Bow Stance and Press (Jǐ 挤) Forward

Shift the body center forward, bend the left leg, straighten the right leg naturally to form a left bow stance; the right hand pushes the left forearm forward, at shoulder height. Keep the arms in a circle. Look straight ahead. (Fig. 53)

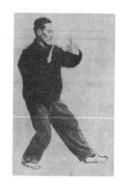

Fig. 52

7.9 Sit Back and Lead Back Hands

Shift the body center back, seat the torso back, bend the right knee, straighten the left leg naturally, and raise the ball of the left foot; turn the left hand down, extend the right hand forward past over the left wrist, and turn the right palm down; part the hands to the left and right, shoulder-width apart. Bend the arms and draw back the hands past the front of the chest to the front of the abdomen, palm slanted down. Look straight ahead. (Fig. 54)

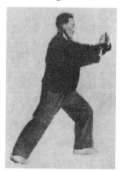

Fig. 53

7.10 Bow Stance and Push (Àn 按) Forward

Shift the body center forward, plant the left foot firmly, bend the left leg into a bow, straighten the right leg naturally to form a left bow stance; push and press the hands in an arc to the front of the body, the wrists shoulder-width apart at shoulder height. The palms are forward, fingertips up. Look straight ahead. (Fig. 55)

Application

This form contains four basic hand techniques of offense and defense of Taijiquan: 1) Péng 掤 ward off; 2) Lǚ 将 roll back; 3) Jǐ 挤 press, and 4) Àn 按 Push.

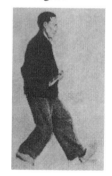

Fig. 54

Péng 掤 means bending the arm to ward off the opponent's attack while observing the opponent's reaction. It looks the same as Part the Wild Horse's Mane, but its application is quite different. Part the Wild Horse's Mane is an attack, applying force with the outside of the arm. Ward Off is a defensive move, warding off the opponent's hand and watching his/her reaction. It involves what is termed "feeling the power" (tīngjìng 听劲).

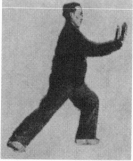

Fig. 55

Lǚ 将 involves using one hand to grab an opponent's wrist and the other hand to grab the elbow, then to pull the opponent's arm back with your hands while turning your body to make the opponent fall. This technique is different from pulling back with power. Rather, roll back makes use of the opponent's power to lead him/her to fall.

Jǐ 挤 means to press the opponent with the forearm when the opponent is going to step back and retreat.

Àn 按 in its original meaning means exerting strength down. But in Taijiquan, we usually first lead and draw the opponent down before exerting strength forward. When the opponent reacts by pulling upward, this brings his/her body center up to unbalance the stance. At that moment, quickly push forward. This alternating strength — called push or push forward — is more effective than just to push forward.

Important Points

• Pay attention in Grasp the Peacock's Tail to the working together of the upper and lower body. Coordinate ward off, press and push with bow stance; coordinate roll back — the stroking and drawing back of the hands — with bending the legs and sitting back. When stepping forward in bow stance and when sitting back, make a complete shift of the body center, keeping the torso relaxed and upright. When bending the legs, lift the head, drop the shoulders, straighten the spine and stretch the back; when seating the legs, relax the waist, draw in the buttocks, bend the knees and lower the hips.

• As stated above, Grasp the Peacock's Tail contains four sections. When finishing each, extend the limbs, focus the power and steady the movements, and make clear the change from empty to solid. However, Taijiquan is characterized by its continuity: The ending of the previous position is the beginning of the next position. That is, no stop exists between positions in the change from empty to solid. Do not stop the power when changing from one position to another; do not end the thought or feeling as the power changes.

• The footwork of this form involves bow step. The width between the feet should be within 4 inches or about 10 centimeters. In Holding a Ball and Drawing in the Foot, try to bring the foot in without landing the toes on the ground.

• When executing ward off (péng 捌), coordinate the movements of separating the hands with turning the body and bending the knee.

When executing roll back (lǚ 将) coordinate stroking back with the turning of the waist. At the end of the movement, keep the hands 45 degrees to the rear at both sides. At the same time, keep the torso straight and the lower body stable.

When executing "sitting back and drawing the hands back," raise the ball of the left foot. Do not straighten the knee and thrust out the abdomen and lean back. At the same time, keep both hands shoulder-width apart and pull them back to the front of the chest, palms down, the elbows slightly drawn outward.

When executing "bow stance and push forward (àn 按)," press the hands forward and up in an arc.

Common Mistakes

● When executing ward off and press, the arms are tense, causing a clamping of the armpits; or they are too lax.

● When stepping forward or sitting back, the heel of the rear leg moves around; the foot is not rooted on the ground as it should be.

● When pressing forward, the hands separate to both sides in an arc, or the palms move up from below in an arc.

● Hands and feet are not coordinated. The feet move faster than the hands or the hands move faster than feet.

8. Yòu Lǎnquèwěi 右揽雀尾 (Grasp the Peacock's Tail on the Right)

8.1 Turn the Body and Part the Hands

Shift the body center back, turn the torso to the right, and move the left toes inward; swing the right hand past the front of the head to the right in an arc, palm outward; the hands are kept on a horizontal line at the both sides of the body. Turn the head and look at the right hand. (Fig. 56)

8.2 Hold a Ball and Draw In the Foot

Bend the left knee, shift the body center to the left, draw the right foot in to the inside of the left foot, with the toes landing on the ground; bend the left hand in front of the left chest, palm down. Bend the right hand in front of the abdomen, palm up. Hands face each other in front of the left ribs as if to "hold a ball." Look at the left hand. (Fig. 57)

8.3 Turn the Body and Step Forward

Turn the torso slightly to the right, move the right foot a step forward to the right, with the heel landing on the ground gently. Look straight ahead. (Fig. 58)

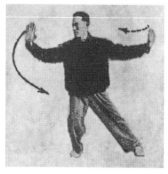 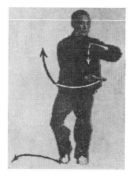 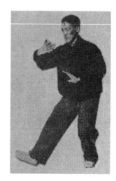

Fig. 56   Fig. 57   Fig. 58

8.4 Bow Stance and Ward Off

Continue to turn the torso to the right; shift the body center forward, plant the right foot firmly, bend the right knee forward into a bow, and straighten the left leg naturally to form a right bow stance; separate the hands, bend the right arm and extend the left arm up before the body, the wrist at shoulder height, palm inward; press the left hand down in an arc to the left side of the hip, palm down and fingers forward. Look at the right hand. (Fig. 59)

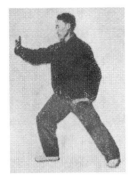

Fig. 59

8.5 Turn the Body and Move the Arm

Turn the torso slightly to the right; extend the right hand forward to the right, and turn the right palm down; at the same time, turn the left arm outward and move the left hand past the front of the abdomen up and forward to the inside of the right forearm, palm up. Look at the right hand. (Fig. 60)

8.6 Turn the Body and Roll Back

Turn the torso to the left; at the same time, both hands stroke down in an arc past the front of the abdomen to the left back. Raise the left hand at the back side of the body until it reaches head level, palm outward; bend the right arm horizontally before the chest, palm inward; shift the body center back, seat the body back, bend the left knee, straighten the right leg naturally. Look at the left hand. (Fig. 61)

8.7 Turn the Body and Put the Hand on the Wrist

Turn the torso to the right, to the direct front; bend the left arm, draw the left hand in front of the chest and place it on the inside of the right wrist, palm forward; the right forearm is still bent before the chest, palm inward, fingers to the left. Look straight ahead. (Fig. 62)

8.8 Bow Stance and Push Forward

Shift the body center forward, bend the right leg, straighten the left leg naturally to

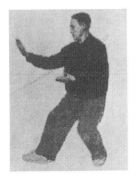

Fig. 60

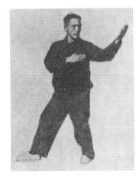

Fig. 61

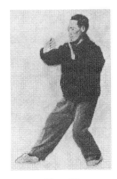

Fig. 62

form a right bow stance; the left hand pushes the right forearm forward in front of the body, at shoulder height. Keep the arms in a circle. Look straight ahead. (Fig. 63)

8.9 Sit Back and Lead Back Hands

Shift the body center back, seat the torso back, bend the left knee, straighten the right leg naturally, raise the ball of the right foot; turn the right hand down, extend the left hand forward past over the right wrist, and turn the left palm down; part the hands to the left and right, shoulder width apart. Bend and pull the arms back to draw the hands to front of the chest then down to the front of the abdomen, palm slanted down. Look straight ahead. (Fig. 64)

8.10 Bow Stance and Press Forward

Shift the body center forward, plant the right foot firmly, bend the right leg into a bow, straighten the left leg naturally to form a right bow stance; push and press the hands in an arc to the front of the body, the wrists at shoulder height, shoulder-width apart. Palms are forward, fingertips up. Look straight ahead. (Fig. 65)

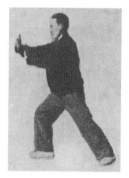 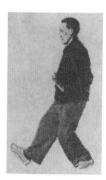 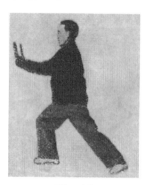

Fig. 63   Fig. 64   Fig. 65

Application

Same as Grasp the Peacock's Tail on the Left.

Important Points

• Move the right hand horizontally in an arc to the right with the turning of the body. The angle between the hands is within 120 degrees. At this time, do not move the left hand to the right with the right hand.

• When turning the body to the right, bend the right knee and seat the body center back, do not raise the body center. At the same time, the ball of the left foot turns inward more than 90 degrees.

• The other points are the same as those of Grasp the Peacock's Tail on the Left.

Common Mistakes

• When turning the body to the right, the ball of the left foot is not drawn inward enough, which makes the right foot step go out in the wrong direction, causing the torso to become tense and to lean.

- The same as that of "Grasp the Peacock's Tail on the Left."

9. Dānbiān 单鞭 (Single Bian)

9.1 Turn the Body and Move the Arms

Shift the body center to the left, turn the torso to the left, and draw the right toes inward; move the left hand past the front of the head in an arc to the left until it reaches the left side of the body, palm outward; move the right hand past the front of the abdomen in an arc to the left until it reaches the left ribs, palm inward. Look at the left hand. (Fig. 66)

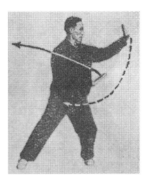

Fig. 66

9.2 Hook the Hand and Draw In the Foot

Turn the torso to the right, shift the body center to the right; bend the right knee, draw in the left foot to the inside of the right foot, with toes landing on the ground; move the right hand up past the front of the head in an arc to the right and change it into a hook at the right front of the body, palm inward, the hook down and the wrist at shoulder height; move the left hand down to the right in an arc past the front of the abdomen until it reaches the front of the right shoulder, palm inward. The eyes follow the movement of the right hand and finally look at the hook hand. (Figs. 67, 68)

9.3 Turn the Body and Step Forward

Turn the torso slightly to the left; move the left foot a step forward to the left, with the heel landing on the ground; move the left hand past the front of the face in an arc to the left, palm inward. Look at the left hand. (Fig. 69)

9.4 Bow Stance and Push Palm

Continue to turn the torso to the left, shift the body center forward; plant the left foot firmly, bend the left leg in a bow, straighten the right leg naturally, the heel pushed

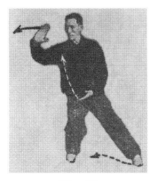

Fig. 67

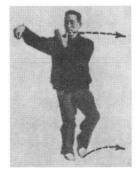

Fig. 68

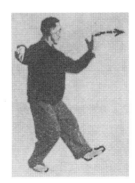

Fig. 69

down and outward, to form a side left bow stance to the front; rotate the left hand past the front of the face and push it forward, the wrist at shoulder height. The left elbow faces the left knee. Look at the left hand. (Fig. 70)

Application

Use your right hook hand to hold the opponent's wrist, then use your left hand to attack as if you were to strike your opponent with a biān.

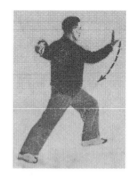

Important Points

Fig. 70

• Face the diagonal within 30 degrees to the left front (Southeast) in bow stance in Single Bian with the width between the feet about 4 inches or 10 centimeters. The direction of the forearm and the direction of the front leg should be the same. When the hand is in a hook form, keep the arm 45 degrees to the rear.

• When moving to the left or right, make a sufficient shift of the body center. Make a clear distinction between empty and solid in the feet.

• When pushing the palm, as the body turns to the left, bend the left leg forward in a bow and turn the left palm hand as it pushes forward. When the left hand reaches the ending point, relax the lower back (waist) and hips, exhale, at the same time, lower the wrist, stretch out the palm and relax the fingers.

• After becoming proficient in these movements, draw in the foot without touching the toes on the ground.

Common Mistakes

• When changing the hand into the hook form, the wrist rotates, forming "a wrist flower;" the five fingers are not closed together at the same time; the wrist is stiff, and the tip of the hook points back.

• When fixing the form, the right heel is not turned enough, causing the hip to loosen and the torso to lean.

• When fixing the form, the chest is thrust out and the waist sinks or the body leans forward.

10. Yúnshǒu 云手 (Move the Hands like Clouds)

10.1 Turn the Body and Loosen the Hook

Shift the body center back, turn the torso to the right; draw the left toes inward (pivoting on the left heel), bend the right leg; move the left hand in an arc to the right past the front of the abdomen until it reaches the front of the right shoulder, palm inward; change the right hook hand into an open-palm hand, palm outward. Look at the right hand. (Fig. 71)

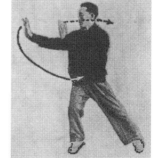

Fig. 71

10.2 Left Move the Hands like Clouds and Stand with Feet Together

Turn the torso to the left, shift the body center to the left; draw the right foot close to the left foot, with the ball of the foot landing on the ground first, then the whole foot firmly rooted. Bend the knees into a half squat, with the two feet parallel and about 8 to 12 inches or 20 to 30 centimeters apart, toes forward; Move the left hand like clouds past the front of the head to the left, turn the palm inward gradually; stop the left palm at the left side of the body, at shoulder height, stop the right hand at the front of the left shoulder. The eyes move with the left hand. (Figs. 72, 73)

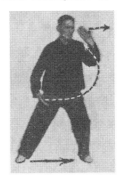

Fig. 72

10.3 Right Move the Hands like Clouds and Stand with Feet Apart

Turn the torso to the right, shift the body center to the right; move the left foot one step to the left, with the ball landing on the ground first, then the whole foot, toes forward; Move the right hand like clouds past the front of the head to the right in an arc, turn the palm outward gradually; at the same time move the left hand like clouds in an arc past the front of the abdomen to the right, turn the

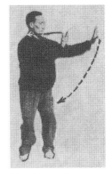

Fig. 73

palm inward gradually; stop the right palm at the right side of the body, at shoulder height, and stop the left hand at the front of the right shoulder. The eyes move with the right hand. (Figs. 74, 75)

10.4 Left Move the Hands like Clouds and Stand with Feet Together

Turn the torso to the left, shift the body center to the left; draw the right foot close to the left foot, with the ball of the right foot landing on the ground first, then the whole foot is rooted. Bend the knees into a half squat, with two feet parallel and 4 to 8 inches or 10 to 20 centimeters apart, toes forward; Move the left hand like clouds past the front of the head to the left, turn the palm inward gradually; stop the left hand at the left side

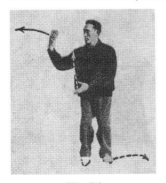
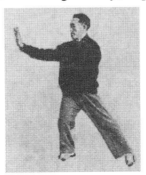
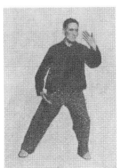

Fig. 74   Fig. 75   Fig. 76

of the body, at shoulder height, stop the right hand at the front of the left shoulder. The eyes move with the left hand. (Figs.76, 77)

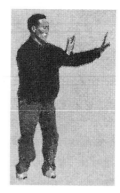

Fig. 77

10.5 Right Move the Hands like Clouds and Stand with Feet Apart

Turn the torso to the right, shift the body center to the right; move the left foot one step to the left, with the ball of the left foot landing on the ground first, then the whole foot is rooted, toes forward; Move the right hand like clouds past the front of the head to the right in an arc, turn the palm outward gradually; at the same time move the left hand like clouds in an arc past the front of the abdomen to the right, turn the palm inward gradually; stop the right hand at the right side of the body, at shoulder height, and stop the left hand at the front of the right shoulder. The eyes move with the right hand. (Figs. 78, 79)

10.6 Left Move the Hands like Clouds and Stand with Feet Together

Shift the body center to the left; draw the right foot close to the left foot, with the ball of the foot landing on the ground first, then the whole foot is rooted. Bend the knees into a half squat, with two feet parallel and about 4 inches or 10 centimeters apart, toes forward; Move the left hand like clouds past the front of the head to the left, turn the palm outward gradually; at the same time move the right hand like clouds in an arc down to the left, and turn the right palm inward gradually; stop the left hand at the left side of the body, at shoulder height, stop the right hand at the front of the left shoulder. The eyes move with the left hand. (Figs. 80, 81)

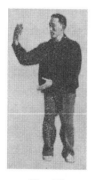
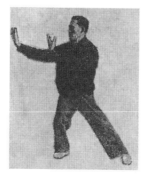
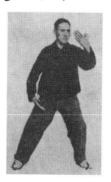
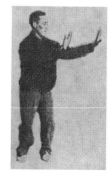

Fig. 78   Fig. 79   Fig. 80   Fig. 81

Application

Move the Hands like Clouds is a defensive movement, using the forearm or hand to deflect the opponent's attack. If the opponent uses his/her left and right hands to attack continuously, use Move the Hands like Clouds to intercept them. Or intercept the opponent's right hand by using the right hand, then thrust the left hand under the opponent's armpit in a splitting attack (liö 挒) on the horizontal to the right.

Important Points

• Use the waist as an axis to direct the movements of hands. Coordinate the movements of the body and hands. Do not let the hands move on their own but rather coordinate their movement with the shifting of the body center, the turning of the waist and the stepping to the side. Coordinate also the hands and feet in movements that are gradual and gentle.

• The stance of this form is Standing with Feet Slightly Apart (Xiǎokāibù 小开步). It requires the feet be parallel, forward, and about 8 to 12 inches or 20 to 30 centimeters apart.

• The footwork is side step. Pay attention to the following four points when executing side steps:

① Master the principle of "point, rise; point, fall" and "rise gently, fall gently" (diǎnqǐ diǎnluò, qīngqǐ qīngluò 点起点落, 轻起轻落。). When executing the side steps, root the feet as each foot supports the body in turn. Make a full body center shift. And make a clear distinction between empty and solid in the two feet. Raise the left foot gently and move it to the left, then gently draw the right foot close to the left.

② Be sure the length of the step is correct. When executing the side step, bend one leg to support the body center, while straightening the other leg naturally and moving it one step to the side.

③ When stepping, do not lean or swing the torso.

④ Do not let the body move up and down. Shift the body center steadily and evenly. Always keep the height of the stance the same.

• Draw overlapping vertical circles with the hands in front of the body with the rotating hands and arms. Bend the arm into a curve when drawing a circle past the front of the face, not be too close to the head. When drawing a circle down, the elbow is slightly bent, the arm naturally straight.

Common Mistakes

• When stepping to the side, the feet are positioned on the ground like the Chinese character for the numeral 8 — 八 — or they are too close to each other.

• There is no change of tension and relaxation in the eyes as they look at the upper hand drawing a circle. The eyes fix on the hand in a stare.

• The movements of the arms are not directed by the waist, causing only the arms to move without a turning of the waist.

• The movements of the lower limbs and the arms are not coordinated, causing a swaying in the waist and hips.

11. Dānbiān 单鞭 (Single Bian)

11.1 Turn the Body and Hook the Hand

Turn the torso to the right, shift the body center on the right leg, and raise the left heel; the right hand draws a circle past the front of the head; rotate the palm and change it into a hook when it reaches the right front of the body; draw a circle down with the left hand to the right past the front of the abdomen and move it "like clouds" until it reaches the front of the right shoulder, and there turn the palm inward. Look at the right hook hand. (Figs. 82, 83)

11.2 Turn the Body and Step Forward

Turn the torso slightly to the left; move the left foot a step forward to the left, with the heel landing on the ground; draw a circle with the left hand to the left past the front of the face, palm inward. Look at the left hand. (Fig. 84)

11.3 Bow Stance and Push the Palm

Continue to turn the torso to the left; shift the body center forward, plant the left foot, bend the left leg, straighten the right leg naturally, with the heel drawn outward, to form a bow stance on the diagonal toward the left front; turn the left hand past the front of the face and push it forward, the wrist at shoulder height; the left elbow facing the left knee. Look at the left hand. (Fig. 85)

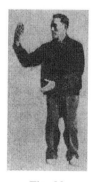 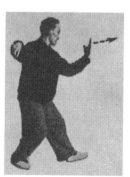 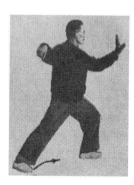

Fig. 82   Fig. 83   Fig. 84   Fig. 85

12. Gāotànmǎ 高探马 (Gauge the Height of the Horse)

12.1 Follow-Up Step and Rotate the Hands

Move the rear foot half a step forward, with the ball of the foot landing on the ground, about one foot's length away from the front foot; loosen the right hook hand, rotate both hands up, and raise up the two arms in front of the body, the elbows slightly bent. Look at the left hand. (Fig. 86)

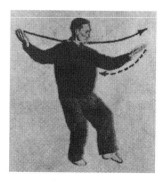

Fig. 86

12.2 Sit Back and Curl the Upper Arm

Turn the torso slightly to the right; shift the body center back, plant the right foot firmly, bend the right leg and seat it back, and raise the left heel; bend the right elbow, curl the right arm to bring the hand to the side of the head, palm slanted down. Look at the left hand. (Fig. 87)

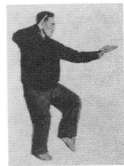

Fig. 87

12.3 Empty Stance and Push the Palm

Turn the torso to the left, move the right shoulder forward; push the right hand forward past the head side, the wrist at shoulder height, palm forward; bend the left arm to bring the left hand to the front of the abdomen, palm up. Look at the right hand. (Fig. 88)

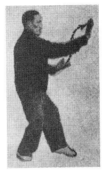

Fig. 88

Application

Turning the left forearm outward to press the opponent's wrist or forearm when he or she punches with the right palm or fist, and then lead it back and down. At the same time, strike the opponent's face with the right hand. Therefore, "Gauge the Height of the Horse" is also called "Strike the Face with the Palm."

Important Points

• Coordinate the movements of Empty Stance and Push the Palm with the turning of the waist and the moving of the shoulder. Keep the body straight, relaxed, and the movements harmonious.

• "Empty Stance and Push the Palm" differ from "Step Back and Curl the Arms" in the following three points:

① In "Step Back and Curl the Arms," Empty Stance and Push the Palm are aligned. That is to say, the front palm and the front leg are on the same side of the body. However, in this form, Empty Stance and Push the Palm is reverse. That is, the front palm and the front leg are on the opposite sides of the body. Therefore, in this form the shoulder moves less than it does in "Reverse Rotating Forearm" to allow a comfortable feeling in the torso.

② In this form, push the palm forward to eye level. Compared to "Step Back and Curl the Arms," in this form the palm is pushed a little higher.

③ In this form, lower the shoulder when drawing the left palm back, rotate the forearm and pull it back and down to draw the elbow to the side of the waist and the hand to the front of the abdomen. However, in "Step Back and Curl the Arms" the hand is drawn to the side of the waist.

Common Mistakes

• When seating the body back, the neck leans the head back to look at the right hand.

- When fixing the form, the legs straighten to raise the body center.
- The right arm is too close to the body, clamping to the ribs and closing the armpit.

13. Yòu Dēngjiǎo 右蹬脚 (Kick with the Right Heel)

13.1 Thread the Hand and Step Forward

Turn the torso to the left; raise the left foot up and move it forward to the left, with the heel landing on the ground; draw the right hand back a little, thread the left hand past the back of the right hand forward to the right, and cross the hands at the wrists. The left palm is slanted up, right palm slanted down. Look at the left hand. (Fig. 89)

13.2 Bow Stance and Separate the Hands

Shift the body center forward, plant the left foot on the ground, bend the left leg into a bow and straighten the right leg naturally; separate the hands to the left and right, palms forward, lift the arms up and outward. Look at the right hand. (Fig. 90)

13.3 Hold in an Embrace and Draw In the Foot

Draw in the right foot to the inside of the left foot, touching the ground with the right toes. Move the hands in arcs to the front of the abdomen until they cross and overlap into a position of holding something, raising the hands in front of the chest, with the right hand on the outside and both palms facing toward the body. Look forward to the right. (Fig. 91)

13.4 Separate the Hands and Heel Kick

Stand on the left leg, bend the right leg and lift it up, draw the right toes up. The right heel kicks forward with force to the upper right slowly; bend the left leg slightly, straighten the right leg as the palms face outward. Extend the arms out on both sides of the body, the elbows slightly bent, the wrists at shoulder height; the right leg and right arm are aligned with each other in a direction of 30 degrees to the front. Look at the right hand. (Fig. 92)

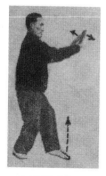 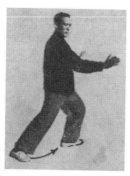 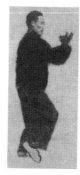 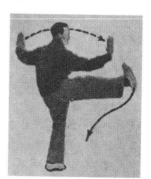

Fig. 89   Fig. 90   Fig. 91   Fig. 92

Application

Intercept an attack with the hands and at the same time kick the opponent.

Important Points

● Heel kick requires leg power as well as flexibility and balance. The points that need to be stressed are "stability" and "coordination." First, stabilize the body center when bringing the right foot in to the left. Beginners can touch their toes to the ground to adjust the body center. Then gradually come to be able to control the body center without the toes landing on the ground when drawing in the foot. To avoid losing balance when lifting up the knee and then kicking, move slowly and steadily rather than suddenly. Basic exercises can improve both stability and flexibility. And to accomplish coordination, pay attention here to the "Six Harmonies" which are:

① "Harmony of threading the hand and bringing the foot in."

② "Harmony of stepping forward and rotating the hands."

③ "Harmony of bending the leg and separating the hands."

④ "Harmony of drawing in the foot and holding in an embrace."

⑤ "Harmony of lifting the knee and lifting up the holding arms."

⑥ "Harmony of heel kick, separating the hands and raising the arms up and out."

If one can achieve the six harmonies, all the movements will be coordinated.

● The arm movements of this form are complicated. In the process of "threading the hand—separating the hands—holding in an embrace—lifting the arms up and out, " the hands twice cross and separate. Make clear the rotation of the forearm and the line on which the circles are drawn.

In the first group of movements, Thread the Hand and Step Forward, the threading of the hand follows the turning of the body, first slightly to the right then stepping forward to the left. The left hand goes forward and upward past the back of the right hand. Have the backs of the hands facing each other, with the wrists crossed, at shoulder height, the elbows slightly bent.

The second group movements, Separate the Hands, and the third group of movements, Hold in an Embrace, involve forming a loop with the arms. When separating the hands, turn the palms inward, at the same time, the hands draw circles in front of the face to left and right, then separate. Next, rotate the palms outward and down without stopping until they overlap in front of the abdomen. Then raise the arms in front of the chest in a position as if holding a ball.

In the fourth group movements, Separate the Hands and Heel Kick, pull the hands apart to the right front and left back in an arc. Do not raise the hands higher than head level. Keep the elbows slightly bent. In the meantime, the body center rises and the supporting leg naturally straightens. The hand work of "thread, separate, hold and lift up" can be selected to practice on its own.

● In this form, look at the left hand when executing the first group movements; at the right hand in the second group movements; to the right front in the direction of heel kick in the third group movements; finally at the right hand in the fourth group.

● When fixing the form, lift the head and keep the waist (lower back) upright with the kicking leg higher than horizontal level. Keep the body center steady. Beginners do not have to kick above horizontal if it is beyond their ability. Students should practice according to their abilities.

Common Mistakes

Beginners can easily make mistakes when executing this form. Some examples:

● The supporting leg is unstable.
● The torso leans forward or back.
● The arms are not at the same level.
● The supporting left leg is bent too much.
● The right arm and kicking right leg aren't aligned with each other.
● The shoulders are tensed and shrugged and the chest is tense. The breath is held.
● The waist is bent and the head lowered.

These are mistakes that can be caused by tension in the body as well as physical limitations. Sort out what the problems are to help correct the mistakes.

14. Shuāngfēng Guàn'ěr 双峰贯耳 (Strike the Opponent's Ears with Both Fists)

14.1 Bend the Knee and Bring the Hands Together

Bend the right knee and draw back the right leg foot, with the toes of the right foot dropping naturally. The left hand draws a circle past the side of the head to the front of the body. Bring both hands together and drop them over the right knee, palms up, fingertips forward. Look straight ahead. (Fig. 93)

14.2 Step Forward and Drop Hands

Step forward to the right, with the right heel landing on the ground, the toes pointing forward 30 degrees to the right; bring the hands to the sides of the waist, palms up. (Fig. 94)

14.3 Bow Stance and Strike with Both Fists

Shift the body center forward, plant the right foot on the ground firmly, bend the right leg into a bow, the left leg naturally straight, to form a right bow stance; change the open-palm hands into fists and swing the fists in curves upward and forward from both sides of the waist until they reach the front of the head with the arms half bent and the fists facing each other as pincers. The fists are a head's width apart. Turn the forearms inward, with the thumb side of the fists slanted down. Look straight ahead. (Fig. 95)

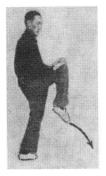
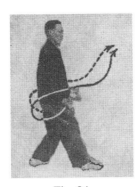
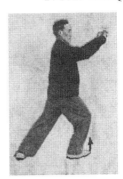

Fig. 93   Fig. 94   Fig. 95

Application

Swing both fists from the sides of the waist in an arc to the upper front to strike the opponent's temples.

Important Points

● Fix the form in the same direction as the direction of the right leg.

● Before the right leg lands on the ground, bend the left leg to lower the body center. Then step forward and land the right foot.

● When striking with both fists, bend the arms slightly in an arc, with power focused on the front of the fists. Keep the thumb sides of the fists slanted down, the body is straight, and the shoulders and elbows down.

Common Mistakes

● The fists are held too tight or too loose.

● When striking with both fists, the arms are straight and the thumb sides of the fist face each other.

● When fixing the form, the shoulders are shrugged and the neck drawn back; the head is lowered and the back bent; the body leans forward which thrusts out the buttocks.

15. Zhuǎnshēn Zuǒ Dēngjiǎo 转身左蹬脚 (Turn and Kick with the Left Heel)

15.1 Turn the Body and Separate the Hands

Shift the body center back, turn the torso to the left; bend and seat the left leg, draw the right toes inward; open the fists, draw a circle with the left hand past the front of the head to the left, bend the arms slightly and as they are raised at each side of the body, palms outward. Look at the left hand. (Fig. 96)

15.2 Draw In the Foot and Hold in an Embrace

Shift the body center to the right, bend and seat the right knee back, bring the left foot to the inside of the right foot,

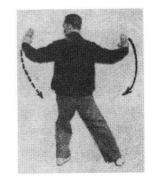

Fig. 96

with the toes landing on the ground; draw circles with both hands down until they cross each other in front of the chest, left hand outside, palms inward. Look straight ahead. (Fig. 97)

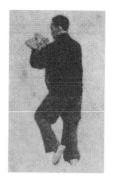
Fig. 97

15.3 Separate the Hands and Heel Kick

Stand on the right leg, bend and raise the left knee, draw the toes of the left foot up, kick forward to the upper left slowly with the left heel; rotate the arms inward until the palms face outward, separate the hands in arcs to the left front and right back with both arms slightly bent and lifted at the sides of the body; straighten the left leg aligned with the left arm. Look at the left hand. (Fig. 98)

Application

Turn the body and intercept the opponent's attack, at the same time kick with the left foot.

Important Points

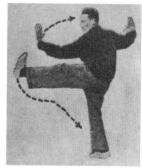
Fig. 98

● When turning the body and separating the hands, keep the torso straight, draw the right foot inward as much as possible. Make a complete shift of the body center. At the same time, separate the hands by drawing circles to both sides. Do not swing the right hand to the left.

● The direction of the left heel kick is opposite to that of the right heel kick. The angle between the direction and the middle axis is about 30 degrees.

● The rest is the same as in "Kick with the Right Heel."

Common Mistakes

● When turning the body, the head lowers, the waist is bent, and the body leans forward.

● When turning the body, the shift of the body center is not complete, leaving no clear distinction between the emptiness and solidity of the two legs.

● The rest is the same as in "Kick with the Right Heel."

16. Zuǒ Xiàshì Dúlì 左下势独立 (Push Down and Stand on the Left Leg)

16.1 Draw In the Foot and Hook the Hand

Bend the left knee and draw the left foot to the inside of the right foot; turn the torso to the right; draw the right arm slightly inward. Change the right hand into a hook; swing the left hand in a circle past the front of the head until it reaches the front of the right shoulder, palm to the right, fingertips up. Look at the right hook hand. (Fig. 99)

16.2 Bend into a Squat and Step Out

Bend the right knee into a half squat, land the left sole on the ground and extend it to the left, then plant the whole foot firmly, and straighten the left leg; drop the left hand at the right ribs. Look at the hook hand. (Fig. 100)

16.3 Crouch Stance and Thread the Hand

Bend the right knee into a squat, turn the torso to the left to form a crouch stance; thread the left hand past the front of the abdomen along the inside edge of the left leg to the left, palm outward, fingertips to the left. Look at the left hand. (Fig. 101)

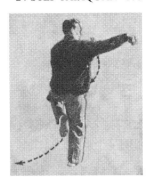

Fig. 99

16.4 Bend the Leg and Raise the Body

Shift the body center onto the left leg and turn the left toes outward. Bend the left knee into a bow, draw the right toes inward, straighten the right leg naturally, and raise the body center up to bow stance level; continue to thread the left hand forward pointing up; rotate the right hook hand inward behind the body, pointing up. Look at the left hand. (Fig. 102)

16.5 Stand on One Leg and Spear Up the Hand

Turn the torso to the left, shift the body center forward; bend the right knee and raise it forward, with the right

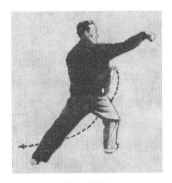

Fig. 100

foot relaxed so that it hangs naturally. Bend the left leg naturally and stand on it to form a left one-leg stance; lower the left hand and press it down at the side of the left hip; change the right hook hand into an open-palm hand and spear it up forward past the side of the body, palm to the left, fingertips up, at eye level. Bend the right arm into an arc, the right elbow in line with the right knee. Look at the right hand. (Fig. 103)

Application

Faced with a left-hand strike, grab hold of the opponent's wrist with the right hook hand, then lower the body, extending the left leg and left hand under the opponent's

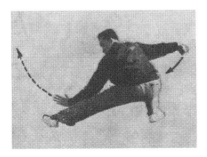

Fig. 101

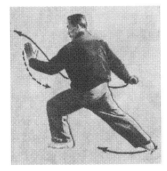

Fig. 102

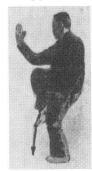

Fig. 103

crotch to throw him/her to the ground.

When the opponent strikes with the left hand, intercept by spearing up the right hand, raise the right knee for a knee-strike.

Important Points

- Pay attention to two key points: The stability of the crouch stance and the shift of the body center. To help maintain the stability of the body during the crouch stance, put the toes of the extended leg and the heel of the bent leg on the same axis at a distance of one leg-length apart. To make it easier to lift one leg while standing on the other when the body center shifts onto the front bow leg, turn the front foot outward and the back foot inward as much as possible.

- Before executing the crouch stance, draw the left foot to the inside of the right leg. Beginners can draw in the left foot with the toes on the ground to stabilize the body center until they gradually progress to the level of drawing in the foot without the toes touching the ground. At the same time, the eyes follow the left hand to the right to look at the right hook hand. Keep the right hook hand 45 degrees to the rear.

- When executing the crouch stance, extend the left leg along the ground to the left. After this is done, bend the right leg into a squat with the left leg straight and both feet rooted on the ground.

- When threading the hand to the left, first bend the left arm then straighten it. Lean the body slightly forward to help complete this movement.

- When fixing the form, circle the right arm up in a curve while lowering the left hand. Press down with the left hand with the left arm slightly bent. Bend the supporting leg with the foot rooted on the ground. Lift the front knee higher than horizontal level. Keep the torso straight and relaxed.

Common Mistakes

- When squatting and stepping out, the eyes look to the left rather than at the right hook hand. Turning the head too early causes the torso to lean.

- When executing the crouch stance, the outer side of the left foot raises up and the right heel raises up instead of having both feet rooted.

- When shifting from the crouch stance to bow stance, the right foot remains rooted rather than allowing the toes to draw inward, which makes the distance between the feet too long. This makes it difficult to bend and raise the left knee. Or the left foot is not turned outward enough, leaving an unsteady support for the one-leg stance that causes the torso to become tense and lean.

- When executing the crouch stance, the right leg is not bent enough, causing a bending of the waist, a raising of the buttocks and a lowering of the head.

17. Yòu Xiàshì Dúlì 右下势独立 (Push Down and Stand on the Right Leg)

17.1 Put the Foot Down and Hook the Hand

Put down the right foot in front of the left foot to the right, with the ball of the right foot landing on the ground; turn the torso to the left, pivot on the ball of the left foot and turn the left foot; form a hook with the left hand and raise it at the left side of the body, to shoulder height; the right hand draws a circle past the front of the head and swings to the front of the left shoulder, palm to the left. Look at the left hand. (Fig. 104)

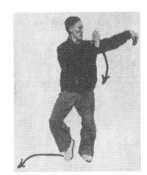

Fig. 104

17.2 Bend into a Squat and Step Out

Draw in the right foot to the inside of the left foot. When the ball of the right foot lands on the ground, extend the right foot to the right along the ground, and straighten the right leg, with the right foot rooted; pull down the right hand to the side of the left ribs. Look at the left hook hand. (Fig. 105)

17.3 Crouch Stance and Thread the Hand

Bend the left knee into a squat, turn the torso to the right to form the right crouch stance; extend the right hand past the front of the abdomen along the inner edge of the right leg to the right, palm outward, fingertips to the right. Look at the right hand. (Fig. 106)

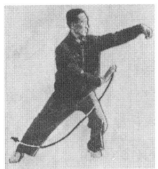

Fig. 105

17.4 Bow Stance and Raise the Body

Shift the body center on the right leg; turn the right toes outward, bend the right knee forward into a bow, draw the left toes inward, straighten the left leg naturally, raise the body center to the bow stance level; continue to thread the right hand forward and spear it up; rotate the left hook hand inward behind the body, pointing up. Look at the right hand. (Fig. 107)

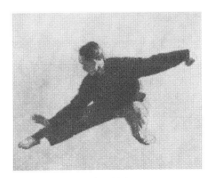

Fig. 106

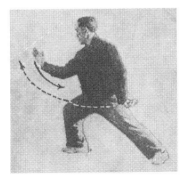

Fig. 107

17.5 Stand on One Leg and Spear Up the Hand

Turn the torso to the right, shift the body center forward; bend the left knee and raise it up to the front, with the toes down. The right leg is slightly bent and supports the body, to form a right one-leg stance; put the right hand down and press it down at the right side of the hip; change the left hook hand into palm, spear it up past the side of the body to the front, palm to the right, finger-tips up, at eye level; bend the left arm into an arc, the left elbow in line with the left knee. Look at the left hand. (Fig. 108)

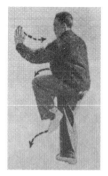

Fig. 108

Important Points

• When executing the first group of movements, bring the right foot about 8 inches or 20 centimeters to the right of the front of the left foot. That is, after the left heel turns inward, the right foot is just at the inside of the left foot.

• When turning the body to the left, keep the body center always on the left leg.

• When extending the right leg, lift the right foot first and then extend it. That is, do not straight away slide the right foot on the ground.

Common Mistakes

• After finishing the first group of movements, the body center shifts to the right leg and then after turning the body, shifts to the left leg.

• The right hand draws a circle down, past the front of the abdomen, swings to the front of the left shoulder.

18. Zuǒyòu Chuānsuō 左右穿梭 (Move the Shuttle Left and Right)
Move the Shuttle — Right

18.1 Step and Hold a Ball

Land the left foot to the left front, with the ball of the foot and toes drawn outward, and turn the torso to the left; rotate the left hand so the palm faces down at chest level, turn the right hand so the palm faces up at abdomen level, keep the hands in front of the left ribs in a position as if to hold a ball. Look at the left hand. (Fig. 109)

18.2 Step Forward and Reverse the Hands

Turn the torso to the right; draw in the right foot, move the right foot on the diagonal forward past the inside of the left foot, with the heel landing on the ground; the right hand draws a circle from below to the upper front; the left hand moves in a circular motion from the upward position down and back, reversing the hands. Look at the right hand. (Fig. 110)

18.3 Bow Stance and Block and Push the Hand

Continue to turn the torso to the right; shift the body center forward, plant the right foot on the ground, bend the right knee into a bow to form a right bow stance; rotate the right hand and block it up until it reaches the upper front corner of the right forehead, palm slanted up; push the left hand to the front of the body, at the nose level. Look at the left hand. (Fig. 111)

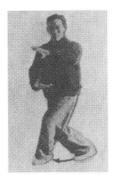 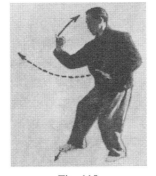 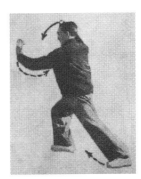

Fig. 109   Fig. 110   Fig. 111

Move the Shuttle — Left (Zuǒ Chuānsuō) 左穿梭

18.4 Turn the Body and Draw the Foot Outward

Shift the body center slightly back, draw the toes and ball of the foot outward, and turn the torso to the right; bring the right hand down in front of the head, draw a circle with the left hand slightly to the left until it reaches the front of the abdomen, and get ready to "hold a ball." Look at the right hand. (Fig. 112)

18.5 Hold a Ball and Draw In the Foot

Keep the hands in front of the right ribs at a position as if to hold a ball; draw the left foot in to the inside of the right foot. Look at the right hand. (Fig. 113)

18.6 Step Forward and Reverse the Hands

Turn the torso to the left; step the left foot on the diagonal forward to the left, with the heel landing on the ground; the left hand draws a circle from below up to the front, the right hand draws a circle back from above to below, reversing the hands. Look at the left hand. (Fig. 114)

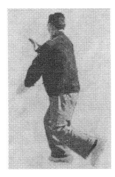 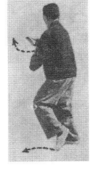 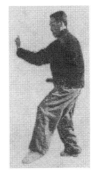

Fig. 112   Fig. 113   Fig. 114

18.7 Bow Stance and Block and Push the Hand

Continue to turn the torso to the left; shift the body center forward, plant the left foot firmly, bend the left knee forward into a bow, to form a left bow stance; rotate the left hand and block it up, and put it up in front of the right forehead; push the right hand to the front of the body, at the nose level. Look at the right hand. (Fig. 115)

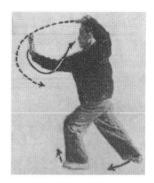

Fig. 115

Application

When faced with a hand attack, intercept with one hand and strike forward with the other.

Important Points

• In Move the Shuttle Left and Right, the bow stance and the push palm are in reverse position (opposite hand and foot forward), with the bow stance and push hand facing the same direction about 30 degrees to the axis. The width between the feet is about 12 inches or 30 centimeters. To stabilize the body center and to relax the torso, do not make the width between the two feet too narrow.

• The hand techniques of this form involve lifting one hand up to intercept while pushing the other hand forward. Bring one hand up in front of the forehead, with power focused on the forearm. Bring the other hand to the front of the ribs or side of the waist to store power, then push it forward with the turning of the waist and the moving of the shoulder.

Common Mistakes

• When keeping the palm at the upper front of the forehead, the shoulders are shrugged and the elbows raised; the torso leans.

• When fixing the form, the direction of pushing the palm and the bow stance are not the same.

• When performing Move the Shuttle — Left, the right toes are drawn outward too much, making it difficult to step forward.

19. Hǎidǐzhēn 海底针 (Needle at the Bottom of the Sea)

19.1 Follow-Up Step and Raise the Hand

Move the right foot half a step forward, with the ball of the foot landing on the ground, about one foot's length away from the front foot; then shift the body center back, bend the right leg and seat it, turn the torso to the right, and raise the left heel; drop the right hand past the right side of the body and then raise it to the right ear, palm to the left toward the ear, fingers forward; the left hand draws a circle to the right until it reaches the front of the abdomen, palm down, finger slanted to the right. Look straight ahead. (Fig. 116)

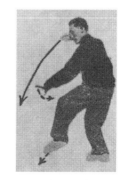

Fig. 116

19.2 Empty Stance and Spear the Hand

Turn the torso to the left, lean the body forward; spear the right hand down from the side of the ear to the front, palm facing left, fingers slanted down; the left hand brushes in an arc past the front of the left knee and presses down at the outer side of the left thigh. Move the left foot slightly forward, with the ball of the foot landing on the ground, to form a left empty stance. Look at the right hand. (Fig. 117)

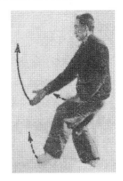

Fig. 117

Application

When faced with a right-hand strike, intercept with the left hand and spear the right hand toward the opponent's groin.

Important Points

● When executing Empty Stance and Spear the Hand, extend the torso while keeping it upright and with a lean forward within 45 degrees.

● The hands movements are: The right hand draws a vertical circle at the side of the body with the turning of the body, the left hand lowers with the turning of the body and draws a horizontal circle past the front of the body and presses down at the side of the left hip. When spearing, focus power into the fingertips.

● In finishing the follow-up step, sit back on the right foot with the turning of the body. Pivot the ball of the right foot and turn the right heel. When fixing the form, the front foot faces directly forward while the right foot turns outward about 45 degrees.

Common Mistakes

● Spearing the Palm can be easily turned into a "chop" or "slicing" motion.

● The movements of the waist and the limbs are not coordinated. The waist doesn't direct and coordinate the movements of other parts of the body.

● When fixing the form, the head lowers, the waist bends; no clear distinction of emptiness and solidity between the two feet.

20. Shǎntōngbì 闪通臂 (Send a Flash Through the Arms)

20.1 Raise the Hand and Draw In the Foot

Keep the torso erect; bend the right knee and support the body with the right leg, and draw in the left foot; raise the right hand up to the front of the body, fingers forward, the palm to the left; bend the left arm and raise it, move the left fingers close to the inside of the right wrist. Look straight ahead. (Fig. 118)

20.2 Bow Stance and Push and Prop Up

Move the left foot one step forward to form a left bow

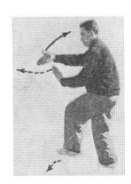

Fig. 118

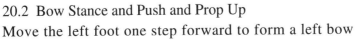

stance; push the left hand to the front of the body, at
the nose level; extend the right hand at the upper side
of the head, palm slanted up; separate the hands and
extend them forward and back. Look at the left hand.
(Fig. 119)

Application

Use your right hand to pull the opponent's right wrist
while using your left hand to attack the opponent's ribs.
Pull and push in a synchronized movement with power
generated through the waist, legs and arms. "Shǎn" means
quick as lightening, "Tōngbì" or "Tōng Bèi" means sending power through the arms or
the shoulder and the back. The whole body acts as one.

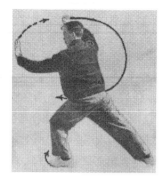

Fig. 119

Important Points

• Coordinate the movements of the arms and legs.

• Align the hands and feet of the bow stance: Keep the feet the correct distance
apart with the front arm and front leg in line with each other. Keep the direction of the
bow stance and the pushing palm directly ahead.

Common Mistakes

• When holding the right hand above the head, the shoulders are shrugged and
elbows raised.

• When fixing the form, the hip turns and body leans, forming a side-bow
stance.

• The movements of the feet are faster than the hands. The movements of the
upper and lower parts of the body are not coordinated.

21. Zhuǎnshēn Bānlánchuí 转身搬拦捶 (Turn the Body, Block and Punch)

21.1 Turn the Body and Draw the Toes Inward

Shift the body center back, bend the right leg and seat it, draw the left toes inward,
and turn the torso to the right; swing the hands to the right, the
right hand draws a circle and swings to the right side of the
abdomen, and the left hand swings to the head side, palms outward.
Look at the right hand. (Fig. 120)

21.2 Seat the Leg and Make a Fist

Shift the body center to the left, bend the left leg and
seat it. Pivot on the ball of the right foot and turn the right
foot straight; the right hand changes into a fist and draws a
circle down to the left then up until it reaches the front of the
left ribs, the palm of the fist down; the left hand is raised to

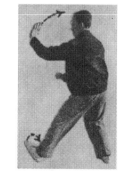

Fig. 120

the upper front of the left forehead. Look straight ahead to the right. (Fig. 121)

21.3 Swing Step and Move the Fist

Bring the right foot to the inside of the left ankle, then step forward, with the right heel landing on the ground, the toes drawn outward; press the right fist forward past the front of the chest, with the palm of the fist up at chest level and the right elbow slightly bent; drop the left hand past the outer side of the right forearm and press down at the side of the left hip. Look at the right fist. (Fig. 122)

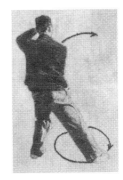

Fig. 121

21.4 Turn the Body and Pull Back the Fist

Turn the torso to the right, shift the body center forward; raise the left foot up; turn the right arm inward, the right fist moves to the right in a curve until it reaches the side of the body with the palm of the fist down and the right arm half bent; turn the left arm outward, and the left hand moves in a curve past the left side to the front of the body, palm slanted up. Look straight ahead. (Fig. 123)

21.5 Step Forward and Palm Block

Move the left foot forward, with the heel landing on the ground; move the left palm to the front of the body to block, at shoulder height, the left palm facing the right, fingers slanted up; rotate the right fist and pull it to the side of the waist, palm of the fist up. Look at the left hand. (Fig. 124)

21.6 Bow Stance and Punch

Turn the torso to the left; shift the body center forward, bend the left leg, plant the left foot, and straighten the right leg naturally to form a left bow stance; the right fist punches out in front of the chest with the right elbow slightly bent, the palm of the right fist to the left, and the thumb-side up; pull the left hand back slightly with the left palm and fingers next to the inside of the right forearm, the left palm facing right. Look at the right fist. (Fig. 125)

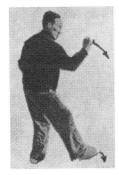
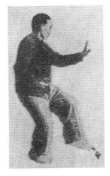
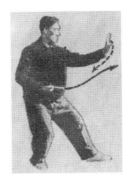
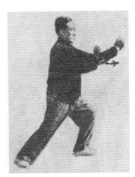

Fig. 122   Fig. 123   Fig. 124   Fig. 125

Application

Faced with a left-hand strike, block down with the right fist, then turn the arm to lead the opponent's hand to the right; when the opponent strikes with the right hand, block with the left palm to push his/her right arm aside, then strike with your right fist.

Important Points

● Turn the Body, Block and Punch includes three different hand techniques: Right fist block, left palm block, and right punch. Make each technique clear.

● As the body turns during each of the three techniques, make a clear distinction between the empty and solid. Keep the change of movements light and agile and the body center steady. When movement changes, pay attention to the shifting of the body center, turning of the feet and bending and extending of the legs. Do not let the body center go up and down. Do not let the torso sway.

Common Mistakes

● When executing the movements of blocking and pulling back the fist, the arms draw circles that are too big and are not coordinated with the turning of the waist.

● When turning the body, the right leg is not bent and seated, causing a throwing out of the hip, raising of the body center and leaning of the torso.

22. Rúfēng Sìbì 如封似闭 (Pull Back then Push, As if to Close)

22.1 Thread the Hand and Turn the Palm

Turn the left hand up and thread it out from under the right forearm to the front; at the same time, change the right fist into an open-palm hand and rotate it up. Extend and raise the crossed hands in front of the body. Look straight ahead. (Fig. 126)

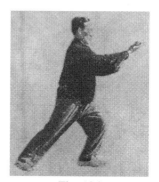

Fig. 126

22.2 Sit Back and Lead Back with the Hands

Shift the body center to the back, bend the right leg and seat it, and raise the left toes up; bend and pull back the arms, leading both hands back while separating them to the front of the chest, shoulder-width apart. Palms face each other on a slant. Look straight ahead. (Fig. 127)

22.3 Bow Stance and Press Palms

Shift the body center forward, bend the left leg into a bow forward, plant the left foot firmly, straighten the right leg naturally to form a left bow stance; rotate the hands and lower them, and push them up and forward past the front of the abdomen,

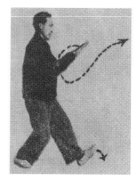

Fig. 127

shoulder-width apart, the wrists at shoulder height, palms forward, and fingers up. Look straight ahead. (Fig. 128)

Application

When the opponent pushes with both hands, intercept by extending the crossed hands forward between the opponent's arms. Then draw the hands back while separating them to lead the opponent into a fall. When the opponent pulls back, press your hands forward to attack.

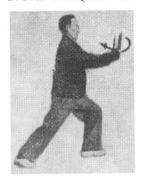

Fig. 128

Important Points

● When sitting back and leading the hands back, bend the elbows, turn the arms and draw the hands back. Do not roll the forearms up. Do not clamp the elbows to the ribs.

● When pressing the palms, keep the hands parallel and move them forward along an arc.

Common Mistakes

● When sitting back and leading the hands back, the right leg is not seated enough. This throws out the hip and makes the torso lean.

● When pressing the palm, the body leans forward.

23. Shízìshǒu 十字手 (Cross Hands)

23.1 Turn the Body and Draw the Foot Inward

Turn the torso to the right, shift the body center to the right, bend the right leg and seat it, and draw the right toes inward; swing the right hand to the front of the head. Look at the right hand. (Fig. 129)

23.2 Bend the Leg into a Bow and Separate the Hands

Continue to turn the torso to the right; turn the right toes outward, bend the right leg into a bow, and straighten the left leg naturally to form a right side-bow stance; the right hand continues to move to the right in a curve until it reaches the right side of the body. Raise both hands so that they are horizontal and extended out to the two sides of the body, palms outward, fingers slanted up. Look at the right hand. (Fig. 130)

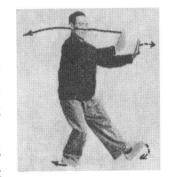

Fig. 129

23.3 Cross Hands

Turn the torso to the left, shift the body center to the left; bend the left leg into a bow,

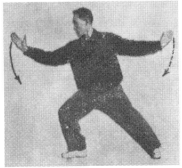

Fig. 130

straighten the right leg naturally, and draw the right toes and ball of the foot inward; move the hands down in curves and cross them before the abdomen, then raise them before the chest, the right hand outside, palms inward; lift up the arms in a circle, with the wrists crossed, to shoulder height. The eyes follow the movements of the hands. (Fig. 131)

23.4 Draw In the Foot and Hold as in an Embrace

Turn the torso to the front; lift the right foot and move it half a step in to the left, with the ball of the right foot landing on the ground first, then the whole foot rooted. The two legs straighten slowly with the body center balanced on both legs, the feet parallel with toes pointing forward, shoulder-width apart, forming a standing feet-apart stance. Cross the hands and keep them in a position as if to hold something before the chest. Look straight ahead. (Fig. 132)

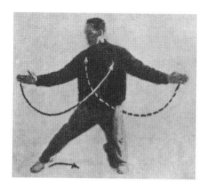

Fig. 131

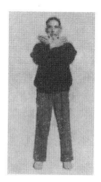

Fig. 132

Application

Both hands are held in front of the chest in a position as if to hold something. This movement is for protection while waiting for a good chance to intercept an attack.

Important Points

• The hands and the waist and the body center move through a wide range in this movement, accompanied by the feet turning in, turning out and drawing in. Coordinate all the movements in one smooth continuous motion without a pause in power.

• When drawing in the foot and placing the hands in a position as if to hold something, keep the torso upright. Do not lean forward and bend the waist. Lift up the arms and extend them in arcs, not too tight. Do not let the arms become too tense.

Common Mistakes

• When turning the torso to the right in the first and second group movements, the movements are not continuous. There is a pause between the movements.

● When shifting the body center from the left to right, the legs stand up straight, the head lowers, the back bends and the torso sways.

● When keeping the hands in a position as if to hold something, the shoulders shrug, the elbows clamp, and the arms are not fully extended.

24. Shōushì 收势 (Closing Position)

24.1 Turn the Palm and Separate the Hands

Turn the arms inward, rotate the hands down and separate them left and right, shoulder width apart. Look straight ahead. (Fig. 133)

24.2 Lower the Arms and Let the Hands Fall

Lower the arms slowly, and lower the hands to the outside of the thighs. Look straight ahead. (Fig. 134)

24.3 Stand with Feet Together

Raise the left foot gently and move it close to the right foot, with the ball of the left foot landing on the ground first, then the whole foot rooted. Return to the Ready Position. Look straight ahead. (Fig. 135)

Important Points

● When executing turning the palms and separating the hands, turn the palms as the hands separate.

● When standing with feet together and returning to the Ready Position, lift the left foot evenly and steadily as in " point, rise, point, fall."

Common Mistakes

● When turning the palms and parting the hands, the wrists turn.

● When lowering the arms and letting the hands fall, the arms bend and the hands press.

● When standing with feet together, the body sways.

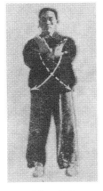
Fig. 133

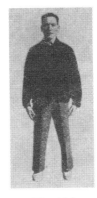
Fig. 134

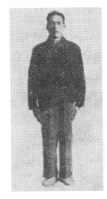
Fig. 135

CHAPTER VII

42-STEP TAIJIQUAN

Sìshíér Shì Tàijíquán   四十二式太极拳

Introduction

The Chinese Martial Arts Research Institute in 1989 organized prominent martial artists, coaches and athletes from all over China to create a series of martial arts sports competition forms in seven areas: Long Fist Boxing, Southern Style Boxing, Taijiquan, Broadsword Play, Swordplay, Cudgel Play and Spear Play. Among the forms created was 42-Step Taijiquan.

While maintaining their respective martial arts traditions, the standard forms in each of the seven areas were designed with competition features such as a prescribed number and sequence of movements in a certain time frame to become compulsory events in Chinese martial arts meets as well as other sports gatherings such as the Chinese National Games, Asian Games, East Asian Games, and Southeast Asian Games. The 42-Step Taijiquan belongs to no specific school, having been drawn from various Taiji styles, so that it is sometimes referred to as "Comprehensive Taijiquan."

42-Step Taijiquan has the following features:

1. It complies with competition rules on number and combinations of techniques and stances, technical standards and time limits.

2. It contains representative movements of different schools of Taijiquan, displaying different styles of Taijiquan and requiring athletes to demonstrate an overall command of skills.

3. Innovative in design, it also reflects inherited traditions of Taijiquan.

4. Beyond helping to popularize Taijiquan as a martial arts sports competition form, 42-Step Taijiquan provides through its beautiful and not-too-difficult movements a good exercise that can help people in general keep fit.

Technical Elements of 42-Step Taijiquan

Order	Forms	Hand shapes	Stances (Bùxíng 步型)	Arm and hand techniques	Footwork (Bùfǎ 步法)	Kick/ balance	Schools
1	Beginnig Position	Zhǎng 掌 Open-palm hand	Kailìbù 开立步 Standing feet-apart stance	Xià'àn 下按 Push down	Kaibù 开步 Feet apart		88-Step
2	Grasp the Peacock's Tail on the Left	Zhǎng 掌 Open-palm hand	Gōngbù, dīngbù 弓步、丁步 Bow stance; T-stance	Péng, lǚ, jǐ, àn, bàozhǎng 掤、捋、挤、按、抱掌 Ward off; roll back; press; push; "hold the ball"	Shàngbù, gēnbù 上步、跟步 Step forward; follow in		Yang, Wu (吴) and Sun styles, and 88-Step
3	Single Bian, Left	Zhǎng, gōu 掌、勾 Open-palm hand; hook	Gōngbù 弓步 Bow stance	Tuīzhǎng, gōushǒu 推掌、勾手 Push palm; hook	Shàngbù 上步 Step forward		Yang Style
4	Lift the Hands	Zhǎng 掌 Open-palm hand	Xūbù 虚步 Empty stance	Héshǒu 合手 Close hands	Niǎnzhuǎnbù 碾转步 Turn on the feet		88-Step
5	White Crane Spreads Its Wings	Zhǎng 掌 Open-palm hand	Xūbù 虚步 Empty stance	Fēnzhǎng 分掌 Separate hands	Huebù 活步 Lift-foot steps		88-Step
6	Brush Aside over the Knee in Reverse Forward Stance	Zhǎng 掌 Open-palm hand	Gōngbù 弓步 Bow stance	Tuīzhǎng, lōuzhǎng 推掌、搂掌 Push; brush aside	Shàngbù 上步 Step forward		Yang Style
7	Turn and Punch	Zhǎng, quán 掌、拳 Open-palm hand; fist	Gōngbù 弓步 Bow stance	Pioquán 撇拳 Strike with the back of the fist	Shàngbù 上步 Step forward		Yang Style
8	Roll Back and Press	Zhǎng 掌 Open-palm hand	Gōngbù 弓步 Bow stance	Lǚ, jǐ 捋、挤 Roll back; press	Shàngbù 上步 Step forward		Yang Style and 48-Step
9	Step Forward, Deflect, Block and Punch	Zhǎng, quán 掌、拳 Open-palm hand; fist	Gōngbù 弓步 Bow stance	Banquán, lánquán, chōngzhǎng 搬拳、拦拳、冲掌 Deflect; block; punch	Jìnbù 进步 Step in (referring to more than one step. More than three steps is xíngbù 行步)		88-Step
10	Pull Back then Push, As if to Close	Zhǎng 掌 Open-palm hand	Dīngbù 丁步 T-stance	Àn 按 Push down	Shàngbù, gēnbù 上步、跟步 Step forward; follow in		88-Step and Sun Style
Sub-total Part I	10	3	5	15	6		

Order	Forms	Hand shapes	Stances	Arm and hand techniques	Footwork	Kick/ balance	Schools
11	Open and Close the Hands	Zhǎng 掌 Open-palm hand	Dīngbù 丁步 T-stance	Kaishǒu, héshǒu 开手、合手 Open and close hands	Niǎnzhuǎnbù 碾转步 Turn on the feet		Sun Style
12	Single Bian, Right	Zhǎng 掌 Open-palm hand	Héngdangbù 横裆步 Side-bow stance	Fēnzhǎng 分掌 Separate hands	Kaibù 开步 Feet apart		Sun Style
13	Fist under Elbow	Zhǎng, quán 掌、拳 Open-palm hand; fist	Xūbù 虚步 Empty stance	Qínshǒu, pīzhǎng 擒手、劈掌 Grab; chop	Diànbù, gēnbù, shàngbù 垫步、跟步、上步 Half-step forward; follow in; step forward		Yang Style
14	Turn the Body and Thrust the Palm	Zhǎng, quán 掌、拳 Open-palm hand; fist	Dīngbù 丁步 T-stance	Tuīzhǎng, lōuzhǎng 推掌、搂掌 Push and brush with palm	Niǎnzhuǎnbù, shàngbù, gēnbù 碾转步、上步、跟步 Turn on the feet; step forward; follow in		Sun Style
15	Jade Maiden Moves the Shuttle Left and Right	Zhǎng 掌 Open-palm hand	Gōngbù 弓步 Bow stance	Jiàzhǎng, tuīzhǎng, píngyúnshǒu 架掌、推掌、平云手 Block up; push the hand; move the hand like clouds on the horizontal	Chèbù, shàngbù, gēnbù 撤步、上步、跟步 Bring the front foot back to the back foot; step forward; follow in		88-Step
16	Kick Right and Left	Zhǎng 掌 Open-palm hand		Bàozhǎng, fēnzhǎng 抱掌、分掌 Hold hands; separate hands	Shàngbù 上步 Step forward	Heel kick	Yang, Sun and Wu styles; 48-Step
17	Conceal the Hand, Bend the Arm and Punch	Quán, zhǎng 拳、掌 Fist; Open-palm hand	Gōngbù, pianmǎbù 弓步、偏马步 Bow stance; side horse stance	Yǎnshǒu, chōngzhǎng 掩手、冲掌 Conceal hand; thrust palm	Cabù 擦步 Move the foot along the ground		48-Step
18	Part the Wild Horse's Mane	Zhǎng 掌 Open-palm hand	Gōngbù, pianmǎbù 弓步、偏马步 Bow stance; side horse stance	Kào, lio 靠、捯 Lean; split	Shàngbù 上步 Step forward		Chen Style
Sub-total Part II	8	2	5	14	7	1	

Order	Forms	Hand shapes	Stances	Arm and hand techniques	Footwork	Kick/ balance	Schools
19	Move the Hands Like Clouds	Zhǎng 掌 Open-palm hand	Xiǎokaibù 小开步 Feet slightly apart	Yúnshǒu 云手 Move hands like clouds	Cèxíngbù 侧行步 Step sideward		Yang Style
20	Stand on One Leg and Hit the Tiger	Quán 拳 Fist	Dúlìbù 独立步 One-leg stance	Jiàquán 架拳 Block up	Tíjiǎo 提脚 Lift foot		Wu (吴) Style
21	Separate the Foot—Right	Zhǎng 掌 Open-palm hand		Bàozhǎng, fēnzhǎng 抱掌、分掌 Bring the hands together; separate hands		Sepa-rate the feet	Yang Style
22	Strike the Opponent's Ears with Both Fists	Quán 拳 Fist	Gōngbù 弓步 Bow stance	Guànquán 贯拳 Roundhouse punch	Shàngbù 上步 Step forward		Yang Style
23	Separate the Foot—Left	Zhǎng 掌 Open-palm hand		Bàozhǎng, fēnzhǎng 抱掌、分掌 Bring the hands together; separate hands		Sepa-rate the feet	Yang Style
24	Turn the Body and Pat the Foot	Zhǎng 掌 Open-palm hand		(Same as above)	Niǎnzhuǎnbù 碾转步 Turn on the feet	Pat the foot	Chen Style; 88-Step
25	Step in and Punch Downward	Quán, zhǎng 拳、掌 Fist; open-palm hand	Gōngbù 弓步 Bow stance	Zaiquán, lōushǒu 栽拳、搂手 Punch downward; brush aside	Jìnbù 进步 Step in		Yang Style
26	Diagonal Flying Posture	Zhǎng 掌 Open-palm hand	Héngdangbù 横裆步 Side-bow stance	Kào 靠 Lean	Kaibù 开步 Feet apart		Wu (吴) Style
27	Single Bian Downward	Zhǎng, gōu 掌、勾 Open-palm hand; hook	Pūbù 仆步 Crouch stance	Chuanzhǎng 穿掌 Thread hand			88-Step
28	Golden Rooster Stands on One Leg	Zhǎng 掌 Open-palm hand	Dúlìbù 独立步 One-leg stance	Tiǎozhǎng 挑掌 Spear up the hand	Tíjiǎo 提脚 Lift foot		Yang Style
29	Step Back and Thread the Open-palm Hand	Zhǎng 掌 Open-palm hand	Gōngbù 弓步 Bow stance	Chuanzhǎng 穿掌 Thread the hand	Tuìbù 退步 Step backward		48-Step; Wu (吴) Style
Sub-total Part III	11	3	5	10	7	2	

Order	Forms	Hand shapes	Stances	Arm and hand techniques	Footwork	Kick/ balance	Schools
30	Press the Palms Down in Empty Stance	Zhǎng 掌 Open-palm hand	Xūbù 虚步 Empty stance	Yazhǎng 压掌 Press palm	Niǎnzhuǎnbù 碾转步 Turn on the feet		Sun Style; 48-step
31	Stand on One Leg and Lift the Hand	Zhǎng 掌 Open-palm hand	Dúlìbù 独立步 One-leg stance	Tuōzhǎng 托掌 Lift hand	Tíjiǎo 提脚 Lift foot		Chen Style; 48-step
32	Lean-in Horse Stance	Quán, zhǎng 拳、掌 Fist and open-palm hand)	Bànmǎbù 半马步 Half horse stance	Kào, cǎi 靠、采 Lean; pull down	Jìnbù 进步 Step in		Push-hands; 48-step
33	Turn the Body with Large Rollback	Quán 拳 Fist	Héngdangbù 横裆步 Side-bow stance	Zhǒu 肘 Elbow	Kaibù 开步 Feet apart		Push-hands; 48-step
34	Grab and Hit in Resting Stance	Quán 拳 Fist	Xiēbù 歇步 Resting stance	Qínshǒu, chōngquán 擒手、冲拳 Grab; punch with fist	Gàibù 盖步 Cross-over step		Xing-yiquan
35	Lower the Body and Thread the Palm-hand	Zhǎng 掌 Open-palm hand	Pūbù 仆步 Crouch stance	Chuanzhǎng 穿掌 Thread the hand	Kaibù 开步 Feet apart		Wu (吴) Style
36	Step Forward and Seven Stars	Quán 拳 Fist	Xūbù 虚步 Empty stance	Jiàquán 架拳 Block up	Shàngbù 上步 Step forward		Yang Style
37	Step Back and Ride the Tiger	Zhǎng, gōu 掌、勾 Open-palm hand; hook		Tiǎozhǎng 挑掌 Spear up the hand	Tuìbù 退步 Step backward	Raise the leg in front and keep balance	Wu (吴) Style; 48-step
38	Turn Around and Make a Lotus Swing Kick	Zhǎng 掌 Open-palm hand		Chuanzhǎng, bǎizhǎng 穿、摆掌 Thread, swing the hands	Kòubù, niǎnzhuǎn bù 扣步、碾转步 Step with toes in; turn on the feet	Swing out the leg	48-Step Bagua-zhang
39	Draw the Bow to Shoot Tiger	Quán 拳 Fist	Gōngbù 弓步 Bow stance	Chōngquán 冲拳 Punch	Shàngbù 上步 Step forward		88-step
40	Grasp the Peacock's Tail on the Left	Zhǎng 掌 Open-palm hand	Gōngbù, xūbù 弓步、虚步 Bow stance and empty stance	Péng, lǚ, jǐ, àn, bàozhǎng 掤、捋、挤、按 Ward off; roll back; press; push down	Shàngbù 上步 Step forward		88-step
41	Cross Hands	Zhǎng 掌 Open-palm hand	Kailìbù 开立步 Standing feet-apart stance	Bàozhǎng 抱掌 Hold hands in embrace	Niǎnzhuǎnbù, bìngbù 碾转步、并步 Turn on the feet; stand upright with feet together		88-step
42	Closing Position	Zhǎng 掌 Open-palm hand	Kailìbù 开立步 Standing feet-apart stance		Bìngbù 并步 Stand upright with feet together		Yang Style
Sub-total Part II	13	3	9	17	9	2	
Total	42	3	12	35	14	5	

Names of the Movements of 42-Step Taijiquan

Part I

1. Qǐshì 起势 (Beginning Position)
2. Yòu Lǎnquèwěi 右揽雀尾 (Grasp the Peacock's Tail on the Right)
3. Zuǒ Dānbiān 左单鞭 (Single Bian, Left)
4. Tíshǒu 提手 (Lift the Hands)
5. Báihè Liàngchì 白鹤亮翅 (White Crane Spreads Its Wings)
6. Lōuxī Àobù 搂膝拗步 (Brush Aside over the Knee in Reverse Forward Stance)
7. Piēshēnchuí 撇身捶 (Turn and Punch)
8. Lǚjǐshì 捋挤势 (Roll Back and Press)
9. Jìnbù Banlánchuí 进步搬拦捶 (Step In, Deflect, Block and Punch)
10. Rúfēng Sìbì 如封似闭 (Pull Back then Push, As if to Close)

Part II

11. Kaihé Shǒu 开合手 (Open and Close the Hands)
12. Yòu Danbian 右单鞭 (Single Bian, Right*)
13. Zhǒudǐchuí 肘底捶 (Fist Under the Elbow)
14. Zhuǎnshēn Tuīzhǎng 转身推掌 (Turn the Body and Thrust the Palm)
15. Yùnǚ Chuansuō 玉女穿梭 (Jade Maiden Moves the Shuttle Left and Right)
16. Yòuzuǒ Dēngjiǎo 右左蹬脚 (Kick Right and Left)
17. Yǎnshǒu Gōngchuí 掩手肱捶 (Conceal the Hands, Bend the Arm and Punch)
18. Yomǎ Fēnzōng 野马分鬃 (Part the Wild Horse's Mane)

Part III

19. Yúnshǒu 云手 (Move the Hands Like Clouds)
20. Dúlì Dǎhǔ 独立打虎 (Stand on One Leg and Hit the Tiger)
21. Yòu Fēnjiǎo 右分脚 (Separate the Foot — Right)
22. Shuangfēng Guàn' or 双峰贯耳 (Strike the Opponent's Ears with Both Fists)
23. Zuǒ Fēnjiǎo 左分脚 (Separate the Foot — Left)
24. Zhuǎnshēn Paijiǎo 转身拍脚 (Turn the Body and Pat the Foot)
25. Jìnbù Zaichuí 进步栽捶 (Step In and Punch Downward)

---

* Danbian单鞭 (Danbian): "Dan" means single. "Bian" here refers to an ancient weapon, an iron rod that is either rectangular in shape or edged as in bamboo, or other patterns. Bian were often used in pairs, hence Danbian means Single Bian.

26. Xiéfēishì 斜飞势 (Diagonal Flying Posture)
27. Dānbiān Xiàshì 单鞭下势 (Single Bian Downward)
28. Jīnjī Dúlì 金鸡独立 (Golden Rooster Stands on One Leg)
29. Tuìbù Chuānzhǎng 退步穿掌 (Step Back and Thrust the Open-palm Hand)

Part IV

30. Xūbù Yāzhǎng 虚步压掌 (Press the Palms Down in Empty Stance)
31. Dúlì Tuōzhǎng 独立托掌 (Stand on One Leg and Lift the hand)
32. Mǎbùkào 马步靠 (Lean-in Horse Stance)
33. Zhuǎnshēn Dàlǚ 转身大捋 (Turn the Body with Large Rollback)
34. Xiēbù Qíndǎ 歇步擒打 (Grab and Hit in Resting Stance)
35. Chuānzhǎng Xiàshì 穿掌下势 (Lower the Body and Thread the Palm-hand)
36. Shàngbù Qīxīng 上步七星 (Step Forward and Seven Stars*)
37. Tuìbù Kuàhǔ 退步跨虎 (Step Back and Ride the Tiger)
38. Zhuǎnshēn Bǎilián 转身摆莲 (Turn the Boby for Lotus Kick)
39. Wāngōng Shèhǔ 弯弓射虎 (Draw the Bow to Shoot Tiger)
40. Zuǒ Lǎnquèwoi 左揽雀尾 (Grasp the Peacock's Tail on the Left)
41. Shízìshǒu 十字手 (Cross Hands)
42. Shōushì 收势 (Closing Position)

Movements and Illustrations of 42-Step Taijiquan

Part I

1. Qǐshì 起势 (Beginning Position)

1.1 Ready Position

Stand with the body straight, feet together, head and neck straight, chin in, chest and abdomen relaxed, arms hanging naturally in light contact with the outside of the thighs. Concentrate the mind and breathe naturally. Look straight ahead. Assume that the direction faced is South. (Fig. 1)

1.2 Step to the Left

Gently step to the left one shoulder-width distance,

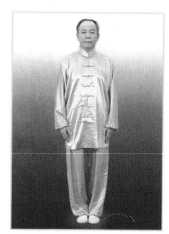

Fig. 1

---

* Shàngbù Qīxīng 上步七星 (Step Forward and Seven Stars): Seven Stars is a reference to the Big Dipper, comparing the outline of the body in this stance to that constellation But, it also could be a reference to the seven stars or "bright spots" of Taijiquan, the seven parts of the body that can be used as weapons: The head, shoulders, elbows, hands, hips, knees and feet.

toes pointing forward. (Fig. 2)

1.3 Raise the Arms Forward

Slowly raise the hands forward and upward to shoulder height, palms down, arms shoulder-width apart, and elbows slightly lowered. (Fig. 3)

1.4 Bend the Knees and Press the Palms Downward

Keep the torso erect; slightly bend the knees to a half squat; gently press the palms downward to the level of the abdomen until the hands are above the knees. When squatting, bend the legs and drop the hips, bend the knees and hips, keeping the buttocks tucked in. Contract and lift the anus. Keep the torso straight. The degree of bending can be different from person to person. When the movement is completed, the body should be in a position of sitting straight in a chair with both hands pressing down gently on an imaginary table in front of the abdomen. The weight falls on the back part of the feet. (Fig. 4)

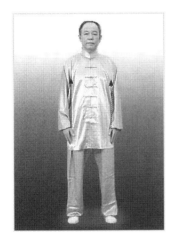
Fig. 2

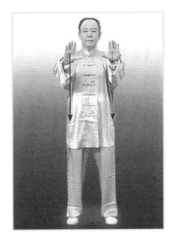
Fig. 3

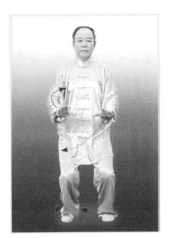
Fig. 4

Important Points

- Keep the body straight, push up with the top of the head, drop the shoulders, relax the chest and abdomen, arms hanging down in light contact with the outer sides of the thighs; concentrate, keep calm, breathe naturally. Look straight ahead.

- When stepping to the side, do not shift the body center too abruptly.

- Lift the wrists when raising the arms, and drop the wrists when pressing down.

- Bend the legs and drop the hips when squatting; bend the knees and hips, keeping the buttocks tucked in and the torso straight. The degree of bending can be different from person to person.

- When the movement is completed, the body should be as if sitting straight up in a chair and with both hands pressing gently on an imaginary table in front of the abdomen. The weight falls on the back of the feet.

Common Mistakes

- When squatting, the torso leans forward, the chest and hips are thrust out; or the abdomen is thrust out and the body leans backward.

- When squatting, the muscles of the torso are tense, and/or the breath is held.

- When standing, the feet are turned out at an angle.

- When pressing down, the arms are bent and dropped abruptly.

2. Yòu Lǎnquèwoi 右揽雀尾 (Grasp the Peacock's Tail on the Right)

2.1 Hold the Ball and Draw In the Foot

Slightly turn out the toes of the right foot and turn the body slightly right at the same time; raise the right arm and bend it in front of the chest, palm facing downward; turn the left hand and sweep it in a curve to the right in front of the abdomen on the right, palm facing up and opposite the right hand as if holding a ball; shift the body center to the right leg and draw the left foot toward the inside of the right foot. Look at the right hand. (Fig. 5)

2.2 Turn the Body and Step Forward

Slightly turn the torso to the left, and move the left foot to the left front, gently landing the heel. (Fig. 6)

2.3 Bow Stance and Ward Off with Left Arm

Keep turning the torso to the left; shift the body center forward to form a left bow stance; at the same time ward off (péng 掤) forward with the left arm, keeping the left hand at shoulder height, palm inward, and fingertips pointing left; lower the right hand to the side of the right hip, palm facing downward, fingertips pointing forward, and arms slightly bent. Look at the left forearm. (Fig. 7)

2.4 Hold the Ball and Draw In the Foot

Slightly turn the torso to the left; draw the right foot to the inside of the left foot;

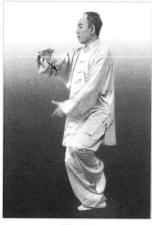

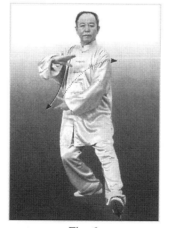

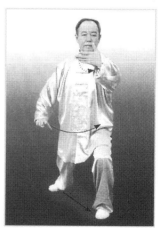

Fig. 5   Fig. 6   Fig. 7

turn the left arm inward and bend it in front of the left chest, turning the left hand downward at chest level with fingertips pointing right; move the right arm to the left in a curve to the front of the left part of the abdomen, palm facing up and fingertips pointing left, forming the "hold a ball" posture. Look at the left hand. (Fig. 8)

2.5 Turn the Body and Step Forward

Slightly turn the torso to the right; gently move the right foot one step to the right front, landing the heel. (Fig. 9)

2.6 Bow Stance and Ward Off with Right Arm

Keep turning the torso to the right; shift the body center forward to form a right bow stance; at the same time ward off with the right arm, bending it slightly and keeping the palm facing the body at shoulder height; lower the left hand to the side of the left hip, palm facing down. Look at the right forearm. (Fig. 10)

2.7 Turn Palm and Sweep Arm

Slightly turn the torso to the right; extend the left hand forward, turning the palm upward at the same time, until it reaches the underside of the right wrist. Look at the right hand. (Fig. 11)

2.8 Roll Back in Back Stance

Shift the body center backward and turn the torso slightly left; roll back (lǚ 挒) with palms downward to the front of the abdomen. Eyes move with the right hand. (Fig. 12)

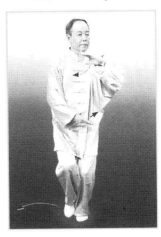

Fig. 8

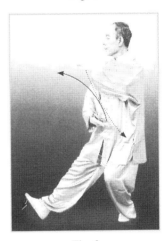

Fig. 9

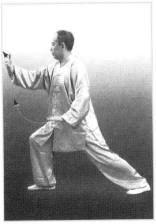

Fig. 10

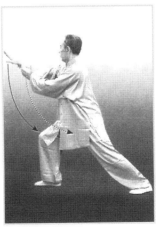

Fig. 11

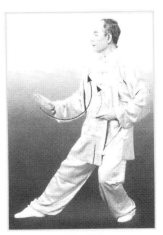

Fig. 12

2.9 Turn the Body and Bring the Hands Together

Turn the right arm outward, bending the elbow so the arm is horizontal to the ground at the front of the chest, right palm facing the body and fingertips pointing to left; turn the left arm inward, left palm facing right, with the palm and fingers on the inside of the right wrist. (Fig. 13)

2.10 Bow Stance and Press Forward

Shift the body center forward to form a right bow stance; press (jǐ 挤) both palms forward together, forming a circle with the arms. Look straight forward. (Fig. 14)

2.11 Back Stance and Ward off (Péng 掤) Backwards

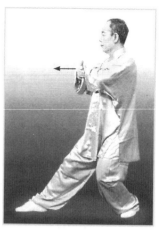

Fig.13

Shift the body center backward and turn the torso slightly right; lift the toes of the right foot; turn the right arm outward, turn the right palm upward, and move the right arm with the elbow bent to the right and back in a horizontal curved line to the front of the right shoulder, in a movement of warding-off; keeping the open-palm left hand on the inside of the right wrist and moving it on the same curved line. Eyes follow the movement of the right hand. (Fig. 15)

Turn the body left; turn in the right toes and land them; move the right palm in a horizontal curve and then bend the arm to move it in to the front of the shoulder. (Fig. 16)

2.12 T-stance and Push the Palm

Turn the body slightly right and shift the body center to the right; draw the left foot to the inside of the right foot and land the toes to form a T-stance; turn the right arm inward, turn the right palm and push (àn 按) it toward the right front, fingers up, wrist at shoulder height, and palm outward; at the same time turn the left palm

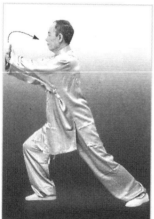
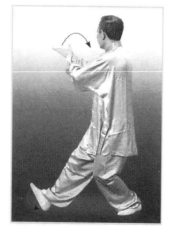
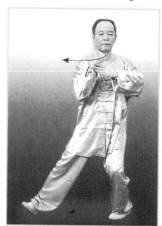

Fig. 14   Fig. 15   Fig. 16

inward, keeping the fingertips on the inside of the right wrist. Look at the right hand. (Fig. 17)

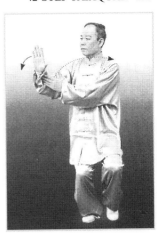

Fig. 17

Important Points

• Shift the body center to the right when holding the ball on the right, turn the torso right and turn the right toes out. Lift the left foot and move it to the inside of the right ankle. Shift the body center forward when holding the ball on the left, turn the torso slightly left, keep the left foot in place, lift the right foot and draw it to the inside of the left ankle.

• When shifting the body center forward after stepping forward, push the back heel down to form a bow stance. When forming a bow stance and when sitting back, do not move the back foot.

• Coordinate the arms, legs and torso in ward off, roll back, press and push through the shifting of the body center and turning of the waist in bow stance and sitting back. Do the hand forms correctly. Be light and nimble when changing from one movement to another, and be smooth and agile in all movements. At the end of the movement, let the power in the arms resist each other and keep the torso straight to show inner strength.

• When shifting from press to push, bend the arms and with the turning of the waist lightly move the arms horizontally in a curve while turning them inward and outward.

• Be relaxed, solid and stable while doing T-stance and Push the Palm, and direct the hands 30 to 45 degrees to the right front.

• Ward off is adapted from 88-Step Taijiquan, roll back and press from Yang Style, push palm from Wu (吴) Style, and the T-stance from Sun Style.

Common Mistakes

• When stepping forward, the foot movement is unsteady with the foot landing heavily.

• When forming a bow stance, the back heel is not thrust down and out; the back leg bends too much; or the outside of the back foot lifts up.

• The body center is shifted too fast, or the legs move faster than the hands.

• When sitting back, the supporting or back leg is too tense; the torso leans forward or backward; and the back foot wobbles.

• The waist does not turn, and the body does not move in a coordinated way.

• The arms tense while holding the ball.

• The T-stance and pushing palm are not done clearly; after pushing the palm, the hook [formed in the next movement] is formed too soon, or after drawing in the left foot to form T-stance, the foot does not land.

• The torso twists and leans to the right too much in T-stance and push palm.

3. Zuǒ Danbian 左单鞭 (Single Bian, Left)

3.1 Hook and Step Forward

Turn the torso slightly to the left; move the left foot forward one step to the left, land the heel; turn the right palm into a hook; and move the left palm to the left in a curve to the front. Look at the left hand. (Fig. 18)

3.2 Continue turning the torso to the left; shifting the body center forward to form a left bow stance; turn the left forearm inward, turn the left palm outward and push forward, keeping the palm forward and wrist at shoulder height. Look at the left hand. (Fig. 19)

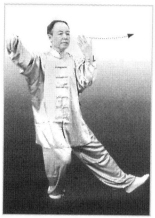

Fig. 18

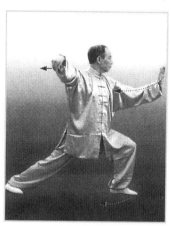

Fig. 19

Important Points

● When moving the foot forward, turn the torso slightly to the left, then move the foot forward to the left.

● When pushing the palm, continue turning the torso to the left, at the same time forming a bow stance.

● When making the bow stance, step about 30 degrees to the left of front, kick down the back leg, turn and straighten it.

● On fixing the form, drop the shoulders and elbows, keep the arms stretched out without losing their force. Keep both wrists at shoulder height.

Common Mistakes

● The torso fails to turn when moving the foot forward, making a side step.

● The palm is not pushed in the same direction as the bow stance, or the back foot fails to kick and turn, thus the palm is pushed to the side.

● The arms are extended too straight and too wide, the chest is thrust out or the shoulders are raised.

● The hooked hand is too high or too low.

● The eyes fail to follow the movement of the left hand.

4. Tíshǒu 提手 (Lift the Hands)

4.1 Turn the Torso and Sweep the Arms

Shift the body center to sit back, turn the torso to the right; turn in the left toes, and sweep the left hand to the right in a horizontal curve. Look at the left hand. (Fig. 20)

4.2 Back Stance (Zuòtuǐ 坐腿) and Draw the Hand

Shift the body center to the left; open the right hook hand, and draw the left hand slightly to the left on a horizontal line. (Fig. 21)

4.3 Empty Stance (Xūbù 虚步) and Put the Hand Next to the Elbow

Turn the torso slightly to the right; lift and turn the right foot, landing the heel; raise the toes, forming a right empty stance; form a vertical palm facing the side with the right hand in front of the body, keeping the fingertips at brow level; bend the left arm to form a vertical open-palm left hand, put the left hand near the inside of the right elbow. Look at the right hand. (Fig. 22)

Important Points

● Turn the waist to lead the left arm in its horizontal sweep to the right; sit back on the supporting leg to lead the arms as they are drawn back at the end of the movement.

● Coordinate the turning of the waist and the lifting and landing of the right foot with the movement of the hands.

● In fixing the form, straighten the torso, push up with the head, lower the shoulders and drop the hips. Bend the arms, extending them fully in curves, elbows in, fingertips slanted upward. The direction at the end faces 45 degrees to the side of the front.

Common Mistakes

● While making the empty stance, the chest thrusts forward, the buttocks thrust backward and the torso leans forward. Or the hips and abdomen thrust forward, and the torso leans backward.

● The arms are limp, or they are bent too much with tension.

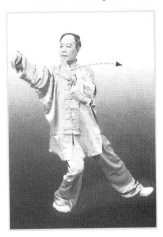

Fig. 20

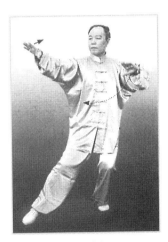

Fig. 21

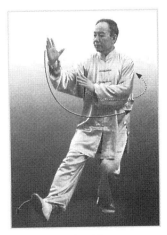

Fig. 22

- The front knee straightens while making the empty stance.
- The back knee points inward or outward too much, in a direction from the direction of the back foot.
- The torso is twisted off line.
- The movements of the hands, feet and waist are not coordinated.

5. Báihè Liàngchì 白鹤亮翅 (White Crane Spreads Its Wings)

5.1 Turn the Body and Separate the Hands

Turn the torso to the left; move the hands down and to the left in a curve, separating them. Look forward. (Fig. 23)

5.2 Step Backward and Hold the Hands Together

Move the right foot slightly backward, turn in the ball of the foot; keep the hands moving down to the left in a curve, and turn them and hold them in front of the left chest, the left hand on top, and the arms bent in arcs. Look at the left hand. (Fig. 24)

5.3 Sitting Stance and Separate the Hands

Shift the body center to the right, turn the torso to the right; move the hands together while raising them to the front of the right shoulder. Look at the right hand. (Fig. 25)

5.4 Empty Stance and Separate the Hands

Turn the torso slightly to the left; slightly draw the left foot inward and touch the ground with the toes, forming a left empty stance; separate the hands in curves, moving the right hand upward and the left hand downward, and raise the right hand to the front of the right forehead, keeping the right palm facing inward; push the left palm to the side of the left hip, the palm downward, and arms are kept curved. Look straight ahead. (Fig. 26)

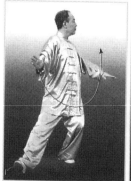 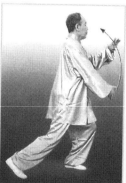 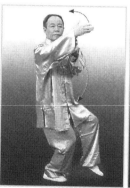 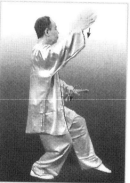

Fig. 23　　　　　Fig. 24　　　　　Fig. 25　　　　　Fig. 26

Important Points

- Move the hands down and to the left in curves while separating them, and turn them, moving them across each other into a position similar to that of holding a ball.

- Move the foot about one foot-length backward, completing the movement at the same time as the hands "hold a ball."
- Coordinate sitting stance and separating of the hands through the turning of the waist.
- Turn the body back toward the front while separating the hands and moving into empty stance.
- When forming an empty stance with the left foot, turn the left foot forward pivoting on the ball of the foot before drawing it inward and touching the ground with the toes.
- When fixing the form, have one hand raised and the other pushed down, in an extended, rounded form.

Common Mistakes
- The torso leans forward when moving the foot backward.
- The arms bend too much so that they do not form a curve.

6. Lōuxī Àobù 搂膝拗步 (Brush Aside over the Knee in Reverse Forward Stance)

6.1 Turn the Body and Sweep the Arms

Turn the torso slightly to the left; with the turn, move the right hand to the left in a curve and then downward passing in front of the head. Look at the right hand. (Fig. 27)

6.2 Sweep the Arms and Draw In the Foot

Turn the torso to the right; with the turn sweep the right hand down, to the right and then upward in a curve until it reaches head level at the right front, the palm slanted upward; sweep the left hand up to the right and then downward in a curve to the side of the right ribs, palm facing down; draw in the left foot toward the inside of the right foot. Look at the right hand. (Fig. 28)

6.3 Bend the Arms and Step Forward

Turn the torso to the left; move the left foot forward, landing the heel lightly; bend the right elbow and draw the right hand to the side of ear, palm facing forward but slanting; move the left hand down in a curve to the front of the abdomen. Look straight ahead. (Fig. 29)

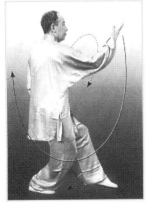

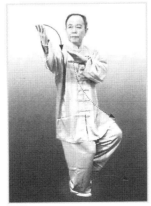
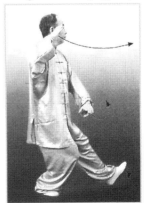

| Fig. 27 | Fig. 28 | Fig. 29 |

6.4 Bow Stance, Brush and Push

Shift the body center forward to form a left bow stance; raise the right hand with fingertips up and push the palm forward, keeping the fingertips at nose level; brush the left hand past the front of the left knee and press it down at the side of the left hip. Look at the right hand. (Fig. 30)

6.5 Turn the Body and Turn the Toes Out

Slightly shift the body center backward, turn the left toes out, and turn the torso to the left; at the same time sweep the right hand to the left in a curve. Eyes move with right hand. (Fig. 31)

6.6 Sweep the Arms and Draw In the Foot

Move the left hand to the left and upward in a curve until it reaches the left front of the body and at head level, palm facing slanted upward; move the right hand to the side of the left ribs, palm downward; draw the right foot to the inside of the left foot. Look at the left hand. (Fig. 32)

6.7 Bend the Arm and Step Forward

Turn the torso to the right; move the right foot forward, landing the heel gently; bend the left arm, moving the left hand to the side of ear, palm facing slanted forward; move the right hand to the right and downward in a curve to the front of the abdomen. Look straight ahead. (Fig. 33)

6.8 Bow Stance, Brush and Push

Shift the body center forward to form a right bow stance; push the left palm forward, keeping the hand upright with fingertips at nose level; brush the right hand around in front of the right knee until it reaches the side of the right hip, palm facing downward. Look at the left palm. (Fig. 34)

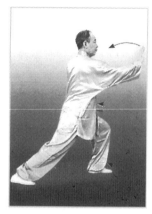

Fig. 30

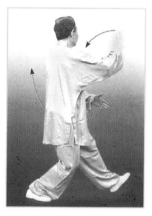

Fig. 31

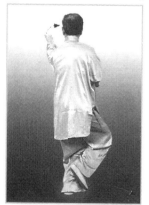

Fig. 32

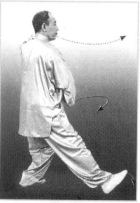

Fig. 33

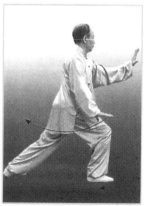

Fig. 34

Important Points

• Do not turn the body too much or sweep the arm in too large an arc, and do not move the right arm past the middle of vertical median line of the body.

• When sweeping the arms and drawing in the foot, turn the torso more than 45 degrees to the right; keep the arms naturally extended and move them lightly when sweeping them across in a curve, moving them to about 30 degrees to the right rear.

• Turn the body before stepping forward to the side.

• While pushing the palm, continue turning the body and moving the shoulder in the same direction. At the end of the movement, drop the shoulders, elbows and wrists; extend the fingers, push the palms and slightly arc in the chest, keeping power in the arms.

• Brush the palm closely over the knee in a curve, not too high or too far from the knee. At the end of the movement, keep the hand by the side of thigh with the palm pressing downward.

• The bow stance of this form features the opposite hand and foot forward. To keep the body center balanced, make the distance between the feet about 12 inches or about 30 centimeters.

• Shift the body center slightly backward when turning the body and turning the toes out, as much as necessary to make it easy for the toes to turn. Coordinate the turning of the body, the drawing in of the foot and the shifting back of the body center.

Common Mistakes

• The sweeping of the arms and the turning of the body are not coordinated; the waist is turned without sweeping the arms, or the waist does not turn enough and the arms sweep too much; the torso is twisted.

• Balance is lost when stepping forward, the movement of drawing in the foot lacks agility, the foot lands too heavily, and the supporting leg is unsteady.

• The arms are too straight or too bent when pushing the palms.

• When making the bow stance, the distance between the feet is too short, or the feet are crossed, causing the body to sway or become tense.

• Turning the body and drawing in the foot are not done at the same time as the shifting of the body center backward, sitting back before turning the waist.

7. Piēshēnchuí 撇身捶 (Turn and Punch)

7.1 Turn the Body and Separate the Hands

Slightly shift the body center backward, turn the right toes out, turn the torso to the right; extend the left hand forward and to the left, palm facing down, turn the right forearm outward, moving the right hand back to the right in a curve. Look at the left hand. (Fig. 35)

7.2 Draw In the Foot and Make a Fist

Draw the left foot to inside of the right foot; make a fist with the left hand, move the fist down in front of the lower abdomen, palm of the fist facing inward, the thumb side of fist toward the right; move the right hand upward and forward in a curve until it reaches inside of the left forearm, palm facing downward. Look forward to the left. (Fig. 36)

7.3 Step Forward and Raise the Fist

Slightly turn the torso left; move the left foot forward one step to the left, landing the heel; raise the left fist to front of face. (Fig. 37)

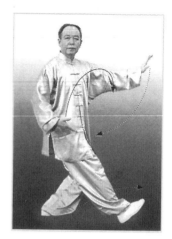

Fig. 35

7.4 Bow Stance and Backhand Strike

Shift the body center forward to form a left bow stance; turn the left fist to strike forward, palm of the fist slanted upward at head level; keep the right hand on the inside of the left forearm. Look at the left fist. (Fig. 38)

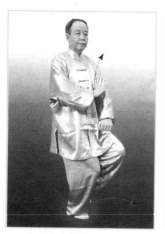

Fig. 36

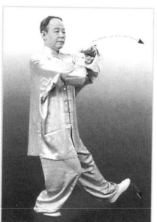

Fig. 37

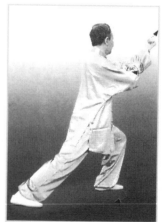

Fig. 38

Important Points

• Coordinate turning the body and separating the hands with shifting the body center backward and turning the toes out. Turn the forearm outward when moving the right hand backward, turning the palm upward.

• Make a fist with the left hand while moving it down, completing the whole movement in front of the abdomen, palm of the fist facing toward the body.

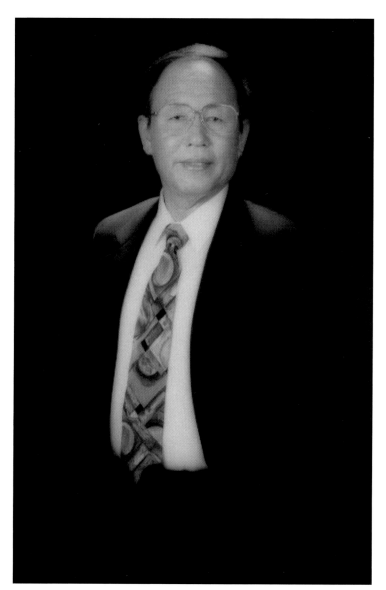

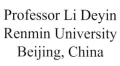

Professor Li Deyin
Renmin University
Beijing, China

A Taijiquan Family of Teachers

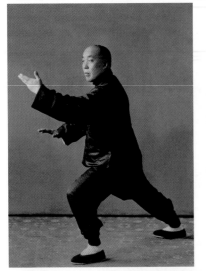

Li Yulin

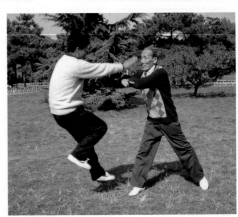

Li Tianji

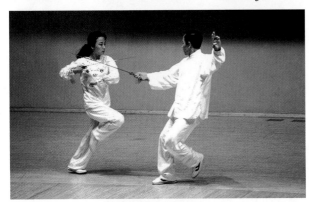

Li Defang and Li Deyin

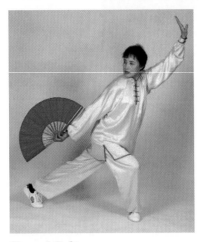

Fang Mishou

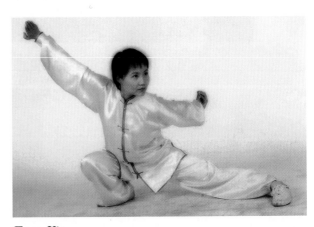

Faye Yip

太極拳

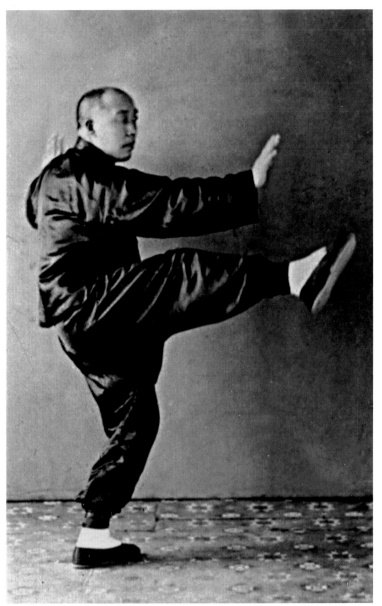
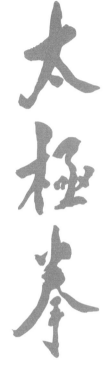

The author's grandfather, Li Yulin, was also his first teacher.

The photographs accompanying the author's explanation of
Yang-Style 81-Step Taijiquan are of Li Yulin circa 1930s,
originally published in a standard Chinese text of that time,
Textbook of Taijiquan.

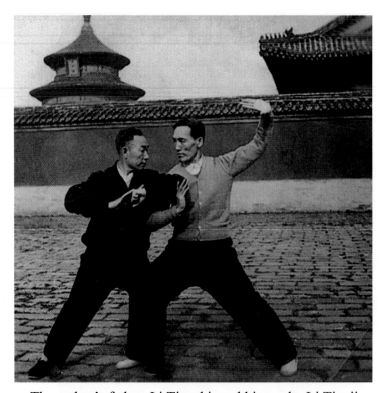
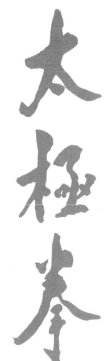

The author's father, Li Tianchi, and his uncle, Li Tianji
(facing camera) perform a two-person Taijiquan routine at
the Temple of Heaven in Beijing.

The photographs accompanying the author's explanation of
24-Step Taijiquan are of Li Tianji, who helped create the
form, from the early days of the People's Republic of China
when 24-Step Taijiquan was first introduced.

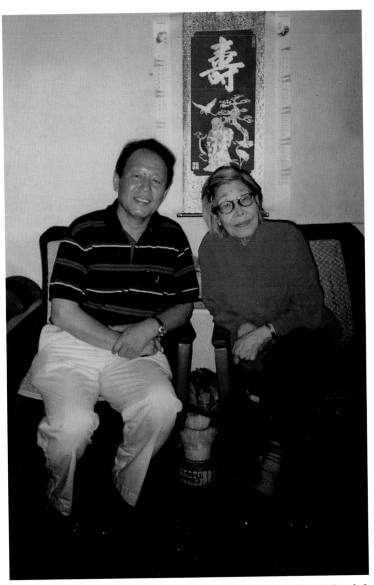
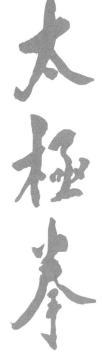

The author with Sun Jianyun, one of the 10 Modern Martial Arts Masters and president of the Sun-style Tajiquan Society, on the occasion of her 80th birthday. Sun is the daughter of Sun Lutang, the founder of Sun-Style Taijiquan.

Li Deyin incorporated movements from Sun and other major Taijiquan styles to create the modern competition 42-Step Taijiquan, which he both explains and demonstrates in this book.

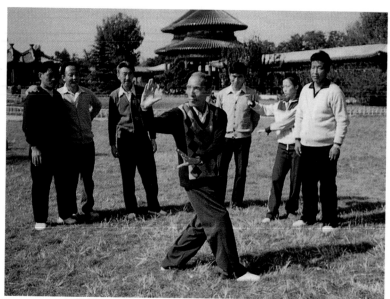

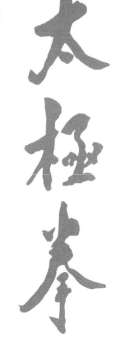

Li Defang (second right) joins her cousin Li Deyin (second left) and others in watching her father, Li Tianji, demonstrate at the Temple of Heaven in Beijing in his later years. A graduate of the Wushu Department of Beijing Normal University, Li Defang today is an instructor for the Sino-Japanese Friendship Association of Taijiquan in Japan.

The photographs accompanying the author's explanation of 42-Step Taiji Sword are of Li Defang.

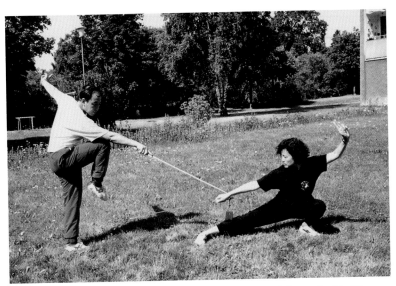

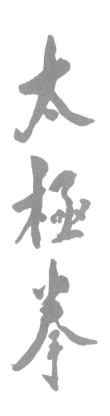

The author practices with his wife, Fang Mishou, in Beijing. Their daughter, Faye Li Yip (Li Hui), who is the great granddaughter of Li Yulin, is the 4th-generation martial arts teacher in the Li family.

The photographs accompanying the author's explanation of 32-Step Taiji Sword are of Faye Yip.

- Do not raise the elbow and shoulder when raising the fist.
- The bow stance and backhand strike with the fist are in a forward direction 45 degrees to the right, the fist at head level.

Common Mistakes

- Raising the elbow and shoulder when raising the fist, leaning the torso. Or turning the forearm without raising the upper arm.
- At the end of movement in the fixed posture, the bow stance is in a different direction from the strike.

8. Lǚjǐshì 将挤势 (Roll Back and Press)

8.1 Turn the Body and Turn In the Foot

Slightly shift the body center backward, turn in the left toes, turn the torso to the right; turn the left fist into an open-palm hand; move the right palm to the right in a horizontal curve and then draw it to inside of the left forearm. (Fig. 39)

8.2 Bend the Leg and Palm Smear

Shift the body center forward, keep turning the torso to the right; smear the right hand from left to the right front in a horizontal curve, palm slanting downward; move the left hand down underneath the inside of the right elbow, palm slanting upward. Look at the right hand. (Fig. 40)

8.3 Draw In the Foot and Roll Back (Lǚ 将)

Two hands stroke downward and backward at the same time, until the left hand reaches the side of the left hip and the right hand is in front of the abdomen; draw the right foot to the inside of the left foot. Look forward to the right. (Fig. 41)

8.4 Step Forward and Put Hands Together

Move the right foot forward to the right, land the heel; at the same time turn the left

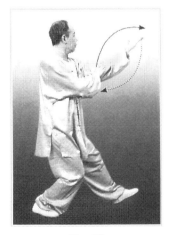
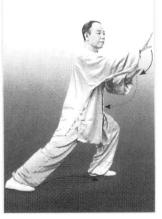
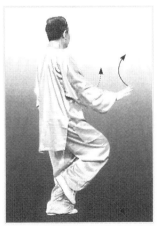

Fig. 39   Fig. 40   Fig. 41

forearm inward and right forearm outward, turn both hands and raise them with elbows bent in front of the chest, palms facing each other. Look straight ahead. (Fig. 42)

8.5 Bow Stance and Press (Jǐ 挤) Forward

Shift the body center forward to form a right bow stance; press both arms forward, forming a circle with the arms, keeping the left fingers at the inside of the right wrist, palm facing outward, fingertips slanting upward; the right palm faces inward, the fingertips pointing left, at shoulder height. Look at the right hand. (Fig. 43)

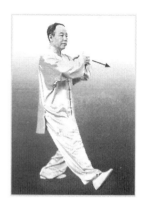

Fig. 42

8.6 Turn the Body and Turn In the Foot

Shift the body center backward, turn in the right toes, turn the torso to the left; turn the right palm upward; move the left hand in a curve over the right forearm. (Fig. 44)

8.7 Bend the Leg and Smear the Hand

Shift the body center forward, continue turning the body to the left; smear the left hand in a horizontal curve from the right to the left front, palm slanting downward; draw the right hand underneath the inside of the left elbow, palm slanting upward. Look at the left hand. (Fig. 45)

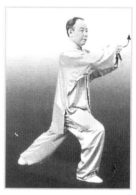

Fig. 43

8.8 Draw In the Foot and Roll Back (Lǚ 捋)

The two hands stroke downward and backward together, until the right hand reaches the side of the right hip and the left hand reaches the front of the abdomen; draw the left foot to the inside of the right foot. Look forward to the left. (Fig. 46)

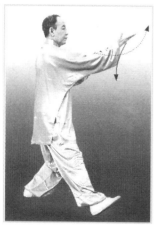

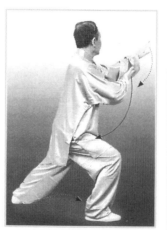

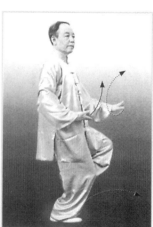

Fig. 44   Fig. 45   Fig. 46

8.9 Step Forward and Put the Hands Together

Move the left foot forward one step to the left, landing the heel; at the same time turn the right forearm inward and the left forearm outward, turn the hands and raise them with the arms bent in front of the chest, the palms facing each other. Look straight ahead. (Fig. 47)

8.10 Bow Stance and Press (Jǐ 挤) Forward

Shift the body center forward to form a left bow stance; press both arms forward, forming a circle with the two arms, keeping the right fingers at the inside of the left wrist, palm facing outward, the fingertips slanting upward; left palm faces inward, at shoulder height, the fingertips pointing right. Look at the left hand. (Fig. 48)

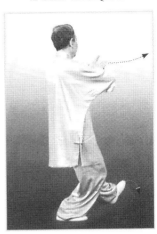

Fig. 47

Important Points

• Turn the body and turn in the foot not more than 45 degrees, and do not shift the body center backward too much. With the turn, draw the hand back in a small curve.

• When smearing the palm, move the hand that is behind over the other forearm and then forward to the left or to the right in a horizontal curve. At the same time bend the leg and turn the waist, keeping all movements coordinated.

• The above two movements should be smooth and agile. Coordinate the movements of waist, legs and hands and complete their movements together.

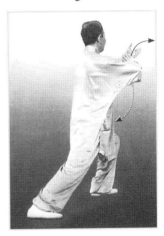

Fig. 48

• Rolling back and drawing in the foot should be coordinated with the turning of the waist.

• As the hands come together, turn the arms, raise the upper arms, bend the forearms horizontally in front of the chest, elbows pointing outward, palms facing each other. Step forward while turning the waist, and complete at the same time landing the heel, turning the body and joining the hands.

• Bow stance and pressing forward should be on a 45-degree angle from the front. Form a circle with the arms.

Common Mistakes

• Smearing the palm faster than making bow stance, leaving the movement of hands and feet uncoordinated.

• Rolling back without turning the waist.

● Stepping forward and placing the hands together without turning the waist, with the result that the body is turned sideways when pressing forward.

● Turning the body and joining the hands together is done earlier than stepping forward, making the movements of the waist and legs uncoordinated.

9. Jìnbù Bānlánchuí 进步搬拦捶 (Step In, Deflect, Block and Punch)

9.1 Turn the Body and Separate the Hands

Shift the body center backward, turn the left toes out, turn the torso to the left; move the left palm downward in a curve, the palm facing upward; extend the right hand forward to the right, palm slanted downward. Turn the head with the torso. (Fig. 49)

9.2 Draw In the Foot and Make a Fist

Shift the body center forward, draw the right foot to the inside of the left foot; move the left palm to the left in a curve and then upward in a curve in front of the body, palm facing downward; make a fist with the right hand and move it downward in a curve to the front of the abdomen, the bottom of the fist facing downward. Look straight ahead. (Fig. 50)

9.3 Step Forward and Deflect with the Fist

Move the right foot forward, landing the heel, the toes pointing out; turn and deflect with the right fist forward to chest level, passing inside of the left arm, bottom of the fist facing upward; with the movement push the left palm downward at the side of the left hip. Look at the right fist. (Fig. 51)

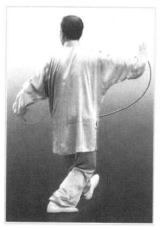 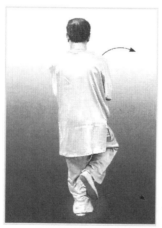 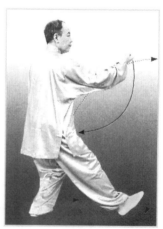

Fig. 49   Fig. 50   Fig. 51

9.4 Draw In the Foot and Fist

Shift the body center forward, turn the torso to the right; turn the right forearm inward, moving the right fist to the right in a curve to the side of the body; turn the left forearm outward, moving the left palm to the left and forward in a curve in front of the body. Look at the left hand. (Fig. 52)

9.5 Step Forward and Block with Palm

Move the left foot forward past the inside of the right foot, landing the heel; withdraw the right fist to the right side of the waist, palm of the fist facing upward; turn the left hand palm downward and block in front of the body. (Fig. 53)

9.6 Bow Stance and Punch

Shift the body center forward to form a left bow stance; the right fist punches forward, the thumb side of fist turned upward, fist at chest level; withdraw the left palm to the inside of the right forearm. Look at the right fist. (Fig. 54)

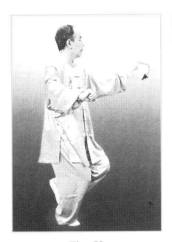 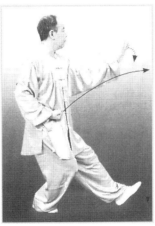 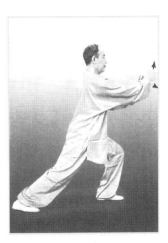

Fig. 52   Fig. 53   Fig. 54

Important Points

• When separating the hands, move them symmetrically in vertical circles in opposite directions. The movement should be done smoothly and in a relaxed way.

• Turn the right open-palm hand into a fist while moving it downward, the palm of the fist facing downward.

• Deflect with the fist at chest level, turn the toes out when moving the left foot forward, land the heel softly, with the knee slightly bent.

• When withdrawing the right fist, turn the torso to the right, turn the forearm inward, turn the palm downward and move it in a curve past the right side of the body, and then turn it outward before drawing it to the waist, turning the palm of the fist up.

• When blocking with the open-palm hand, turn the left arm outward, move the left hand to the left and forward in a curve to the front of the body, then turn it inward, turning the palm to slant toward the side and downward.

• When punching, lean the right shoulder slightly forward, drop the shoulders and elbows, push up with the head, have the chest slightly arced in and the torso extended.

- Make the bow stance about 8 inches or about 20 centimeters wide.

Common Mistakes

- Turning the torso too much when stepping forward, making the body face front.

- Leaning the torso forward when deflecting with the fist and stepping forward.

10. Rúfēng Sìbì 如封似闭 (Pull Back then Push, As if to Close)

10.1 Thread and Turn the Palm

Move the left hand past the right forearm from underneath, palm facing upward; at the same time turn

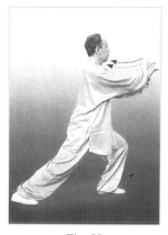

Fig. 55

the right fist into an open-palm hand and turn the right palm upward. (Fig. 55)

10.2 Sitting Stance and Draw the Hands Back

Sit back with the torso, shifting the body center backward; tilting the left toes up; part the two hands, bend the arms, turn them inward and draw them to the front of the chest, shoulder-width apart, palms slanted facing each other. (Fig. 56)

Turn the palms downward and move them in front of the abdomen. Look straight ahead. (Fig. 57)

10.3 T-Stance and Push Forward

Shift the body center forward, draw the right foot behind and to the side of the left foot about 4 inches or 10 centimeters behind it, touching the ground with the toes, forming a right T-stance; push the palms forward, keeping them shoulder-width apart, palms facing forward, wrists at shoulder height. Look straight ahead. (Fig. 58)

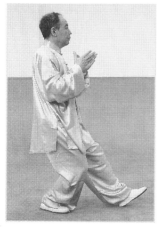 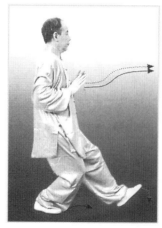 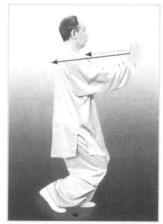

Fig. 56   Fig. 57   Fig. 58

Important Points

● After threading the left hand, cross the two hands and turn them upward.

● When drawing the hands backward, bend the arms toward the body while turning the arms inward, turn both hands, part them and draw them to the front of the abdomen, passing the chest.

● Shift the body center backward fully, bend the leg, drop the hips, relax the knee and hip joints; keep the torso straight and natural.

● When pushing the palms, shift the body center forward and at the same time draw in the right foot. Land the ball of the right foot about 8 inches or 20 centimeters to the side of the left foot and about 8 inches or 20 centimeters behind it, toes pointing front but a little off center.

● At the end of movement, keep the torso and arms extended.

Common Mistakes

● When making a sitting stance, the torso leans forward and tenses, or the leg is not bent enough, the body center rises, and the torso leans backward.

● When drawing the hands back, the palms turn upward, and the elbows are bent but not drawn back.

● When making the T-stance, a clear distinction is not made between empty and solid.

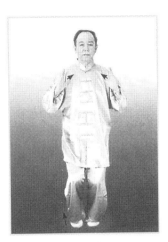

Fig. 59

Part II

11. Kaihé Shǒu 开合手 (Open and Close the Hands)

11.1 Turn the Body and Open the Hands

Turn the body to the right by first pivoting on the ball of the right foot and then pivoting on the left heel, stand firmly on both feet ready to make a T-stance; turn the two palms to face each other, fingertips pointing upward, and draw them to the front of the chest, palms shoulder-width apart. Look straight ahead. (Fig. 59)

11.2 T-Stance and Close Hands

Move the hands toward each other until they are head-width apart, palms facing each other. The eyes look through the space between hands. When closing the hands, make a T-stance by shifting the body center to the left leg and lifting the right heel. (Fig. 60)

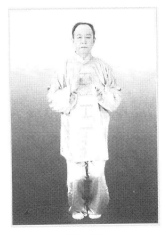

Fig. 60

Important Points

• When turning the body, turn the right heel inward and land the foot, then turn left toes 90° inward, turn the torso to the right, keeping the feet parallel.

• When opening the hands first bend the arms to draw them in front of the chest, hands upright and palms facing each other, head-width apart, and then separate them to the left and right. This whole movement should be completed together with turning the body.

• When closing the hands, drop the wrists and extend the palms, keeping the palms facing each other; slightly arc in the chest, exhaling at the same time.

• When closing the hands put more of the body center on the left leg, lift the right heel to form a right T-stance.

Common Mistakes

• When turning, the body sways, the feet move in a tense and disconnected way; the body center shifts too much.

• When opening and closing the hands, the fingers and wrists are too loose, the elbows and shoulders are raised, the chest is thrust out, the arms or palms turn.

12. Yòu Danbian 右单鞭 (Single Bian, Right)

12.1 Turn the Hands and Step to the Side

Turn the body slightly to the right; move the right foot to the right one step, landing the heel; turn the arms inward, palms facing out, with the web between thumb and index finger of each hand facing each other. Look at the left hand. (Fig. 61)

12.2 Side-Bow Stance and Part the Hands

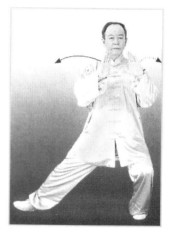

Fig. 61

Shift the body center to the right to form a right side-bow stance; separate the hands, moving them to the right and left on a horizontal line, and turn the palms to face outward, the fingers pointing upward. Look at the left hand. (Fig. 62)

Important Points

• Turn the body about 30 degrees to the right, slightly extend the arms and turn palms forward.

• Be light and easy when stepping to the side, landing the heel first.

• When separating the hands, stretch out the bent arms and turn the palms to face outward.

• Do not turn the torso too far when making the side-bow stance.

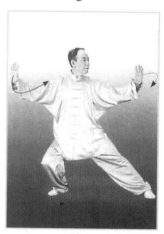

Fig. 62

Common Mistakes

• When making the side-bow stance, the bent leg turns too much inward or outward, turning the torso too far, or the knees and toes point in different directions.

• When making the side-bow stance, the feet turn out too much, or the extended leg is bent too much. A clear distinction is not made between the empty and the solid in the stance.

• When stepping to the side, the ball of the foot lands first, or the heel kicks against the ground before stepping out.

• When separating the hands, the arms push forward and sweep horizontally before separating.

• The torso leans forward or to the side.

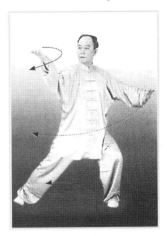

Fig. 63

13. Zhǒudǐchuí 肘底捶 (Fist Under the Elbow)

13.1 Turn the Body and Sweep the Hands

Shift the body center to the left, turning the right toes inward and the torso slightly to the left; turn the right forearm outward, turn the palm upward, and swing the right hand in a curve to the front of the right shoulder as the right hand turns outward; move the left hand left-downward in a curve. Look at the right hand. (Fig. 63)

13.2 Draw In the Foot and Hold the Ball

Shift the body center to the right, turn the body to the right; draw the left foot to the inside of the right foot; turn the right hand and draw it to the front of the right chest, palm facing downward; turn the left forearm outward, turn the left palm upward and move it to the right in a curve passing in front of the abdomen until it reaches under the right hand, as if holding a ball. (Fig. 64)

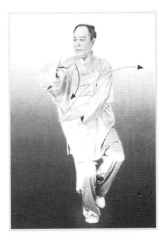

Fig. 64

13.3 Step Forward and Separate the Hands

Turn the torso to the left; move the left foot forward to the left, landing the heel, toes turned outward; move the left hand upward and to the left in a curve passing underneath the right forearm, hand at head level and palm facing inward; move the right hand downward in a curve passing in front of the left chest to the side of the right hip. Look at the left hand. (Fig. 65)

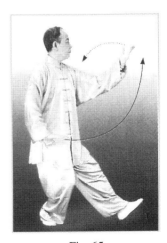

Fig. 65

13.4 Follow In and Grab

Continue turning the torso to the left, shifting the body center forward; move the right foot forward half a step, landing the right ball of the foot behind the left foot; turn the left arm inward and palm outward, move the left hand to the left and downward in a curve to the left side of the body; turn the right arm outward, and move the right hand to the right and forward in a curve to the front of the body, palm slanted upward at head level. Look straight ahead. (Fig. 66)

13.5 Step Forward and Chop

Shift the body center to the right leg, keep the right foot firmly on the ground, move the left foot forward, landing the heel and tilting the toes up to form a left empty stance; draw the left hand back, start to turn it sideways and upright at the left side of the waist, move it up past the right wrist, and chop forward, fingertips at brow level; turn the right hand into a fist, the thumb side of the fist upward, and draw it under and to the inside of the left elbow. Look at the left hand. (Fig. 67)

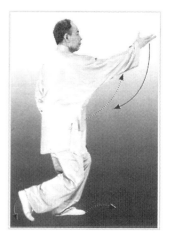

Fig. 66

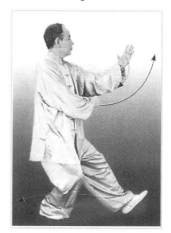

Fig. 67

Important Points

• Be smooth with the whole movement, and turn the waist to lead the movement of the hands.

• Turn the body before moving the back foot forward.

• When pulling back, turn the right arm outward and sweep it forward, then turn it inward and make an upright fist, the thumb-side facing upward.

• When chopping, turn the left hand outward and draw it to the waist, palm facing upward, then turn it inward to be a side-facing upright palm before chopping. At the same time, slightly turn the waist to the left and to the right.

Common Mistakes

• The back foot is moved forward in the wrong direction, or the body is not turned enough.

• The back foot moves backward instead of forward.

• The chopping hand is swept too much horizontally so that it does not move in a vertical circle.

• The turn of the arms and waist is not coordinated with the movement of the hands.

• At the end, the movement is too relaxed or too tense.

• While doing the empty stance, the knees are straight, the chest thrust out, the body leans forward or buttocks protrude backward.

14. Zhuǎnshēn Tuīzhǎng 转身推掌 (Turn the Body and Thrust the Palm)

14.1 Turn the Body and Raise the Hand

Draw the left foot behind the right foot, landing the ball of the foot; turn the right fist into an open-palm hand and raise it until the wrist is at shoulder height, palm facing upward; turn the left hand and move it downward to the front of the right chest, palm facing downward. Look at the right hand. (Fig. 68)

With the right heel and the ball of the left foot as pivots, turn the body about 90 degrees to the left, keeping the body center on the right leg; while turning, slightly roll and draw in the right hand, and move the left hand a little downward. Look straight ahead. (Fig. 69)

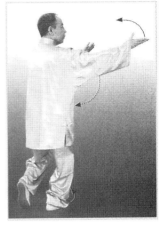

Fig. 68

14.2 Step Forward and Draw In the Hand

Move the left foot forward and a little to the left, landing the heel; draw the right hand to the side of the right ear, palm facing frontward and downward; move the left hand to the left in a curve. Look straight ahead. (Fig. 70)

14.3 T-Stance and Push the Palm

Shift the body center forward, turn the waist and turn the shoulders in the same direction; draw the right foot behind the inside of the left foot, landing the ball of the foot to form a right T-stance; push the right hand forward, palm facing forward, fingertips at the level of the tip of the nose; the left hand brushes aside and over the left knee, and presses down by the side of the left hip. Look at the right hand.(Fig. 71)

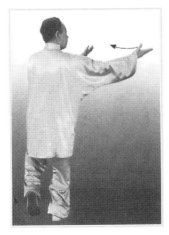
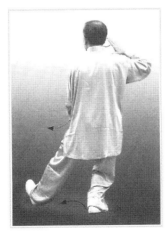
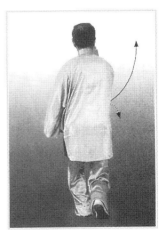

Fig. 69   Fig. 70   Fig. 71

14.4 Turn the Body and Raise the Hand

Turn the body toward the right to the rear with the left heel and the ball of the right foot as pivots, keeping the body center on left leg; turn the left arm outward and raise it upward and forward to the left, the palm facing upward at head level; move the right palm downward to the front of the left side of the chest, palm facing downward. Look at the left hand. (Fig. 72)

14.5 Step Forward and Draw Back the Hand

Move the right foot forward to the right, landing the heel; draw the left hand to the side of the left ear, palm facing forward and downward; lower the right hand to the front of the abdomen. Look straight ahead. (Fig. 73)

14.6 T-Stance and Push Palm

Shift the body center forward, turn the waist and turn the shoulders with it, draw the left foot up behind the inside of the right foot to form a left T-stance; push the left hand forward, palm facing forward, fingertips at the level of the tip of the nose; brush aside with the right hand over the right knee and press the right palm down by the side of the right hip. Look at the left hand. (Fig. 74)

Important Points

● This form is adapted from Roll the Arms Back of Sun-style Taijiquan. Turn the body and move the feet in a direction that is side-forward; the whole pattern of movement of both feet should be in a "Z" line.

● When turning the feet against the ground, first turn the front foot with heel as pivot and then turn the back foot with the ball of the foot as pivot. The weight can be shifted between the two feet, but not too much either way.

● In the movement of drawing back the hands, bend the arms but not the wrists or hands.

● Push the palm forward 90 degrees from the direction of the arm and hand of the previous movement. Do not move the hand too high or too far when brushing aside over the knee; stop it at the side of hip.

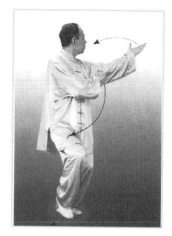

Fig. 72

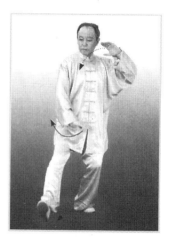

Fig. 73

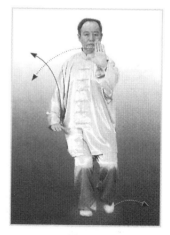

Fig. 74

- Turn the body and step forward in an agile, smooth way.
- Finish the drawing in of the back foot at the same time as the pushing of the palms. When moving the back foot forward, land it about 8 inches or 20 centimeters behind the inside of the supporting foot.

Common Mistakes

- Abruptly speeding up the movement when turning the body and stepping forward.
- Shifting the body center too far when turning the feet against the ground, so that the body sways and movement hesitates.
- When turning the feet against the ground, the feet are too close, making it hard to turn the body.
- When stepping forward, the feet move straight forward in a "T" line instead of a "Z" line.
- Bending the leg without drawing in the foot when pushing the palms, resulting in a "bow stance and push palm."

15. Yùnǚ Chuɑnsuō 玉女穿梭 (**Jade Maiden Moves the Shuttle Left and Right**)

15.1 Turn the Body and Extend the Hand

Turn the torso to the right; move the left foot half a step backward; turn the left arm outward, move the left hand to the right in a curve in front of the right chest, turning the palm upward; extend the right hand forward in front of the body, passing over the left forearm, the right palm slanted downward, and wrist at shoulder height. Look at the right hand. (Fig. 75)

15.2 Step Backward and Stroke Backward

Turn the torso to the left, shifting the body center to the left leg; draw the right foot to the inside of the left foot, toes touching the ground; stroke the hands forward, downward and backward, stopping the left hand by the side of the left hip and right hand in front of the abdomen. Eyes follow the hands. (Fig. 76)

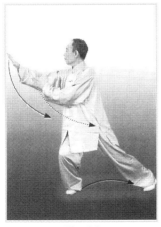

Fig. 75

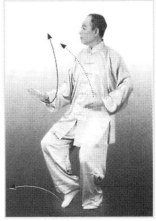

Fig. 76

15.3 Step Forward and Bring the Hands Together

Move the right foot forward to the right, landing the heel; turn both forearms, raising the hands to bring them close to each other in front of chest, the right palm facing inward, the fingertips pointing to the left, and left palm facing outward, the fingers resting on the inside of the right wrist. Look at the right hand. (Fig. 77)

15.4 Move the Back Foot Forward and the Hand Horizontally

Shift the body center forward, turning the torso to the right; at the same time move the left foot up behind and on the inside of the right foot, landing the ball of the foot;

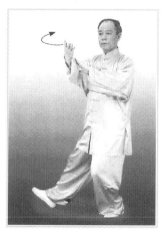

Fig. 77

move the right hand from left to forward in a horizontal curve, turning the palm upward; at the same time turn the left hand with the movement of the right hand. Eyes follow the right hand. (Fig. 78)

15.5 Sit Back and Move the Hand Horizontally

Land the left foot fully, turning the torso to the left; bend the right elbow and turn it inward, moving the right hand to the right and back in a horizontal curve. Look at the right hand. (Fig. 79)

15.6 Step Forward and Draw In the Hands

Turn the torso to the right; move the right foot one step forward to the right, landing the heel; turn the right hand inward until the wrist bends backward over the front of the right shoulder, palm slanted upward; at the same time move the left hand back in a curve to the left side of the waist. Look straight ahead. (Fig. 80)

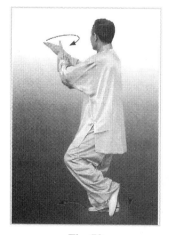
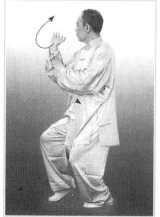
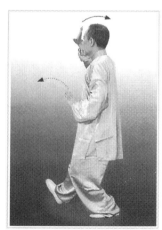

Fig. 78　　　　　　　Fig. 79　　　　　　　Fig. 80

15.7 Bow Stance and Block and Push

Shift the body center forward to form a right bow
stance, turning the torso to the right; block with the right
hand above and in front of the right forehead, palm slanted
upward; push forward the left hand to the front of the body,
palm facing forward, fingertips at level of the tip of the
nose. Look at the left hand. (Fig. 81)

15.8 Turn In the Foot and Draw In the Hand

Shift the body center backward, turn in and lift the
right toes, turning the torso to the left; turn the right forearm outward, turn the right hand and move it downward
in front of the body, palm facing upward, the right wrist at

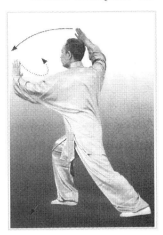

Fig. 81

shoulder height; move the left hand to the right in a curve and draw it back to the inside
of the right elbow, palm facing down. Look at the right hand. (Fig. 82)

15.9 Bend the Leg and Smear with the Hand

Shift the body center forward, landing the right foot firmly on the ground, and
continue turning the torso to the left; thread the left hand across over the right
forearm and smear it from right to left in a curve; draw the right hand beneath the
inside of the left elbow, the palms facing each other on a slant. Look at the left
hand. (Fig. 83)

15.10 Draw In the Foot and Stroke Backward

Turn the torso to the right; draw the left foot to the inside of the right foot; stroke
with both hands downward and backward, stopping the right hand by the side of the
right hip and the left hand in front of the abdomen. Eyes follow the movement of hands.
(Fig. 84)

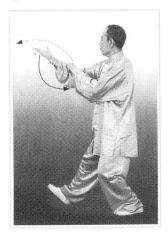
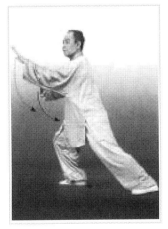
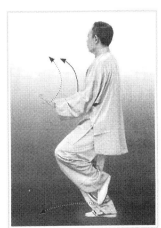

Fig. 82   Fig. 83   Fig. 84

15.11 Step Forward and Put the Hands Together

Move the left foot forward to the left, landing the
heel; turn both forearms, raise the hands up to the front
of the chest, left palm facing inward, its fingertips pointing to the right, right palm facing outward, its fingertips
resting on the inside of the left wrist. Look at the left
hand. (Fig. 85)

15.12 Move the Back Foot Forward and the Hand
Horizontally

Shift the body center forward, turning the torso to the
left; at the same time move the right foot up behind the
inside of the left foot, landing the ball of the foot; move

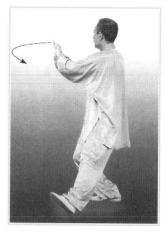

Fig. 85

the left hand from right to forward in a horizontal curve, turning the palm upward; at
the same time turn the right hand with the movement of the left hand. Look at the left
hand. (Fig. 86)

15.13 Sit Back and Move the Hand Horizontally

Land the right foot fully, turning the torso to the right; bend the left elbow and
turn it inward, moving the left hand to the left and backward in a horizontal curve.
Look at the left hand. (Fig. 87)

15.14 Step Forward and Draw In the Hands

Turn the torso to the left; move the left foot one step forward, landing the heel; turn
the left hand inward until wrist bends back over the front of the left shoulder, palm
slanted upward; at the same time move the right hand back to the right side of the waist
in a curve. Look straight ahead. (Fig. 88)

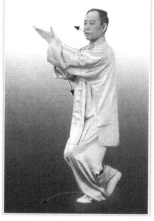

Fig. 86

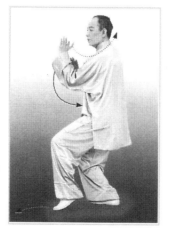

Fig. 87

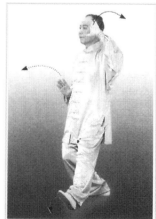

Fig. 88

15.15 Bow Stance and Block and Push

Shift the body center forward to form a left bow stance, turning the torso to the left; block with the left hand over the front of the left forehead, palm slanted upward; move the right hand to the front of body, palm facing forward, fingertips at the level of tip of the nose. Look at the right hand. (Fig. 89)

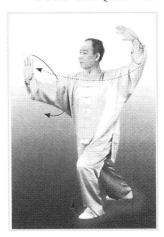

Fig. 89

Important Points

● Do the movement in a smooth and flexible way, and move the feet in a "Z" line.

● When turning the body and extending the hand, move the left foot to the left, landing the inside of the ball of the foot first.

● When stepping forward and putting the hands together, step forward on the diagonal, and put the hands together in front of the chest on the left (or right).

● When moving the hands horizontally, draw a horizontal curve starting from the front of the left shoulder to the front of the right shoulder, at the same time turning the waist and sweeping the hands like clouds. While doing this movement, extend or bend the arms as necessary. Relax the shoulders, elbows and wrists.

● When stepping forward and drawing in the hand, separate the hands, drawing one hand to the waist while turning the other hand inward and bending the arm, raising the hand with the elbow until it reaches head level, and turning the palm forward and upward. Turn the waist slightly to the front.

● The direction of the bow stance and the pushing of the palm should be 45 degrees on the diagonal. For reverse forward step in bow stance, place the feet about 12 inches or 30 centimeters apart.

Common Mistakes

● When turning the body and extending the palm, the left foot moves straight forward.

● At the end of the movement, the bow stance is too narrow, the torso is twisted; the pushing palm and bow stance are in different directions.

16. Yòuzuǒ Dēngjiǎo 右左蹬脚 (Kick Right and Left)

16.1 Turn In the Foot and Draw In the Hand

Shift the body center backward, turn in the left toes and turn the torso to the right; turn the left arm outward, turn the left hand and move it down in front of the body, palm facing upward, wrist at shoulder height; move the right hand to the left in a curve before drawing it to the inside of the left elbow, palm facing downward. Look at the left hand. (Fig. 90)

16.2 Bend the Leg and Separate the Hands

Shift the body center forward, turn the torso to the left; thread the right hand across and over the left forearm and then extend it upward and to the right in a curve; move the left hand downward and to the left in a curve to the waist. Turn the head together with the torso. (Fig. 91)

16.3 Draw In the Foot and Hold in an Embrace

Turn the torso to the right; draw in the right foot to the inside of the left foot; move the right hand downward to the

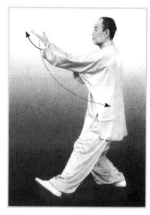

Fig. 90

left and upward in a curve; move the left hand to the left upward and then to the right in a curve, overlap the wrists in front of the chest crossing the hands as if holding something, the right hand on the outside and both palms facing toward the body. Look forward to the right. (Fig. 92)

16.4 Kick and Part the Hands

Slightly bend the left leg to stand firm, bend the right knee and lift the right leg, slowly kick the right foot forward at an angle of about 30 degrees to the right, tilting the toes upward, with the heel higher than waist level; separate the hands in curves, one forward to the right and the other to the left, palms facing outward, wrists at shoulder height, arms extended, elbows slightly bent, and the right arm just above the right leg. Look at the right hand. (Fig. 93)

16.5 Step Forward and Thread the Hand

Bend the right leg, and move the right foot downward to the right side in front, landing the heel; turn the right forearm outward, turning the right hand upward and moving it a little

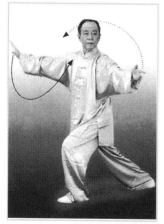

Fig. 91

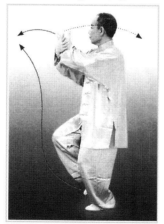

Fig. 92

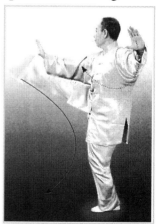

Fig. 93

inward; move the left hand downward, past the waist and then forward and upward in a curve to the inside of the right elbow, palm facing downward. Look at the right hand. (Fig. 94)

16.6 Bend the Leg and Separate the Hands

Shift the body center forward, plant the right foot on the ground, turn the torso to the right; thread the left hand across and over the right forearm and then extend it upward and to the left in a curve; move the right hand downward and to the right in a curve to the side of the waist. Turn the head together with the torso. (Fig. 95)

16.7 Draw In the Foot and Hold in an Embrace

Turn the torso to the left; draw the left foot to the

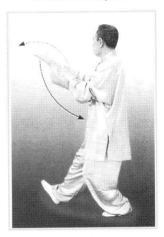

Fig. 94

inside of the right foot; move the left hand downward, to the right and then upward in a curve; move the right hand to the right, upward and then to the left in a curve, cross the wrists in front of chest in a position of holding something, left hand on the outside, both palms facing the body. Look forward to the left. (Fig. 96)

16.8 Kick and Separate the Hands

Slightly bend the right leg, standing firmly, bend the left knee and lift the left leg, slowly kick the left foot forward about 30 degrees to the left, tilting the toes upward, with the heel higher than waist level; separate both hands in curves, one forward to the left and the other to the right, palms facing outward, wrists at shoulder height, arms extended, elbows slightly bent, and the left arm directly over the left leg. Look at the left hand. (Fig. 97)

Important Points

● In this form, the hands separate in two ways: In the movement of crossing the hands, the hands move in the same direction in a vertical circle; or they move out in

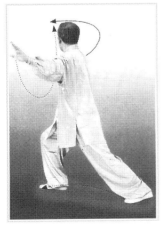
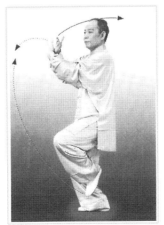
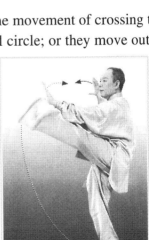

Fig. 95   Fig. 96   Fig. 97

opposite directions in vertical circles. Do both in a smooth, flowing and natural circular motion coordinated with the turning of the waist and arms; do not raise the hands higher than head level; kick the foot in about the same direction as the vertical circle made by the front hand, or about 30 to 45 degrees on the diagonal from the front.

- When holding the hands in an embrace, fully extend the arms so they make a circle.
- When kicking, keep the torso upright, drop the shoulders, arc in the chest, extend the arms with the palms facing outward, fingertips pointing upward.
- After the right kick, step forward in the same direction as the kick, keeping the feet about 8 inches or 20 centimeters apart in width. When threading the hand, turn the right palm upward, and keep the left palm facing downward when moving it downward and threading it forward.

Common Mistakes

- When kicking and separating the hands, the head is lowered, the waist bent, the torso leans backward, the legs are bent, the direction of the front arm and the kick are different; one hand is higher than the other; the arms are either too bent or too extended; the arms straighten and the chest thrusts out to form a straight line.
- The kick is not high enough, and the body center is not steady.

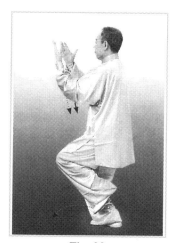

Fig. 98

17. Yǎnshǒu Gōngchuí 掩手肱捶 (Conceal the Hand, Bend the Arm and Punch)

17.1 Draw In the Foot and Bring the Hands Close Together

Bend and draw in the left lower leg and put the left foot down next to the inside of the right foot; turn the arms outward, bring the hands close together in front of head, keeping them head-width apart, palms facing inward. Look at the palms. (Fig. 98)

17.2 Step with the Foot Skimming the Ground and Press the Hands Down

Draw the left toes up, move the left foot to the left side without lifting the heel, the torso slightly turned to the right; turn the arms inward, turn the hands and move them downward, cross them, left palm over right palm, on the right side of the lower abdomen, palms both facing downward. Look at the hands. (Fig. 99)

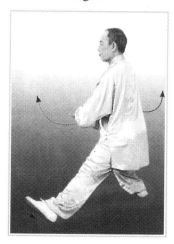

Fig. 99

17.3 Horse Stance and Separate the Hands

Turn the torso to the front, shifting the body center to the left to balance on both legs; pull the hands apart to both sides, keeping them at shoulder height, turn the fore-arms inward, and turn the hands outward. Look straight ahead. (Fig. 100)

17.4 Conceal the Hand and Gather Power

Shift the body center to the right, slightly turn the torso to the right, turn the arms outward, moving the elbows toward each other, sweep the left hand to the front of the body, palm upward and at shoulder height; turn the right open-palm hand into a fist, bend the arm to draw the fist to the front of chest, palm facing upward. Look at the left hand. (Fig. 101)

17.5 Bow Stance and Punch

Shift the body center to the left, turning the torso to the left; turn the waist and shoulder in the same direction to form a left bow stance; turn the right fist forward while punching, with the palm of the fist turned down; draw the left open-palm hand backward until it touches the left side of the abdomen, fingertips pointing to the right. Look at the right fist. (Fig. 102)

Important Points

● When drawing in the foot and bringing the hands together, do not land the left foot. Move the hands close to each other in front of the head, palms facing inward, and head-width apart.

● When skimming the foot along the ground, keep the inside of the left heel on the ground and extend it sideways, first lightly and then forcefully. Turn the torso to the right, slightly lower the body center, press the hands downward with the one over the other.

● When turning the body and separating the hands, relax the torso and turn it to the front, slightly raising the body center, and relax the arms and raise them to the sides until they are horizontal.

● When concealing the hand and gathering power,

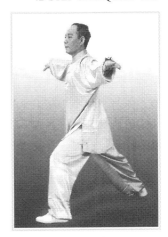

Fig. 100

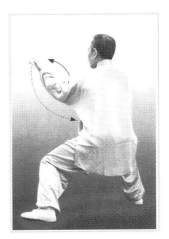

Fig. 101

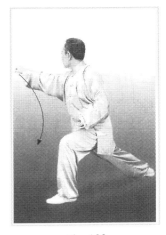

Fig. 102

shift the body center to the right to form a side-horse stance, turn the torso to the right, arc in the chest and arch the back, move the elbows toward each other and turn the hands, rotating the arms outward with power. Extend the left arm to the front of the body, put the fingers of the left hand together, open the "tiger's mouth" (Hǔkǒu 虎口) or the web between the thumb and index finger, palm stretching out; bend the elbow of the right arm and press it against the ribs, make a fist with the right hand, turn it upward and move it to the inside of the left elbow. Contract the whole body and exhale, storing up energy, ready to release it.

- When punching into bow stance, abruptly speed up the movement, turn the waist to the left, kick the leg, extend the torso, snap the punch forward on the diagonal with a vibrating power in the right fist. Punch fast in one movement, joining energy (qì 气) and power (lì 力). After punching, relax the right arm and fist, stretch the elbow, focus the power in the front of the fist, which is at shoulder height, and turn the palm of the fist downward; draw the left palm to the abdomen, four fingers pointing to the right and thumb upward. While turning the waist put force into the feet and turn them sharply, the left toes slightly outward and the right heel slightly extended to form a bow stance with feet basically parallel toward the West.

Common Mistakes

- The release of strength is too stiff and tense without elasticity or explosive power.

- Power is in the right arm only, so the arm moves independently rather than in coordination with the waist, legs and the torso.

- Not enough energy is put into concealing the hand and gathering power.

- The fist punches in a curved line, thus becoming a kind of uppercut or round house punch.

- After concealing the hand, the right fist is drawn back once more, and the torso turns to the right to gather power again, breaking the flow of energy.

18. Yomǎ Fēnzōng 野马分鬃 (Part the Wild Horse's Mane)

18.1 Turn the Waist and Twist the Hand Around

Turn the torso to the left; turn the right fist into an open-palm hand and move it downward to the front of the abdomen in a curve, palm facing downward; twist the left hand pivoting on the thumb and turning the four fingers downward. (Fig. 103)

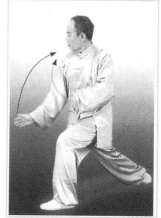

Fig. 103

18.2 Form a Circle with Arms and Wind the Hands Around

Shift the body center to the right, turn the torso to the right; turn the right arm inward, turn the right palm outward, and move the hand upward and to the right in a curve, bend the right arm in front of the right shoulder, thumb pointing downward and four finger-tips to the left; turn the left arm outward, turn the left hand to face inward, touching the inside of the right forearm with back of the left hand and fingers, and move the left hand together with right forearm in a curve, forming a circle with the arms. Look at the right hand. (Fig. 104)

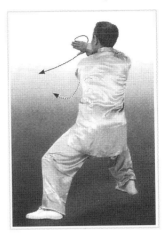

Fig. 104

18.3 Turn the Waist and Twist the Hand

Shift the body center to the left, turn the torso to the left; twist the right arm outward and left arm inward, cross the hands, both of them facing forward to the left, fingertips pointing outward; turn them horizontally in front of abdomen, power springing from the waist and abdomen. Look at the hands. (Fig. 105)

18.4 Fold and Sweep the Hands

Turn the waist and abdomen back to the right and then to the left; move the hands from right to left in an arc, both of them facing downward, cross and sweep them in front of the abdomen, and slightly extend the left hand forward. Look at the left hand. (Fig. 106)

18.5 Lift the Foot and Palm

Shift the body center to the right, turn the waist to the right; move the hands to the

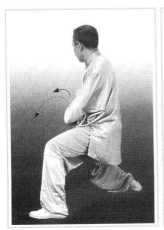

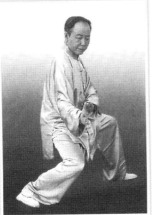

Fig. 105

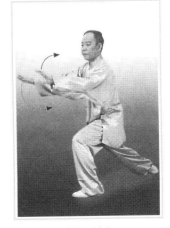

Fig. 106

right in a curve and part them, turning the left hand to the right. Look at the left hand. (Fig. 107)

Shift the body center backward, lift the left leg, bending the left knee; turn the left arm outward, lift the left hand over the left knee, palm facing upward; move the right hand to the right and upward in a curve until the hand is horizontal on the right side of body at shoulder height, palm facing to the right. Look straight ahead. (Fig. 108)

18.6 Step Forward and Draw In the Hand

Move the left foot forward; draw the left hand back, slightly bending the left arm. Look straight ahead. (Fig. 109)

18.7 Bow Stance and Thread the Slanting Palm-Hand

Shift the body center forward to form a left bow stance; thread the left hand slanting forward, palm facing upward, fingertips pointing forward, left wrist at shoulder height; push the right palm to the right side of the body, palm facing outward, fingertips slanting upward, wrist at shoulder height; look at the left hand. (Fig. 110)

18.8 Turn the Body and Turn the Foot Outward

Shift the body center backward, turn the left toes outward, turn the torso to the left; turn the left arm inward, turn the left palm outward and push it outward, slightly bending the arm; also turn the right arm outward, and slightly lower the right hand and draw it toward the body. Look at the left hand. (Fig. 111)

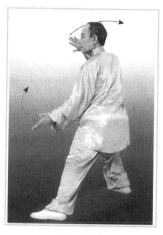

Fig. 107

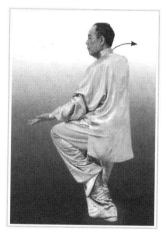

Fig. 108

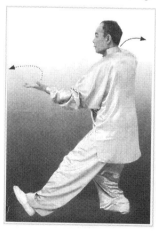

Fig. 109

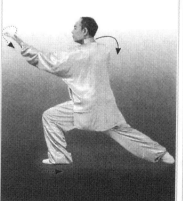

Fig. 110

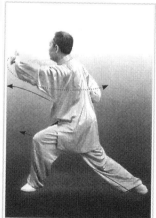

Fig. 111

18.9 Lift the Foot and Hand

Shift the body center forward, turn the torso to the left; lift the right leg in front, bending the right knee; move the right hand downward in a curve, and lift it forward past the side of the body until it reaches over the right knee, palm facing upward; sweep the left hand to the left in a curve until it is horizontal at the side of body, palm facing outward, and fingertips slanting upward to the side. Look at the right hand. (Fig. 112)

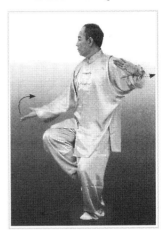

Fig. 112

18.10 Step Forward and Draw In the Hand

Move the right foot forward; draw the right hand back, slightly bending the right arm. Look forward. (Fig. 113)

18.11 Bow Stance and Thread the Slanting Palm-Hand

Shift the body center forward to form a right bow stance; thread the right hand slanting forward, palm facing upward, fingertips pointing forward, right wrist at shoulder height; push the left palm to the left side of the body, palm facing outward, fingertips slanting upward to the side, wrist at shoulder height; look at the right hand. (Fig. 114)

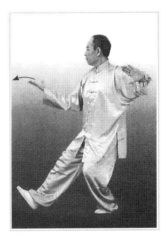

Fig. 113

Important Points

● Relax the torso a little bit after the punch, move the right wrist and waist to the right in a short curve. Then turn the torso to the left, change the right fist into an open-palm hand, press the fingers together, bend the wrist, stretch the web between the thumb and index finger; turn the right forearm outward and move it downward in a curve. Keeping the left hand on the abdomen, bend the left wrist downward and turn the fingers. At the same time lift the left side of the waist and the abdominal muscles, and lower the right side so that the waist, abdomen and arm are coiled.

● When forming a circle with the arms and twisting the hand, turn the left arm outward, place the back of the left hand on the right wrist, push power upward in the little finger; turn the right arm inward, bend the

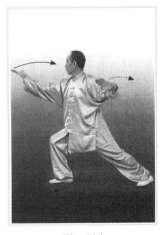

Fig. 114

arms and turn elbows outward, keeping right hand level to the ground in front of the right shoulder, turning the base of the thumb downward with force, four fingers pressed together and extended. At the same time slightly turn the heel of the right foot inward, turn the waist to the right, drop the shoulders, slightly arc in the chest and inhale.

● When twisting the hands, turn the torso to the left, and turn the hands at the same time in opposite directions, move them downward in curves until they are level to the ground in front of abdomen, bend and draw the left forearm and right upper arm close to the torso, turn the waist and abdominal muscles to the left before releasing power, then slightly lower the body center while exhaling sharply, and in an instant stop the whole movement.

● After the sudden stop of the turning the hands movement, relax the waist, abdomen and arms; return the body to its relaxed state and let the torso recover a little before continuing to turn the waist and move the hand to the left. This recovery and resumption of movement produced by energy in tensing and relaxing is called "folding" (zhédié 折叠).

● When lifting the foot, do not lift the toes or drag them on the ground. Draw the foot to the front of the fibula of the supporting leg, which is half bent.

● When stepping forward, slightly draw the forearm back.

● When the threading the slanting hand, turn the forearm outward and extend it forward, the four fingers pressed together and pointing forward, the thumb away from the index finger; turn the back arm inward and raise it horizontally behind the side of body, wrist bent, hand horizontal, with the palm pushing and facing outward.

Common Mistakes

● When winding the hands, the arms are turned without force, and without coordination with the movements of the waist and abdominal muscles.

● When twisting the hands, the hands make a patting movement downward.

● When twisting the hands, force is put only into the arms, without coordination with movements of the waist and legs.

● The outside of feet come off the ground, or the feet wobble.

● When doing "folding," the body sways too far.

● When lifting the foot, a one-leg stance is made.

● When threading the slanting palm-hand, the torso is turned too far to make a side-bow stance.

Part III

19. Yúnshǒu 云手 (Move the Hands Like Clouds)

19.1 Turn the Body and Sweep the Hands

Shift the body center to the left, turn in the right toes, turn the torso to the left; turn the right forearm inward, tilt the right wrist back, turn the right hand to the right, and move the right hand to the left in front of the right shoulder; push the left palm slightly to the left, palm facing to the left. Look at the right hand. (Fig. 115)

19.2 Turn the Body and the Hands

Shift the body center to the right, turn the torso to the right; turn the left heel on the ground; turn the right palm

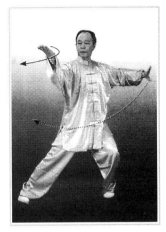

Fig. 115

outward, and move the right hand to the right side of the body, keeping it horizontal; move the left hand down from the left to pass in front of the abdomen, and then to the right in a curve, turning the palm upward. Eyes follow the movement of the right hand. (Fig. 116)

19.3 Turn the Body and Move the Hands Like Clouds to the Left

Shift the body center to the left, turn the torso to the left; move the left hand up from the right and to the left in a curve, passing in front of the face, palm facing inward, fingertips at eyebrow level; move the right hand downward, passing in front of the abdomen, and to the left in a curve like clouds, turning the hand from outward to inward. Eyes follow the movement of the right palm. (Fig. 117)

19.4 Stand Upright with Feet together and Turn the Hands

Continue turning the torso to the left; draw the right foot to the inside of the left foot and land it, feet parallel, pointing forward, 8-10 inches or about 20 centimeters apart; move the hands like clouds to the left side of the body, gradually turning the left

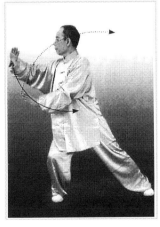

Fig. 116

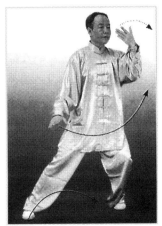

Fig. 117

palm outward, and turning the right palm inward when it reaches the inside of the left elbow. Look at the left palm. (Fig. 118)

19.5 Turn the Body and Move Hands Like Clouds to the Right

Shift the body center to the right, turn the torso to the right; move the right palm from the left in a curve to the right, passing in front of face, fingertips at eyebrow level; move the left palm downward, passing in front of the abdomen, and to the right in a curve like clouds. Look at the right palm. (Fig. 119)

19.6 Stand Upright with Feet Together and Turn the Hands

Continue turning the torso to the right; move the left foot to the left side, keeping toes pointing forward; move the hands like clouds to the right side of the body, gradually turning the right palm outward, and turning the left palm inward when it reaches the inside of the right elbow. Look at the right palm. (Fig. 120)

19.7 Turn the Body and Move Hands Like Clouds to the Left

Shift the body center to the left, turn the torso to the left; move the left palm to the left in a curve like clouds passing in front of the face; move the right palm downward, passing in front of the abdomen, and to the left in a curve like clouds. Eyes follow the movement of the left palm. (Fig. 121)

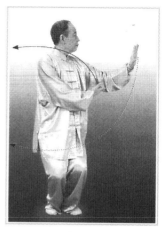

Fig. 118

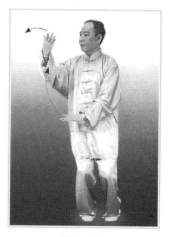

Fig. 119

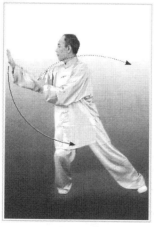

Fig. 120

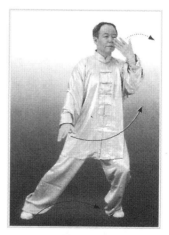

Fig. 121

19.8 Stand Upright with Feet Together and Turn the Hands

Continue turning the torso to the left; draw the right foot in to the inside of the left foot and land it, feet parallel and 8-10 inches or about 20 centimeters apart, toes pointing forward; move the hands like clouds to the left side of body, gradually turning the left palm outward, and turning the right palm inward when it reaches inside the left elbow. Look at the left palm. (Fig. 122)

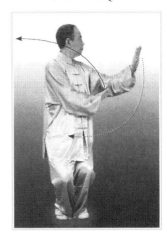

Fig. 122

19.9 Turn the Body and Move Hands Like Clouds to the Right

Shift the body center to the right, turn the torso to the right; move the right hand from left to right in a curve, passing in front of the face, fingertips at eyebrow level; move the left palm downward, passing in front of the abdomen in a curve like clouds. Look at the right palm. (Fig. 123)

19.10 Separate the Feet and Turn the Hands

Continue turning the torso to the right; move the left foot to the left side, keeping the toes pointing forward; move the hands like clouds to the right side of the body, gradually turning the right palm outward, and turning the left palm inward when it reaches the inside of the right elbow. Look at the right hand. (Fig. 124)

19.11 Turn the Body and Move Hands Like Clouds to the Left

Shift the body center to the left, turn the torso to the left; move the left palm to the left in a curve like clouds passing in front of the face; move the right palm downward, passing it in front of the abdomen and to the left in a curve like clouds. Eyes follow the movement of the left palm. (Fig. 125)

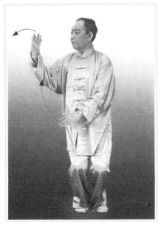
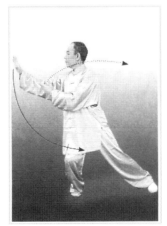
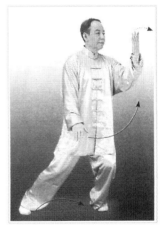

Fig. 123   Fig. 124   Fig. 125

19.12 Turn In the Foot and Turn the Hands

Continue turning the torso to the left, draw the right foot to the inside of the left foot and land it, turning in the toes by about 45 degrees, feet parallel, toes pointing forward, and 18-10 inches or about 20 centimeters apart; move hands like clouds to the left side of the body, gradually turning the left palm outward, and turning the right palm inward when it reaches inside of the left elbow. Look at the left hand. (Fig. 126)

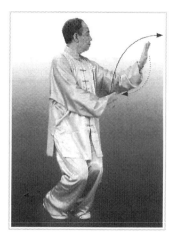

Fig. 126

Important Points

• When sweeping the hands to the left, bend the wrist and relax the hands, following the turn of the waist. Sweep the hands about 45 degrees.

• When turning the body and hands, move the right hand in a short arc, sinking the wrist, turn the forearm inward, turn the right palm outward, sweep the right palm to the right, keeping it horizontal, and turning it vertical while lowering the wrist when it reaches the side of the body. At the same time slightly turn the left heel inward, toes pointing straight forward.

• When moving hands like clouds, move the arms and hands with the turn of the waist. Keep the arms half bent, and move the hands in vertical circles that cross each other. Have the upper hand not higher than head, and the lower hand not lower than the crotch. Eyes follow the movement of the upper hand.

• When moving the feet apart and together, move the foot gently and with agility, landing the ball of the foot first, and then the whole foot with the shift of the body center. Keep the body center steady, and do not move the body up and down or sway it. When bringing the feet together, keep them slightly apart.

• Do not turn the hand abruptly. Gradually turn the arm and turn the hand after it passes the front of the body, and at the same time move the foot. Coordinate the movements of the waist, hands and feet.

• When the feet move together for the last time, turn in the ball of the back foot when landing it.

Common Mistakes

• Moving the hands without the coordination of the turning of the waist. Moving the arms without first turning the waist, or turning the waist too early, making the torso sway.

• Abruptly moving the foot or turning the palm, breaking the flow of energy.

• When turning the body and moving the hands, the right hand is tensed.

- When moving the hands, the elbow and shoulder on the side of the hand on top are raised, the heel of the palm is relaxed, or the arm is tensed and bent, bringing the hand too close to head.
  - After moving the feet together, the toes point outward.
  - The torso leans forward, or the chest and buttocks are thrust out.

20. Dúlì Dǎhǔ 独立打虎 (Stand on One Leg and Hit the Tiger)

20.1 Step Back and Extend the Hand

Shift the body center to the right, move the left foot backward one step, bend the right knee forward; turn left palm upward and move it downward in a curve, stopping it in front of the abdomen; turn the right palm downward, thread it across and over the left forearm, and extend the right hand forward to the front of the body, wrist at shoulder height. Look at the right hand. (Fig. 127)

20.2 Sitting Stance and Separate the Hands

Shift the body center to the left, turn the torso to the left; turn in the right toes; move the hands downward, passing in front of the abdomen, and then to the left in a curve. Eyes move in the same direction as the turning of the torso. (Fig. 128)

20.3 Stand on One Leg and Upward Block

Gradually make fists of the open-palm hands, move the left fist upward passing the side of body to the front and above the left forehead, keeping the arm bent, palm of the fist facing outward, and the thumb side of the fist slanted downward; bend the right arm and draw the right fist to the front of the left chest, palm of the fist facing inward and the thumb side of the fist upward; slightly bend the left leg, stand firmly, bend the right leg and lift it, drawing the right foot to the front of the crotch, lifting up and turning in the toes; turn the head forward to the right. Look straight ahead. (Fig. 129)

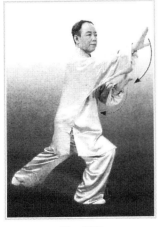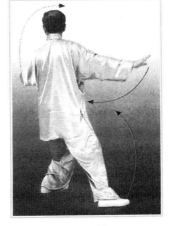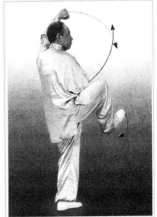

| Fig. 127 | Fig. 128 | Fig. 129 |

Important Points

● When forming a side-bow stance, move the left foot backward, about 45 degrees to the right.

● When lifting the foot and standing on one leg, shift the body center backward, lift the right toes, lift the right leg before bending the knee, and move the right foot in a curve to the front of the crotch. At the same time, separate the hands while moving them downward in a curve.

● The standing on one leg is adapted from the Wú (吴) Style. Lift the thigh high, turn the knee outward, and draw the calf inward, lifting up the toes. The angle between the thigh and the lower leg should be about 90 degrees.

● When separating the hands, turn the torso to the left, and then to the right when blocking up. At the end of the movement, keep the torso straight, facing forward on the diagonal. Block up with left fist above the front of the left forehead, draw the right fist to the side of body, arm bent, about a fist-width from the left ribs. The thumb sides of the fists face each other. Keep the arms half bent and fully extended. Turn the head to look straight ahead.

Common Mistakes

● When lifting the foot, the movement is cumbersome; the foot is dragged on the ground or kicked off the ground.

● When standing on one leg, the right leg is not bent enough so the calf is not drawn inward enough, or the leg is lifted without drawing a curve with the right foot.

● When stepping backward, the feet cross each other; the foot steps back too far to the side; and the right hand is not extended far enough.

● The hands are not separated clearly, the separating of the hands is confused with rolling back, or the body fails to turn to the left.

21. Yòu Fēnjiǎo 右分脚 (Separate the Foot — Right)

21.1 Lower the Toes and Hold in an Embrace

Slightly turn the torso to the right; draw the right foot inward, letting the toes drop; change the fists into open-palm hands and cross them in front of the chest as if holding something, right hand on the outside, and both palms facing inward. Look ahead to the right. (Fig. 130)

21.2 Lift the Foot and Separate the Hands

Extend the top of the right foot, slowing kick with toes forward to the right, keeping the kick above waist level; move the hands at the same time, one forward to the right and the other to the left, palms facing outward, fingertips pointing upward, wrists at shoulder height, arms raised, elbows slightly bent, right arm extending directly over the right leg. Look at the right hand. (Fig. 131)

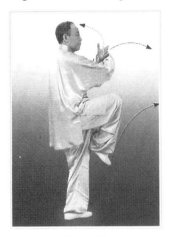

Fig. 130

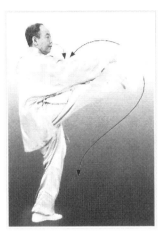

Fig. 131

Important Points

● When the arms are in the position of holding something, form a circle with the arms, hands crossing on a slant, right hand on the outside, and wrists at shoulder height. When separating the hands, turn the forearms inward, turn the palms outward, and pull them apart in curves, the top of the curve not higher than the top of the head. Separate the arms until they form about a 135-degree angle, keeping them slightly bent. Drop the shoulders, elbows and wrists, and slightly arc in the chest.

● The direction of the foot that is lifted is about 30 degrees on the diagonal from the front, and the right hand points in the same direction as right foot.

● At the end of movement, extend the torso and arms, slightly lift the body center and keep steady.

Common Mistakes

● When raising the foot, the head is lowered, the waist bent, the torso leans backward, the legs bend, hands and feet move in different directions, the hands are not kept at the same height, the arms are extended or bent too much, or the arms are extended to form a straight line.

● The foot is not raised high enough, and the body center is not balanced.

22. Shuāngfēng Guàn'or 双峰贯耳 (Strike the Opponent's Ears with Both Fists)

22.1 Draw In the Foot and Bring the Hands Together

Bend the right knee and draw in the calf, letting the toes drop; bend the elbows and turn the arms outward, move the arms close to each other in front of chest, move the hands past the front of the face in a curve and lower them parallel directly above the right knee, and turn the palms upward. Look straight ahead. (Fig. 132)

22.2 Land the Foot and Make Fists

Land the right foot in front of the body, landing the heel; lower the hands to either side of the waist, gradually making fists, palm of the fists facing upward. Look straight ahead. (Fig. 133)

22.3 Bow Stance and Strike with Both Fists

Shift the body center forward to form a right bow stance; at the same time strike with the fists in arcs upward and forward to ear level, fists head-width apart, the thumb side of the fists slanted downward, and the arms half bent in the shape of pincers. Look straight ahead. (Fig. 134)

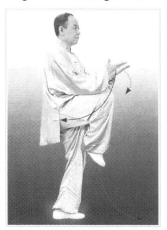 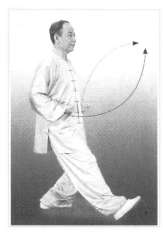 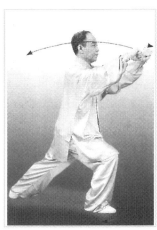

Fig. 132   Fig. 133   Fig. 134

Important Points

● When drawing in the foot, bend the knee while keeping the thigh steady. Turn the hands and move them toward each other until they are 4 inches or about 10 centimeters apart.

● When landing the right foot, bend the supporting left leg and lower the body center. Lower the right foot to the inside of the left ankle, then move the right foot forward one step and land the heel gently.

● The direction of striking with the fists is the same as the direction in which the right leg was raised, both hands and feet in a 30 degree angle on the diagonal from the front. Bend the arms into curves with the fists opposite each other like pincers. The fists should be at head level and head-width apart.

Common Mistakes

● When striking with the fists, the elbows and shoulders are raised, or the head is lowered.

● The foot lands heavily and on a straight line.

23. Zuǒ Fēnjiǎo 左分脚 (Separate the Foot — Left)

23.1 Turn the Body and Separate the Hands

Shift the body center backward, turn the right toes outward, turn the torso to the right; change the fists into open-palm hands and pull them to the right and left, both palms facing outward. Look at the left hand. (Fig. 135)

23.2 Draw In the Foot and Hold in an Embrace

Shift the body center forward, draw the left foot to the inside of the right foot, slightly turn the torso to the left; move the hands from both sides downward and inward in curves, cross them in front of the abdomen, raise them in front of chest as if holding something, left hand on the outside, both palms facing inward. Look forward to the left. (Fig. 136)

23.3 Lift the Foot and Separate the Hands

Slightly bend the right leg and stand firmly, raise the left leg, bending the left knee, and slowly kick the left toes upward and forward to the left (a 90-degree angle from the direction the body faced at the starting form), extending the top of the foot, with the foot above waist level; separate the hands, moving one hand forward to the left and the other to the right in curves, palms facing outward, wrists at shoulder height, arms raised, elbows slightly bent, and the left arm extending directly over left leg. Look at the left hand. (Fig. 137)

Important Points

● Coordinate turning the body, shifting the body center backward and turning the right toes outward while at the same time separating the hands.

● Lift the foot in the advance direction (90 degrees from the direction of Beginning Position).

● Put the left hand outside the right when in the position of holding something.

Common Mistakes

Same as those in Separate the Foot — Right.

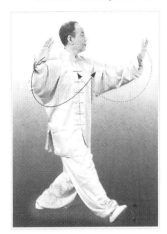

Fig. 135

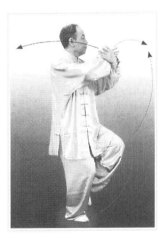

Fig. 136

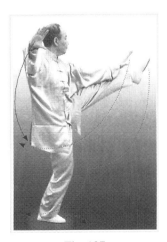

Fig. 137

24. Zhuǎnshēn Pāijiǎo 转身拍脚 (**Turn the Body and Pat the Foot**)

24.1 Turn the Body and Land the Foot

Bend the left leg and start to lower it, turn the body to the right around to the back pivoting on the ball of the right foot; with the turning of the body, turn the left toes in and land them on the ground; lower the hands in curves from both sides of the body toward the front of the abdomen, turn the forearm outward, palms facing each other on a slant. Turn the head together with the body. (Fig. 138)

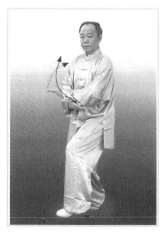

Fig. 138

24.2 Turn the Body and Hold in an Embrace

Shift the body center to the left, continue turning the body back to the right (moving sideways toward the direction in which the left foot was separated in the previous movement); at the same time turn the right foot straight, touching the ground with the toes; cross the hands, right hand on the outside, raise and hold the arms as if holding something in front of the chest. Look forward to the right. (Fig. 139)

24.3 Separate the Hands and Pat the Foot

Support the body with the left leg while kicking up the right foot, extending the top of the foot; turn the forearms inward and palms outward; move the right hand forward to pat the top of the right foot at head level; move the left hand backward in a curve, raising it horizontally on the left side of body, wrist at shoulder height. Look at the right hand. (Fig. 140)

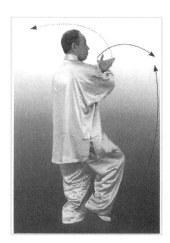

Fig. 139

Important Points

• Land the foot while turning the body. At the same time lower the hands and cross them in front of the abdomen to facilitate the turning of the body.

• When landing the left foot, turn in the toes and land the ball of the foot and then the whole foot. Shift the body center to the left leg, lift the right heel and turn the right foot on the ground.

• Separating the hands and kick at the same time. Pat the top of the right foot with the right hand.

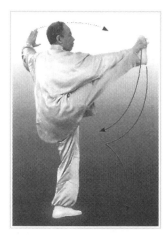

Fig. 140

Common Mistakes

● Landing the foot and bringing the hands together are not coordinated with the turning of the body. The foot lands before the bringing together of the hands and the turning of the body.

● When landing the foot, the left foot turns outward and then inward and then the body turns, in an attempt to gain more power.

● When patting the foot, the head lowers, the waist bends, the wrist behind bends, the pat misses the foot, or the supporting leg is bent too much.

25. Jìnbù Zāichuí 进步栽捶 (Step In and Punch Downward)

25.1 Turn the Body and Land the Foot

Bend the left knee, bend the right leg and land it in front, toes turned outward; turn the torso to the right, shift the body center forward; turn the forearms outward, move the left hand upward and to the right in a curve, turning the palm to the right; turn the right hand and lower it to the waist level, palm facing upward. Turn the head together with the torso. (Fig. 141)

25.2 Draw In the Foot and Sweep the Arms

Continue turning the torso to the right; keep moving the right hand upward in a curve to the back right, and move the left hand to the right ribs in a curve, passing in front of the head. (Fig. 142)

25.3 Step In and Make a Fist

Move the left foot forward one step, landing the heel, turn the torso slightly to the left; move the right hand to the right and upward in a curve, bend the elbow and make a fist, draw the fist to the side of the right ear, the palm of the fist facing downward; move the left hand downward in a curve to the front of the abdomen. Look forward and downward. (Fig. 143)

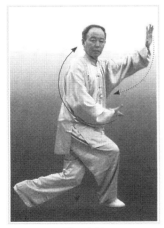
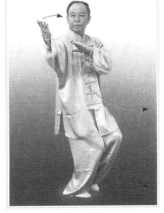
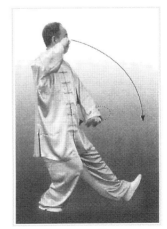

Fig. 141   Fig. 142   Fig. 143

25.4 Bow Stance and Punch Downward

Turn the torso to the left; slightly lean the body forward, shift the body center forward to form a left bow stance; punch forward and downward with the right fist, stopping the fist at abdomen height, the front of the fist facing forward and downward, thumb toward the left; sweep the left hand over the left knee to the side of the left hip, palm facing downward. Look at the right fist. (Fig. 144)

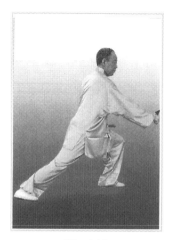

Fig. 144

Important Points

• Bend the leg before landing the foot, keep the thigh lifted, bend the supporting leg, land the right foot one step forward, landing the heel, turning the toes outward.

• The movement of sweeping the arms here is the same as in Brush Aside over the Knee in Reverse Forward Stance [Movement 6: Lōuxī Àobù 搂膝拗步].

• Make a fist while bending the arm and draw the fist to the side of the head, the thumb side of fist toward the body, the palm of the fist facing forward.

• When punching downward, slightly turn the right shoulder forward, the fist is a little higher than the knee, lean the torso forward not more than 45 degrees, keeping the neck straight. When making the bow stance, the width between the feet is about 8 inches or 20 centimeters.

Common Mistakes

• The foot lands heavily and in a straight line.

• The wrist bends when making a fist.

• The waist bends and the back hunches when punching downward.

26. Xiéfēishì 斜飞势 (Diagonal Flying Posture)

26.1 Turn the Body and Separate the Hands

Shift the body center backward, turn the left toes outward, turn the torso to the left; turn the right fist into an open-palm hand and move it upward and to the right in a curve, move the left hand to the left in a curve, separating the hands. (Fig. 145)

26.2 Draw In the Foot and Hold the Hands

Draw the right foot to the inside of the left foot, move the left palm upward and to the right in a curve, bend the

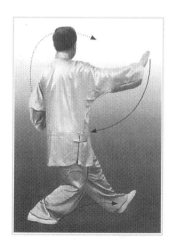

Fig. 145

arm in front of the chest, palm slanted downward; move the right hand downward and to the left in a curve, bend the right arm in front of the abdomen, right palm slanted upward; cross the arms in an embrace, left forearm on top. Look at the left hand. (Fig. 146)

26.3 Step to the Side and Cross the Arms

Slightly turn the torso to the right; move the right foot to the right side one step, landing the heel. Look at the left hand. (Fig. 147)

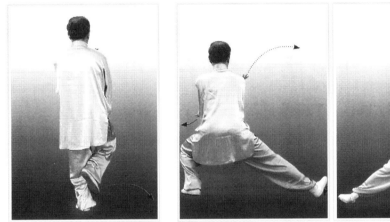
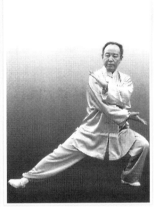

Fig. 146   Fig. 147

26.4 Lean the Body and Shoulder to the Side

Shift the body center to the right, turn the torso to the left to form a right side-bow stance; lean the right shoulder to the right; extend the right hand forward to the right and lower the left hand forward to the left, the right hand a little above the head, palm slanted upward; the left hand at hip level, palm slanted downward. Eyes follow the movement of the left hand. (Fig. 148)

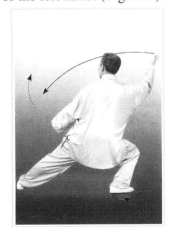
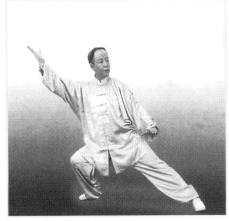

Fig. 148

Important Points

• When separating the hands, turn the right fist into an open-palm hand and move it upward and to the right in a curve, and move the left palm downward and to the left in a curve.

• When stepping sideways and crossing the arms, move the right foot to the right side and a little backward, landing the heel first, and slightly turning the torso to the right. At the same time, thrust right palm to the left and downward. Cross the arms, one slanting upward and the other slanting downward. Keep the legs steady.

• When leaning the body and the shoulder to the side, first raise the right arm in front of the body, at the same time lean the right shoulder to the side, leaning the torso with it, and separate and extend the arms in opposite directions on the diagonal. Turn the right arm outward, right palm slanted upward. Turn the left arm inward, pushing the left palm on a slant downward. The extended arms form an angle of about 120 degrees.

• When leaning the body and shoulder to the side, lean the torso, keep the head and the torso upright and relaxed, chest slightly arced in, back rounded, shoulders down and head upright. This movement is adapted from the Wú (吴) Style, which requires that the leaning of the torso be straight while leaning the shoulder to the side.

Common Mistakes

• When stepping to the side, the heel brushes the ground, or the body turns while advancing.

• When crossing the hands, the armpits are open.

• When making a side-bow stance, the feet turn too far outward, forming a T-stance.

• When leaning the body to the side, the torso bends to the side.

• When leaning the body and shoulder to the side, the power is not focused in the right place, confusing the movement with turning the waist and sweeping the arms outward. The leaning of the body is not led by the leaning of the shoulder.

• When extending the arms, the chest is thrust out and arms straightened, forming a diagonal line with the arms.

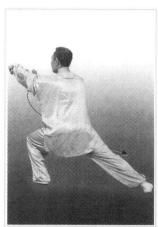

27. Danbian Xiàshì 单鞭下势 (Single Bian Downward)

27.1 Hook the Hand and Sweep the Hand

Shift the body center to the left, turn the torso to the left; slightly push the right heel outward; hook up the left hand and lift it to the left side of body, wrist at shoulder height; move the right hand to the left in a curve, passing the front of the head, to the inside of the left elbow. Eyes follow the movement of the right hand. (Fig. 149)

Fig. 149

27.2 Crouch Stance and Thread the Hand

Fully bend the left leg, stretch out the right leg, turn the torso to the right, forming a right crouch stance; lower the right hand, pass it in front of the abdomen and thread it to the right along the inside of the right leg, turning palm from inward to outward, fingertips pointing to the right. Look at the right hand. (Fig. 150)

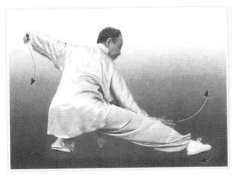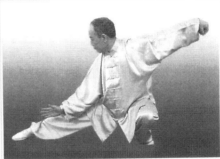

Fig. 150

Important Points

• When hooking the hand and sweeping the hand, lift the left hand and hook it up, turn the right hand inward and sweep it to the left, turn the torso to the left, and thrust the right heel slightly outward against the ground.

• When threading the hand, lower the right hand and turn it outward, palm facing outward and fingertips pointing to the right, and gradually straighten the bent arm until the hand reaches the inside of the right ankle. Extend the arms, the hooked hand at head level, fingertips pointing downward.

Common Mistakes

• When making the crouch stance, the supporting leg is not bent enough, the head is lowered, the waist bends and the buttocks protrude.

• When making the crouch stance, the right leg is bent, the outside of the right foot is lifted off the ground, or the right heel is off the ground, or the left heel is off ground.

• The back arm is either too bent or too straight, or the hooked hand is too high or too low.

28. Jīnjī Dúlì 金鸡独立 (Golden Rooster Stands on One Leg)

28.1 Bow Stance and Spear Up the Hand

Shift the body center to the right, turn the torso to the right; turn the right toes outward, turn in the left toes, bend the right leg, and kick-straighten the left leg naturally; raise the right hand to the front of the body, palm vertical and facing to the side with the wrist at shoulder height; turn the left arm inward and lower it behind the body, top of the hook pointing upward. Look at the right hand. (Fig. 151)

28.2 Stand on One Leg and Spear Up the Hand

Shift the body center forward, turn the torso to the right; bend the left knee and lift the left leg upward in front of the body, let the toes drop naturally, and stand on the right leg, which is slightly bent, to form a right one-leg stance turn the left hook hand into an open-palm hand, spear it forward and upward, passing the side of body, until it is vertical and facing sideways, fingertips at brow level; turn the right hand and push it downward at the side of the right hip. Look at the left hand. (Fig. 152)

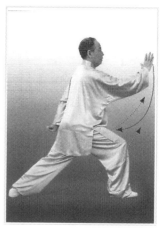
Fig. 151

28.3 Land the Foot and Push the Palm Downward

Slightly bend the right leg, land the left foot behind the inside of the right foot, shift the body center backward; turn the left hand and lower it, and stretch the right hand downward. (Fig. 153)

28.4 Stand on One Leg and Spear Up the Hand

Turn the torso to the left; bend the right knee and lift the right leg upward in front of the body, let the right toes drop naturally, and stand on left leg, which is slightly bent to form a left one-leg stance; push the left hand downward by the side of the left hip; make the right hand vertical palm facing sideways and raise it to the front of the body until the fingertips reach brow level. Look at the right hand. (Fig. 154)

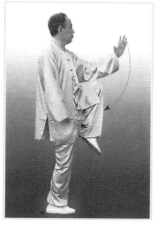
Fig. 152

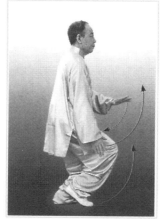
Fig. 153

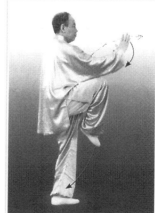
Fig. 154

Important Points

• When making a bow stance and spearing up the hand, shift the body center forward, turn right toes outward and turn in the left toes.

● When lifting the foot, turn the waist, bend the knee and draw in the foot before lifting it. Do not drag the left foot on the ground or press it against the ground before lifting it.

● When standing on one leg and spearing up the hand, relax the torso, turn the waist and shoulder forward and to the side. Bend the arm into a curve, bend the wrist and extend the hand, drop the shoulders and elbows, making the web between the index finger and thumb opposite the tip of the nose, and the knee opposite the elbow.

● When landing the foot, turn the waist and bend the leg, and land the ball of the foot first. Do this movement gently and completely.

Common Mistakes

● When bending the leg, the feet do not turn on the ground, which makes the lifting of the foot and one-leg stance unsteady, and the movement is awkward.

● When lifting the foot, the movement is heavy, the toes drag on the ground or abruptly kick off the ground.

● When standing on one leg, the body is tense, the stance is unsteady, or the leg and the waist bend, the lower leg comes forward, or the toes tilt upward.

● When landing the foot and pressing the palm downward, the waist is not turned, and the foot makes a heavy landing.

● When spearing up the hand and pushing the palm downward, the arms, hands and wrists are too tensed or too relaxed,

● When spearing up the hand, the palm turns forward.

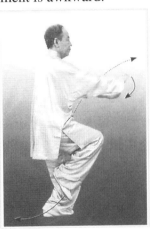

Fig. 155

29. Tuìbù Chuanzhǎng 退步穿掌 (Step Back and Thrust the Open-Palm Hand)

Slightly bend the left leg, move the right foot backward one step, kick-straighten the right leg naturally; bend the left leg, and turn the left foot straight pivoting on the ball of the foot, forming a left bow stance; turn the left arm outward, turn the left palm upward and draw it to the waist, and thrust it across and over the right forearm, until the wrist reaches shoulder height; turn the right arm inward, the flat palm pressing downward until it is underneath the left elbow. Look at the left hand. (Figs. 155, 156)

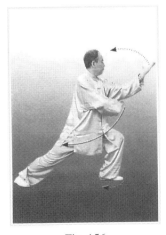

Fig. 156

Important Points

• Bend the supporting leg, turn the torso to the right, move the right foot backward passing the inside of the left foot. Land the ball of the foot first, then turn the left foot straight pivoting on the ball of the foot to form a left bow stance.

• Turn the left hand and thrust it upward to head level, and turn the right hand and push it downward to chest level.

Common Mistakes

• When stepping backward, the torso leans forward, the right lower leg is lifted up behind, or the supporting leg is not bent.

• When making a left bow stance, the front foot is not turned straight forward, but the toes are left pointing outward; or the feet cross and the back leg is bent.

• The legs move faster than the hands, making the movements of the torso and lower body uncoordinated.

Part IV

30. Xūbù Yazhǎng 虚步压掌 (Press the Palms Down in Empty Stance)

30.1 Turn the Body and Raise the Hand

Shift the body center backward, turn in the left toes, turn the torso to the right and backward; draw the right open-palm hand to the front of the abdomen; raise the left hand over and at the side of the left forehead. Turn the eyes with the body and look straight ahead. (Fig. 157)

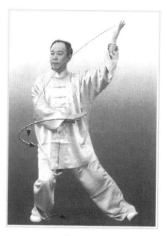

Fig. 157

30.2 Press the Palms Down in Empty Stance

Shift the body center to the left leg, lift the right foot, turn the right toes forward, and touch the ball of the foot on the ground, forming a right empty stance; relax the torso and drop it down with a slight lean of the torso forward; move the left hand downward from above and stop it down over the front of the right knee, fingertips pointing to the right; push the right palm downward by the side of the right hip, fingertips pointing forward. Look forward and downward. (Fig. 158)

Important Points

• When turning the body, make sure the left foot is turned inside enough; turn the right heel inside and lift the right foot and step slightly to the right to form a right empty stance.

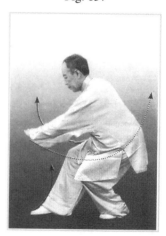

Fig. 158

- When pushing the palms downward, turn the waist and move the shoulder in the same direction, bend the legs and drop the hips. Lean the torso forward 30 degrees to 45 degrees. Keep the body straight. Press the hands down in front of the body.

Common Mistakes

- When turning the feet, the left toes are not turned in enough, or the right foot is not moved. When making an empty stance, the torso is not kept straight, or the legs are tensed.

- When pressing the palm downward, the torso leans forward too much, the back is hunched, the waist is bent, or the torso is rotated too much, or the hands stop on the right side of the body.

- Failing to make a distinct pressing movement with the palms, moving the hands downward in a curve to the right side of the body.

31. Dúlì Tuōzhǎng 独立托掌 (Stand on One Leg and Lift the Hand)

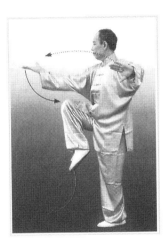

Press the left foot against the ground, slightly bend the left leg and stand firmly, bend the right knee and lift the right leg, dropping the toes, forming a left one-leg stance; turn the right hand and lift it to the front of the body, palm facing upward and the wrist at chest height; move the left hand to the left and upward in a curve, extend it at the side of the body, wrist at shoulder height, palm facing outward, and fingertips slanted upward. Look at the right hand. (Fig. 159)

Important Points

- Before lifting the right foot to stand on one leg and

Fig. 159

then lifting the hand, first rotate the waist and kick the left leg to lift the body center. Start the movement from the waist and supporting leg and send it to the hands and right foot, until the movement extends throughout the whole body.

- At the end of the movement, extend the front arm, and keep the left arm at the side, curved and extended, keep the torso straight, lift the head, drop the shoulders, slightly arc in the chest and round the back, relax the waist and lift the right leg, keep the supporting leg stable, and press the toes against the ground.

- Bend the left wrist and push the left palm outward, turn the web between the thumb and index finger forward, palm facing outward. Lift the right hand in front of the body, hands are at shoulder height.

Common Mistakes

- The arms are too limp and too bent, the torso is not stretched out.

● When making a one-leg stance, the supporting leg is bent too much, the lifted leg sticks out, and the toes tilt upward.

32. Mǎbùkào 马步靠 (Lean-In Horse Stance)

32.1 Land the Foot and Move the Hand Downward

Land the right foot in front of the body, turning the toes outward, shift the body center forward, turn the torso to the right; turn the right arm inward, turn the right palm down and move the hand downward; turn the left arm outward, move the left palm upward and to the right in a curve. Look straight ahead. (Fig. 160)

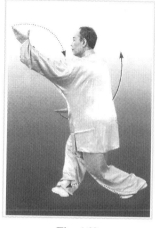

Fig. 160

32.2 Draw In the Foot and Swing the Arm

Draw the left foot to the inside of the right foot, continue turning the torso to the right; turn the right palm upward, and move it to the right in a curve and lift it by the side of the body, hand at head level; turn the left hand into a fist, and lower it in front of the right abdomen, the palm facing downward, the thumb side of the fist inward. Look at the right palm. (Fig. 161)

32.3 Lean in Half Horse Stance

Turn the torso to the left; move the left foot one step forward to the left side; lower the left fist and sweep it to the left side of the body (Fig. 162); slightly shift the body center forward to form a half-horse stance; turn the left arm inward and press the arm with force to the left front, the thumb side of the left fist toward the body, the knuckles facing downward, in front of the left knee; bend the right hand and draw the palm in to the left arm to assist its press forward, palm facing to the left, fingers resting on the inside of the left forearm. Look to the left front. (Fig. 163)

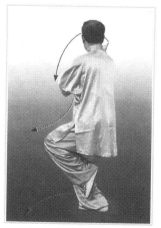

Fig. 161

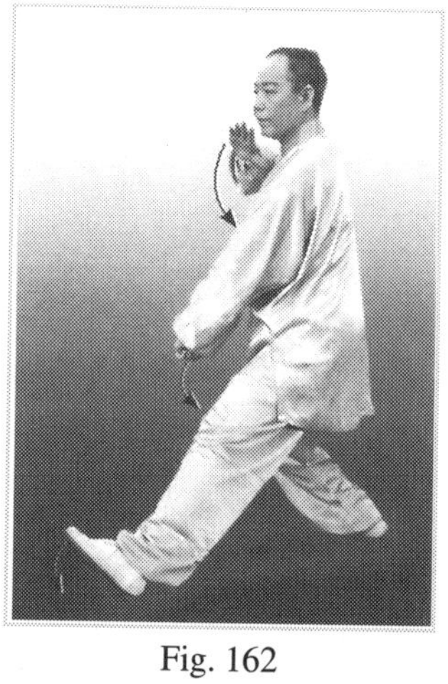

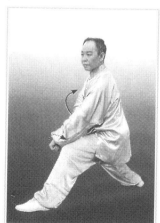

Fig. 162

Fig. 163

Important Points

• When landing the right foot, bend the right leg, step forward and land the foot in front of the body, turn the torso to the right, turn the toes outward, and land the heel first.

• When sweeping the arms, move the arms in vertical circles across each other. The movement is the same as in Brush aside over the Knee in Reverse Forward Stance (Movement 6 Lōuxī Àobù 搂膝拗步). When the left hand moves in front of the right shoulder, make a fist, the palm downward, its thumb side facing into the body.

• The direction of the advance of the left foot is 45 degrees left of the front. Land the heel fist and at the same time shift the body center forward and then land the whole foot to form a half horse stance.

• When leaning forward, generate the power from the waist and legs, the strength is in the lower abdomen, the whole movement is fast and integrated, and the breath is sharply exhaled. Bend the legs and squat, pull the thighs outward, slightly lower the body center, turn the rear leg inward and kick against the ground, slightly bend the left leg. Slightly turn the torso to the left, the direction of the lean is forward on the diagonal in the same direction as the left foot. Turn in the left arm and slightly bend it, put the left fist over or to the inside of the left knee, the knuckles downward, and the palm of the fist inward. The power is always on the outside of the left upper arm.

Common Mistakes

• At the beginning of the movement, when landing the right foot, the right hand is not turned and moved downward; or the right hand is moved to the left and downward in a circular motion, or the shape of the hand is not precise enough.

• The power is not generated through the waist and legs.

• The arms are too bent when they sweep, sending the power into the elbow.

• The press to the side is made in either horse stance or bow stance.

• When pressing, the torso leans forward too much.

33. Zhuǎnshēn Dàlǚ 转身大捋 (**Turn the Body with Large Rollback**)

33.1 Turn the Foot and Hands

Shift the body center backward, turn the left toes up and out; turn the left fist into an open-palm hand, turn the left arm outward and right arm inward, turn the palms outward at the same time, and slightly draw them toward the body. Look at the hands. (Fig. 164)

33.2 Move the Feet Together and Lift the Hands

Turn the torso to the left and shift the body center forward; draw the right foot to the inside of the left foot,

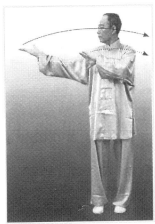

Fig. 164

the feet parallel and pointing forward, the body center stays mainly on the left leg and is raised a little; turn the left arm inward, bend the left elbow and raise the left hand up to the front of the chest, forming a flat hand with the palm facing outward; turn the right arm outward and lift it out from the right side of the body at shoulder height, palm upward. Look at the right hand. (Fig. 165)

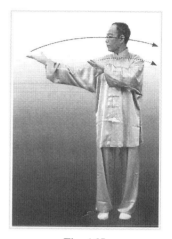

Fig. 165

33.3 Turn the Body with Large Rollback

Turn the right heel outward pivoting on the ball of the foot, and turn the body to the left; with the movement of the body, the hands make a wide stroke to the left in a movement level to the ground to the front of the body. (Fig. 166)

Continue to turn the torso to the left; move the left foot back on the diagonal one full step, landing it with the toes pointing outward, bending the right leg; the right hand with the palm facing out on the diagonal is at the head level; the left hand is next to the inside of the right elbow with the palm facing the elbow. Look at the right hand. (Fig. 167)

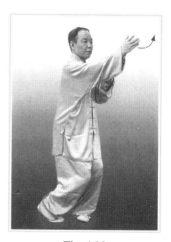

Fig. 166

33.4 Side-Bow Stance and Roll the Elbow Down

Continue to turn the torso to the left, shift the body center to the left; push the right heel outward and straighten the right leg naturally to form a left side-bow stance; the hands continue to stroke in a movement level to the ground to the left and gradually make fists, turn the left arm to the left, move the left fist to the left in a curve, and draw the left fist to the waist, the palm facing upward; bend the right arm, turn it outward, roll and press the elbow down in the front of the body, the right fist at the chest level, and the palm slanted upward. Look at the right fist. (Fig. 168)

Important Points

● This movement comes from 48-Step Taijiquan where it evolved from the Wide Rollback and Push Hands of the Yang-style Taijiquan, mainly composed of such hand techniques as roll back (lǚ 捋) , bump with the body (kào 靠) , elbow strike (zhǒu 肘), split (liè 挒), and pull

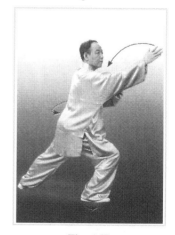

Fig. 167

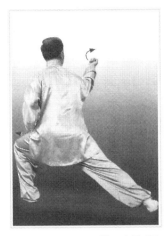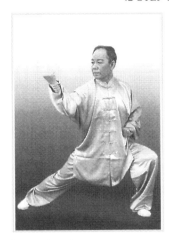

Fig. 168 (Front and rear views)

down (cǎi 采). This movement includes two techniques: 1. Turning the body and roll back and 2. Rolling the elbow.

- When turning the feet and the open-palm hands, the strength should change from tensed to relaxed and from solid to empty. After pressing with force in the previous movement (Movement 32), relax the body, and then sweep the body back in a short arc like a spring uncoiling. Turn the left foot outward, turn the torso to the left, relax both arms, turn and draw them back to the left, allowing the wrist to bend and wind. In this movement, at the beginning, the left arm turns outward and then comes back inward, and the right arm first turns outward and then comes back outward. Then both arms move upward, the feet come together, and the open-palm hands turn and lift up.

- After the feet come together, raise the body center, turn the body to the direction of the Beginning Position (South) with the body center resting on the left leg. The right palm faces upward and the left palm forward.

- When turning the body with a wide stroke, pivot on the ball of the right foot and turn the right heel outward, keep turning the torso to the left. Bend the right knee, and move the left foot back one step on the diagonal (Northwest corner) to the right, landing the inside of the ball of the foot.

- When rolling the elbow, shift the body center to the left, straighten the right leg, push the right heel outward to form a left side-bow stance. At the same time, turn the torso to the left, turn the left fist outward and draw it to the waist, the palm facing upward. Turn the right fist outward also, roll the right forearm and press it downward, using the joint-twisting [fǎnguānjié 反关节] technique to seize and twist the opponent's arm to the side.

Common Mistakes
- The feet are not parallel when the feet are brought together, but rather are turned in.

- When turning the hands, they move in a curve too far backward.
- When rolling the elbow, the torso is not turned to the left, or the right arm is drawn back straight.
- When making the side-bow stance, the toes are turned outward too much, forming a T-stance.
- The feet move around, the turning is not distinct, or the body center is unsteady.

34. Xiēbù Qíndǎ 歇步擒打 (Grab and Hit in Resting Stance)

34.1 Turn the Body and Arms

Turn the torso to the right, shift the body center to the right; turn the right arm inward, bend the elbow and push it upward, put the right fist in front of the right forehead, the palm facing outward; turn the left arm inward, thread the left fist behind the left side of the body, the palm facing backward. Look straight ahead. (Fig. 169)

34.2 Turn the Body and Grab

Turn the torso to the left; turn the left toes outward, shift the body center forward; lower the right fist past the side of the body, turn the wrist and draw the fist to the waist, the palm of the fist facing upward; change the left fist into an open-palm hand, and move it forward in a curve, turning the palm to the right. Turn the head with the body, and look straight ahead. (Fig. 170)

34.3 Punch in Resting Stance

Move the right foot past the front of the left foot and land the right foot to the left of the front of the body, cross the legs and squat to form a resting stance; make a fist with the left hand, and draw it to the front of the abdomen, the palm of the fist facing downward, the web between the thumb and the index finger facing toward the body; punch with the right fist forward and downward, past over the left forearm, stopping the right fist at the abdomen level, the palm of the fist facing upward. Look at the right fist. (Fig. 171)

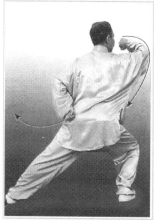
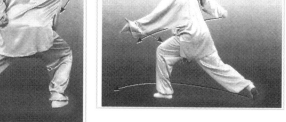
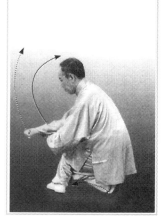

Fig. 169   Fig. 170   Fig. 171

Important Points

● This movement evolved from the "Small Grab and Hit" of the Chen-style Taijiquan and the movement of "Lazy Dragon Lying Across the Road" from the combination forms of punching in Xingyiquan [a kind of Chinese martial arts based on the fighting movements of 12 different animals]. The stance is high resting stance, the step is a cross-over step, and the hand techniques involve grabbing and punching forward and downward.

● In the first movement, do not turn the torso more than 90 degrees, make fists with the hands and turn them inward, the right fist not higher than the head, and the left fist not lower than the hips.

● When grabbing, turn the left toes outward, turn the torso to the left, move the left hand in an arc to the left front of the body, turn the palm to the right, and after making a fist, turn the palm of the fist downward.

● When punching in resting stance, make a cross-over step with the right foot forward to the left side, landing the right heel first and forming a high resting stance with the legs half bent. Punch the right fist forward and downward, the palm of the fist facing upward, the fist at the abdomen level. Rest the left fist underneath the right forearm, the palm facing downward. Lean the torso slightly forward.

Common Mistakes

● The legs are not crossed tightly when making resting stance.

● When turning the body and arms, the torso is turned to the right too much, and the fists are moved too far.

● When punching, the fists are at chest level.

35. Chuānzhǎng Xiàshì 穿掌下势 (Lower the Body and Thread the Palm-Hand)

35.1 Draw In the Foot and Lift the Hands

Turn the torso to the right; draw the left foot to the inside of the right foot; turn the fists into open-palm hands, turn the right arm inward, and the palm outward, the fingertips pointing to the left, lift the hand to the front of the chest; turn the left arm and left palm outward, the fingertips pointing to the left, and raise the hand to the left side of the body. Look at the left hand. (Fig. 172)

35.2 Step Sideways and Sweep the Hands

Turn the torso to the right; bend the right leg into a squat, and extend the left leg to the left side; move the hands upward and to the right in an arc, passing the front

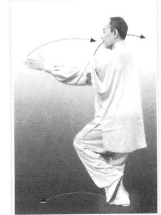

Fig. 172

of the face, to the right side of the body, turning the palms slanted downward, the fingertips pointing upward to the right, raise the right hand to the right side of the front, the palm at head level; bend the left arm and sweep the left hand to front of the right shoulder at shoulder height. Look at the right hand. (Fig. 173)

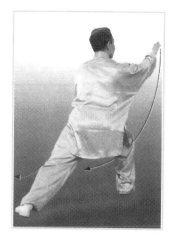

Fig. 173

35.3 Crouch Stance and Thread the Hands

Bend the right leg to a full squat, straighten the left leg, and turn the torso to the left, forming a left crouch stance; revolve the hand, turning the fingertips to the left, and thread the hand past the front of the abdomen and along the inside of the left leg to the left, the left hand in front, palm facing outward, and the right hand behind the left hand, palm facing inward. Look at the left hand. (Fig. 174)

Important Points

• When drawing in the foot and lifting palms, lift the body center back to the height of a bow stance. Turn the hands sideways and lift them no higher than shoulder height, the fingertips pointing to the left.

• When sweeping the hands down, turn the torso to the right, sweep the hands to the right past the front of the body no higher than the head. When extending the left foot to the left side, land the inside of the ball of the foot first, keeping a width of one foot's distance between the two feet.

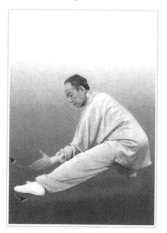

Fig. 174

• When threading the hands, bend the wrists and rotate the hands, turn the left palm outward and the right palm inward so that both hands have the thumb side up, all the fingertips pointing to the left as the hands thread along the inside of the left leg.

Common Mistakes

• The range of movement is too small when the hands are lifting and/or sweeping.

• When the hands begin the sweep, the torso is not turned to the right, or the eyes are not on the right hand.

• When threading the hands, the wrists and hands are not turned distinctly.

• The range of threading the hands is not long enough; or only the left hand threads out, the right hand remaining at the waist.

• When doing the crouch stance, the head is lowered, the waist is bent, the hips are lifted, or the right leg is not fully bent.

36. Shàngbù Qīxīng 上步七星 (Step Forward and Seven Stars)

36.1 Bend the Leg and Lift the Hand

Shift the body center forward, turn the torso to the left; turn the left toes outward, and the right toes inward, straighten the right leg, and bend the left leg; lift the left palm forward and upward, the wrist at the shoulder height, the palm facing to the right, the fingertips slanted upward; slightly pull the right hand backward and put it by the side of the right hip. Look at the left hand. (Fig. 175)

36.2 Empty Stance and Block Up with the Fists

Step forward with the right foot, landing the ball of the foot to form a right empty stance; make a fist with the left palm and draw it slightly in toward the body, the palm of the fist toward the body; make a fist with the right hand and block it forward and upward, the palm of the fist facing outward; cross the wrists, put the fists across each other in front of the body, the fists at the shoulder height, the right fist on the outside and with the arms rounded. Look at the left fist. (Fig. 176)

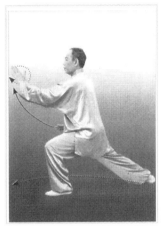

Fig. 175

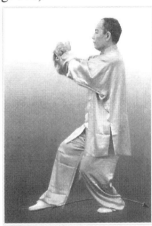

Fig. 176

Important Points

• When bending the leg and lifting the hands, shift the body center forward, bend the left leg, turn the left toes outward, straighten the right leg, and turn in the right toes.

• When blocking up with the fists, cross the fists at the shoulder height. The right fist is on the outside and the left fist on the inside. Half bend the elbows and round the arms, lower the shoulders and let the elbows hang. Slightly arc in the chest and extend the back.

Common Mistakes

• When bending the leg, the feet do not turn enough.

• When lifting the hands, the right hand is drawn backward too much.

- When drawing in the back foot and stepping forward with the right foot, the movement is not light and smooth, but rather the right foot drags or kicks off against the ground.

- The empty stance is too tense or strong, the back leg and foot do not turn outward enough.

- When blocking up with the fists, the elbows drop so that the arms are pressed against the body.

37. Tuìbù Kuàhǔ 退步跨虎 (Step Back and Ride the Tiger)

37.1 Step Back and Open the Fists

Step back and to the right with the right foot; open the fists. Look at the hands. (Fig. 177)

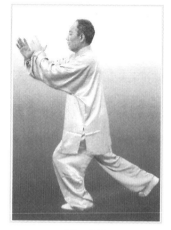

Fig. 177

37.2 Turn the Body and Sweep the Hands

Turn the torso to the right, shift the body center backward; move the right hand downward to the right in a curve to the side of the right hip, palm facing downward; turn the left hand to the right together with the body, and move the left hand slightly to the right in a curve, palm facing to the right. Turn the head slightly to the right, and look forward to the right. (Fig. 178)

37.3 Bring the Feet Together and Sweep the Hands

Draw in the left foot slightly backward, landing the ball of the foot in front of the right foot; turn the torso to the left, slightly lower and bend the body down; move the right hand upward in a curve, past the face and then to the left and downward in a curve, and stop it by the outside of the left leg, the palm facing outward. The eyes follow the movement of the body, look to the left at the right hand. (Fig. 179)

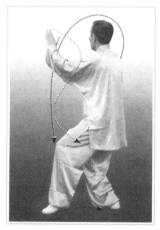

Fig. 178

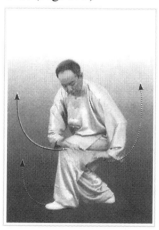

Fig. 179

37.4 Lift the Leg and the Hands

Kick the right foot against the ground, and stand firmly on the right leg, lift the left leg forward, with the knee slightly bent, extend the foot, and turn the toes a little inward; lift the right hand forward and upward with a flick of the wrist to form a side straight open-palm hand, the wrist at the shoulder height; the left hand turns into a hook and lifts at the same time to the left, the hand at the shoulder height, the tip of the hook pointing downward, and the torso is turned to the left. Look forward to the left. (Fig. 180)

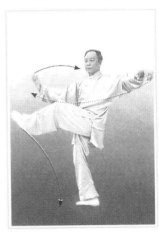

Fig. 180

Important Points

• When turning the body and sweeping the palms, turn the body about 45 degrees to the right. When sweeping the palms, first lower the right hand in a curve, then sweep the hands across each other, the left palm facing to the right and the right palm facing downward.

• When drawing in the left foot backward, press the ball of the back foot against the ground, turn the torso to the left, and slightly lower the body center. At the same time continue to sweep the hands across each other to the outside of the left leg, the right palm facing outward and the left palm facing downward.

• Let the turning of the body lead the sweeping of the hands.

• When fixing the movement, keep the torso straight and upright, turned about 45 degrees to the left. Stand firm on the right leg, and raise the left leg forward and upward. Slightly bend the knee, keep it above the waist, extend the top of the left foot, turn the ball of the foot inward as if the left foot were coming in toward the body. The right arm and the left leg should be raised in the same direction as the "Step Forward and Seven Stars."

Common Mistakes

• When sweeping the hands, the torso is not turned.

• At the end of the movement, the left leg and right hand are lifted forward over 30 degrees to the right.

• The right arm and the left leg are lifted in different directions.

• When lifting the right hand forward, the palm faces forward instead of sideways.

• The left leg straightens as it is lifted.

• At the end of the movement, the torso leans backward or is not straight enough.

38. Zhuǎnshēn Bǎilián 转身摆莲 (**Turn the Body for Lotus Kick**)

38.1 Turn the Foot In and Sweep the Hands

Lower the left foot in front of the body, landing the heel first, turn the toes inward and turn the torso to the right; turn the right arm inward and the right palm downward, bend the elbow and draw it horizontally to the right; open the left hook hand, turn the palm upward, and sweep the hand forward horizontally to the side of the body from behind. The head turns with the body. Look straight ahead. (Fig. 181)

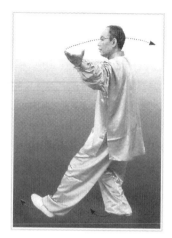

Fig. 181

38.2 Turn the Body and Thread the Hand

Turn the body to the right and backward pivoting on the balls of the feet; sweep the left hand to the front of the body, palm facing upward at head level; turn the right hand downward, and thread it past the front of the chest and underneath the left elbow to the left. The head turns with the body. Look straight ahead. (Fig. 182)

38.3 Turn the Body and Sweep the Palm

Continue to turn the torso to the right to the opposite direction of "Step Forward and Seven Stars;" rest the weight on the left leg to form a right empty stance; after threading the right hand, move it upward and to the right in a curve, and at the same time turn the forearm inward and the palm to the right, the fingertips pointing upward; put the hand on the right side of the body, the wrist at shoulder height; turn and move the left hand from the inside of the right arm downward, and draw it to front and below the right shoulder, the palm also facing to the right. Look at the right hand. (Fig. 183)

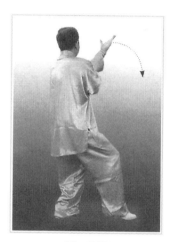

Fig. 182

38.4 Sweep the Leg and Pat the Foot

Turn the torso to the left; lift the right heel (Fig. 184).

Continue to turn the torso to the left, lift the right foot and sweep it to the left, upward and to the right in a fan-shaped arc, extending the top of the foot; turn the torso to the

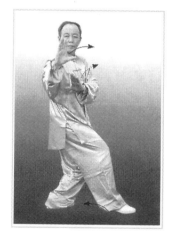

Fig. 183

left; sweep the palms horizontally from right to left, and pat the top of the right foot first with the left hand and then with the right hand in front of the head. Look at the hands. (Fig. 185)

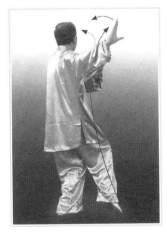

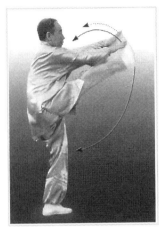

Fig. 184

Fig. 185

Important Points

● When turning the foot inward, turn the torso to the left, landing the heel in front of the body, the toes turned inward. When turning the body, turn both feet, the left foot pivoting on the heel, and the right foot pivoting on the ball of the foot.

● When sweeping and threading the hands, first turn the right hand inward and draw the palm to the right in a small circular motion, and then turn the hand outward and move it to the left passing underneath the left elbow in an arc, and then to the right side of the body, passing the face, the palm facing to the right at shoulder height; turn the left hooked-hand outward and open it, sweep it past the face in a curve to the front of the right shoulder, and turn the left hand inward and lower it to under the inside of the right elbow, the palm facing to the right. The wrists are lowered, the fingers are extended, the webs between the thumbs and index fingers are open, the shoulders are relaxed and the hips are lowered. This movement is adapted from "sweep and brace with palms" from Baguazhang.

● When sweeping the leg and patting the foot, slightly lean the torso forward. Sweep the right leg from the left side of the body upward and to the right in an arc, bend the wrist and then straighten it, sweep the palms from right to left, and pat the top of the right foot. After patting the foot, bend the right knee and lift the leg to the right side of the body.

Common Mistakes

● When turning the body, the body center is lifted, or the torso sways or looses its strength.

● When doing the lotus kick, the head ducks down, the waist bends, or the leg bends.

● After patting the foot, the right leg is not bent with control or kept lifted in a stable manner in a rush to land the foot.

39. Wāngōng Shèhǔ 弯弓射虎 (Draw the Bow to Shoot Tiger)

39.1 Bend the Leg and Draw In the Foot

Draw in the foot, bend the right knee and lift the right leg to the front of the body, the toes lowered, and stand firmly on the left leg; turn the torso to the left; continue to sweep the palms to the left, stopping the left palm by the left side of the body, stop the right hand in front and under the left shoulder, both palms facing downward at the shoulder height. Look at the left hand. (Fig. 186)

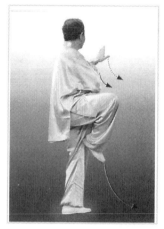

39.2 Turn the Body and Land the Foot

Lower the right foot forward to land on the right side,

Fig. 186

turn the torso to the right; lower both hands in a curve. Look at the hands. (Fig. 187)

39.3 Sweep the Hands and Make Fists

Shift the body center forward, turn the torso to the right; sweep the palms downward and to the right in a curve to the right side of the body, and at this point make fists, the palms of the fists facing downward. Look at the right fist. (Fig. 188)

39.4 Bow Stance and Punch Forward

Turn the torso to the left; bend the right leg and naturally straighten the left leg to form a right bow stance; punch with the left fist forward to the left past the face, the fist at nose level, the palm of the fist slanted forward, and the thumb side of the fist slanted downward; at the same time bend the right elbow and punch with the right fist forward to the left until it reaches the front of the right forehead, the palm of the fist facing outward, and the thumb side of the fist slanted downward. Look at the left fist. (Fig. 189)

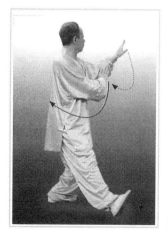

Fig. 187

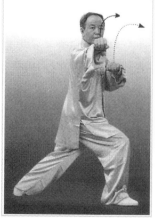

Fig. 188

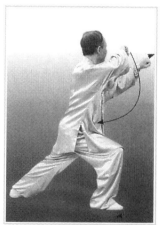

Fig. 189

Important Points

- The direction of landing foot is forward and 45 degrees to the right.

- While turning the body, move the hands downward in a curve, and make fists when they reach the right side of the body, the palms of the fists facing downward, the shoulders relaxed.

- After making fists, bend the arms. Punch with the left fist passing the front of the nose forward to the left, and at the same time punch with the right fist forward and to the left until it reaches the front of the right forehead. Turn both arms inward, fists facing each other.

- On fixing the movement, have the right bow stance directed forward and 45 degrees to the Southeast, turn the torso slightly to the left and lean the torso forward slightly, and turn the head to the direction of the punch.

Common Mistakes

- When punching, the waist is twisted, the hips are turned, the right knee is turned inward, forming a side-bow stance, or the head is tilted to the side when turning the waist.

- The right fist blocks in an upward motion.

- The range of sweeping the palms is not long enough, or the waist and head do not turn to the right with them.

- The right leg bends too much.

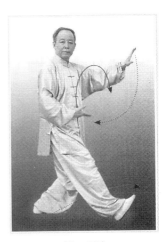

Fig. 190

40. Zuǒ Lǎnquèwoi 左揽雀尾 (Grasp the Peacock's Tail on the Left)

40.1 Turn the Body and Separate the Hands

Shift the body center backward, turn the right toes outward and lift them up, turn the torso to the right; open the fists, extend the left hand to the left; turn the right hand and move it downward in a curve to the waist, the palm facing upward. Turn the head naturally with the body. (Fig. 190)

40.2 Draw In the Foot and "Hold a Ball"

Shift the body center forward, draw the left foot to the inside of the right foot; move the right hand under to the right and then turn and move it upward in a curve; move the left hand downward to the right in a curve, "hold a ball" in front of the chest and abdomen, the palms facing each other. Look at the right hand. (Fig. 191)

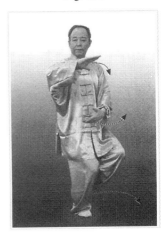

Fig. 191

40.3 Turn the Body and Step Forward

Turn the torso slightly to the left; step forward with the left foot, landing the heel; slightly separate the palms. Look straight ahead. (Fig. 192)

40.4 Bow Stance and Ward Off to the Left

Shift the body center forward, landing the whole left foot to form a left bow stance; ward off forward with the left forearm, the left palm facing the body at shoulder height; push the right hand down to the side of the right hip, the palm facing downward. Look at the left hand. (Fig. 193)

40.5 Turn the Hands and Sweep the Arms

Slightly turn the torso to the left, turn the left palm downward and extend the hand a little forward; turn the right palm upward, and move it upward and forward in a curve, passing the front of the abdomen, and extend it underneath the inside of the left forearm. Look at the left hand. (Fig. 194)

40.6 Back Stance and Roll Back

Turn the torso to the right, shift the body center backward; stroke downward with the palms past the front of the abdomen and then move them backward to the right and upward in a curve, until the right hand is at the shoulder height, the palm slanted forward; bend the left arm and sweep the left hand to the front of the right chest, the palm facing toward the body. Look at the right hand. (Fig. 195)

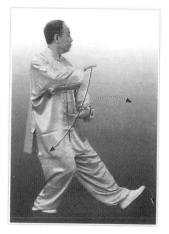

Fig. 192

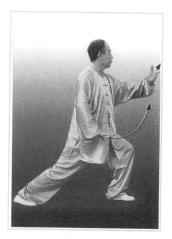

Fig. 193

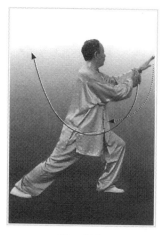

Fig. 194

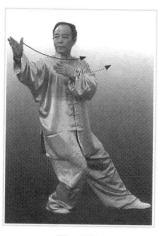

Fig. 195

40.7 Turn the Body and Put the Hands Together

Turn the body to the left to face the front; bend the right elbow and put the right palm and fingers onto the inside of the left wrist; bend the left arm horizontally in front of the chest, the palm facing toward the body, the fingertips pointing to the right. Look straight ahead. (Fig. 196)

40.8 Bow Stance and Press Forward

Shift the body center forward to form a left bow stance; press the arms forward, keep the arms in a circle, rest the right palm and fingers on the inside of the left wrist at the shoulder height. Look at the left forearm. (Fig. 197)

40.9 Back Stance and Draw the Hands

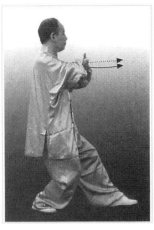

Fig. 196

Extend the right hand outward over the left palm, separating the hands, keeping them at the shoulder height, both palms turned downward; sit back, shift the body center backward, and tilt up the left toes; bend the elbows, draw the palms backward to the front of the chest and then down to the front of the abdomen, the palms facing forward and downward. Look straight ahead. (Fig. 198)

40.10 Bow Stance and Push Forward

Shift the body center forward to form a right bow stance; push the hands parallel upward and forward, the wrists at shoulder height, the palms facing forward, the fingertips pointing upward, the wrist dropped and the hands relaxed. Look straight ahead. (Fig. 199)

Important Points

When turning the body and separating the hands, turn the right toes outward, turn the torso to the right and shift the body center backward all at the same time.

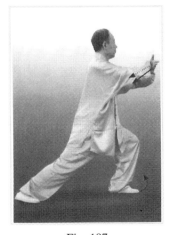
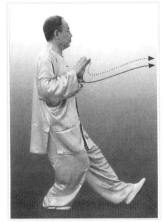
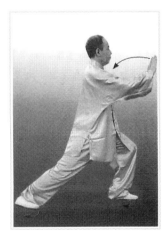

Fig. 197   Fig. 198   Fig. 199

Common Mistake

The body center is not shifted backward with the turning of the body and foot.

41. Shízìshǒu 十字手 (Cross Hands)

41.1 Turn the Body and Turn the Foot Inward

Shift the body center to the right, turn the torso to the right, turn the left toes inward and the right toes outward; with the movement of the body, sweep the right hand to the right to front of the face, the palm facing outward; move the left hand to the left side of the body, the palm also facing outward. Eyes move with the right hand. (Fig. 200)

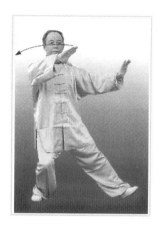

Fig. 200

41.2 Turn the Body and Separate the Hands

Continue to extend the right toes outward, shift the body center to the right, continue to turn the torso to the right, and naturally straighten the left leg; sweep the right hand to the right side of the body, lift the hands to horizontal level at either side of the body, the elbows slightly bent, and the palms facing forward. Eyes move with the right hand. (Fig. 201)

41.3 Turn the Body and Hold the Hands in Embrace

Shift the body center to the left, turn the right toes inward, turn the torso to the left; move the palms downward and toward the body in a curve, cross the hands in front of the abdomen, and lift the hands as if to hold something in front of the chest, the right palm on the outside, and both palms facing toward the body. Look at the hands. (Fig. 202)

41.4 Draw In the Foot and Hold the Hands in Embrace

Draw in the right foot parallel with the left foot at shoulder-width, the toes pointing forward in a feet apart stance; immediately turn the torso to the front, slowly straightening the legs; hold the hands in front of the body, keeping them crossed on a slant, the palms facing toward the body at shoulder height. Look at the hands. (Fig. 203)

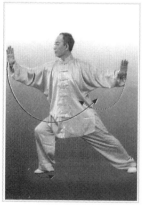

Fig. 201

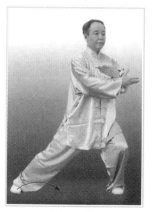

Fig. 202

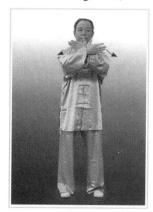

Fig. 203

Important Points

● Do not pause between the movements of shifting the body center to the right, turning the toes, separating the hands and turning the torso to the right. Turn the right toes outward while changing the right leg from empty to solid, so that the movement can be done in a continuous and steady manner.

● When separating the hands and raising them to either side of the body, drop the shoulders and elbows and bend the wrists, the palms facing forward and the fingertips slanted upward.

● When holding the hands, bend the arms in a circle with the right hand on the outside.

Common Mistakes

● There is a break in the movement between shifting the body center to the right and turning the right toes outward.

● When bringing the palms together, the head lowers, the waist bends, and the torso leans forward.

● When holding the palms, the elbows drop, the arms bend too much and the arms are too tight against the body.

42. Shōushì 收势 (Closing Position)

42.1 Separate and Raise the Hands

Turn the forearms inward, turn the hands while separating them so they are parallel and apart at shoulder width, the palms facing forward and downward. Look straight ahead. (Fig. 204)

42.2 Lower the Arms

Slowly lower the hands to either side of the thighs, relax the shoulders and drop the arms, the torso naturally straight. Look straight ahead. (Fig. 205)

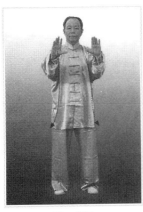 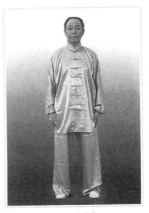

Fig. 204   Fig. 205

42.3 Draw In the Foot and Bring the Feet Together

Draw the left foot to the side of the right foot, feet together, the toes pointing forward, the body naturally straight, breathe naturally and regularly. Look straight ahead. (Fig. 206)

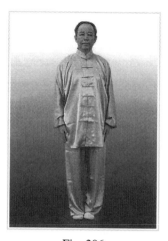

Fig. 206

Important Points

● When separating and raising the hands, turn the arms inward and the palms downward.

● When lowering the arms, lower them slowly with control.

● After bringing the feet together, return to the beginning position.

● Make this a flowing, steady movement.

Common Mistakes

● The closing is done in a manner that is too relaxed, lacking concentration.

● When lowering the arms, the arms are bent, the palms are pressed down, or the chest or abdomen is thrust out.

● When drawing in the foot, the torso leans or sways.

● The feet are brought together with the toes turned outward.

CHAPTER VIII
42-STEP TAIJI SWORD
Sìshíèr Shì Tàijíjiàn 四十二式太极剑

Introduction

Following the creation of 42-Step Taijiquan, the Chinese Martial Arts Research Institute organized experts to create a Taiji sword competition form, which was completed in 1991 as 42-Step Taiji Sword [The sword or jiàn 剑 is a double-edged sword with a tassel attached to its handle.] As a standard competition form, 42-Step Taiji Sword meets all martial arts competition requirements in terms of specifications, number of movements, degree of difficulty and length of time. Original in design and composition, 42-Step Taiji Sword incorporates the cream of Yang-style, Wu (吴)-style, Chen-style and other styles of Taiji sword as well as Wudang Taiji Sword. It also contributes to the traditional spirit of Taiji Sword through gentle, slow and flowing movements that embody stillness in motion (dòng zhōng yù jìng 动中寓静), hardness in gentleness (gangreu xiangjì 刚柔相济) and emphasize the use of mind (yì 意) over physical power(lì 力). The whole set of 42 steps contains 22 kinds of sword techniques, 10 kinds of stances, three ways of exerting power and many kinds of footwork and balanced postures — all arranged in a way that not only makes the form suitable for those interested in athletic competition but also enjoyable for those interested in it as an exercise for general physical fitness. The 42-Step Taiji Sword has been widely welcomed by all Taiji Sword practitioners.

Names of the Movements of 42-Step Taiji Sword

Part I
1. Qǐshì 起势 (Beginning Position)
2. Bìngbù Diǎnjiàn 并步点剑 (Stand with the Feet Together and Point the Sword)

3. Gōngbù Xuējìan 弓步削剑 (Bow Stance and Cut with the Sword)

4. Tíxī Pījiàn 提膝劈剑 (Lift the Knee and Chop with the Sword)

5. Zuǒ Gōngbù Lán 左弓步拦 (Left Bow Stance and Block)

6. Zuǒ Xūbù Liao 左虚步撩 (Left Empty Stance and Slice Upward)

7. Yòu Gōngbù Liao 右弓步撩 (Right Bow Stance and Slice Upward)

8. Tíxī Pongjiàn 提膝捧剑 (Lift the Knee and Hold the Sword)

9. Dēngjiǎo Qiáncì 蹬脚前刺 (Kick and Stab Forward)

10. Tiàobù Píngcì 跳步平刺 (Jump Step and Stab with a Flat Sword)

11. Zhuǎnshēn Xiàcì 转身下刺 (Turn the Body and Stab Downward)

Part II

12. Gōngbù Píngzhǎn 弓步平斩 (Bow Stance and Chop with Flat Sword)

13. Gōngbù Bēngjiàn 弓步崩剑 (Bow Stance and Snap the Sword)

14. Xiēbù Yajiàn 歇步压剑 (Rest Stance and Press the Sword)

15. Jìnbù Jiǎojiàn 进步绞剑 (Step In and Circle to Entwine with the Sword)

16. Tíxī Shàngcì 提膝上刺 (Lift the Knee and Stab Upward)

17. Xūbù Xiàjié 虚步下截 (Empty Stance and Intercept Downward)

18. Zuǒyòu Píngdài 左右平带 (Draw with the Flat Sword Left and Right)

19. Gōngbù Pījiàn 弓步劈剑 (Bow Stance and Chop with the Sword)

20. Dīngbù Tuōjiàn 丁步托剑 (T-Stance and Lift the Sword)

21. Fēnjiǎo Hòudiǎn 分脚后点 (Separate the Feet and Point Backward)

Part III

22. Pūbù Chuanjiàn 仆步穿剑 (Crouch Stance and Thread the Sword)

23. Dēngjiǎo Jiàjiàn 蹬脚架剑 (Kick and Block Up with the Sword)

24. Tíxī Diǎnjiàn 提膝点剑 (Lift the Knee and Point the Sword)

25. Pūbù Héngsǎo 仆步横扫 (Crouch Stance and Sweep to the Side)

26. Gōngbù Xiàjié 弓步下截 (Bow Stance and Intercept Downward)

27. Gōngbù Xiàcì 弓步下刺 (Bow Stance and Stab Downward)

28. Zuǒyòu Yúnmǒ 左右云抹 (Smear the Clouds Left and Right)

29. Gōngbù Pījiàn 弓步劈剑 (Bow Stance and Chop with the Sword)

30. Hòujǔtuǐ Jiàjiàn 后举腿架剑 (Lift the Leg Behind and Block Up with the Sword)

31. Dīngbù Diǎnjiàn 丁步点剑 (T-Stance and Point the Sword)

32. Mǎbù Tuījiàn 马步推剑 (Horse Stance and Push the Sword)

Part IV

33. Dúlì Shàngtuō 独立上托 (Stand on One Foot and Lift Up)

34. Jìnbù Guàdiǎn 进步挂点 (Forward Step, Hook, and Point)
35. Xiēbù Bēngjiàn 歇步崩剑 (Resting Stance and Snap the Sword)
36. Gōngbù Fǎncì 弓步反刺 (Bow Stance and Reverse Stab)
37. Zhuǎnshēn Xiàcì 转身下刺 (Turn the Body and Stab Downward)
38. Tíxī Tíjiàn 提膝提剑 (Lift the Knee and the Sword)
39. Xíngbù Chuānjiàn 行步穿剑 (Walking Step and Thread the Sword)
40. Bǎituǐ Jiàjiàn 摆腿架剑 (Swing Out the Leg and Block Up with the Sword)
41. Gōngbù Zhícì 弓步直刺 (Bow Stance and Stab Straight)
42. Shōushì 收势 (Closing Position)

Movements and Illustrations of 42-Step Taiji Sword

Ready Position
Stand with feet together, toes pointing forward; relax the chest and the back; keep the body straight and let the arms hang naturally at the sides of the body. Change the right hand into the sword-fingers form, with the right palm inward toward the thigh; the left hand holds the sword, with the left palm facing back; the sword is held straight against the back of the left arm, with the tip of the blade upward. Assume that the direction faced is South. Look straight ahead. (Fig. 1)

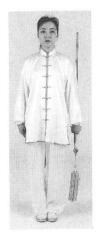

Important Points
Hold the body naturally straight. Lift the head and neck, draw in the chin slightly, relax and lower the shoulders, and breathe naturally. Concentrate.

Fig. 1

Common Mistakes
● The chest is thrust out and the knees are locked, and the body is tense.

● The sword is held on a slant, the blade touches the body.

Part I

1. Qǐshì 起势 (Beginning Position)
1.1 Stand with Feet Apart

Lift the left foot and move it half a step to the left, shoulder-width apart; keep the body center balanced on both feet. At the same time, bend the arms slightly and turn them slightly inward, with each hand 4 inches or about 10 centimeters away from the side of the body. Look straight ahead. (Fig. 2)

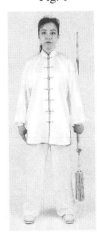

Fig. 2

1.2 Lift the Foot and Hold the Sword

Straighten the arms naturally and draw them to the left front until they reach shoulder height, palms downward; then turn the torso slightly to the right; with the turning of the body swing the right sword-fingers to the right until they reach the right front. Then bend the right elbow and move the right hand in an arc to the front of the abdomen, the right palm upward; the left hand holding the sword swings to the right, then bend the left elbow and move the left hand to the front of the body, with the wrist at shoulder height, the left palm downward; the palms face each other; at the same time, shift the body center to the left and bend the left leg into a half squat. Lift and draw in the right foot to the inside of the left foot. (Do not touch the right foot to the ground.) Look straight ahead. (Figs. 3, 4)

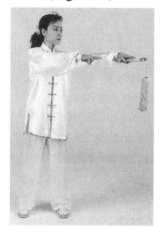

Fig. 3

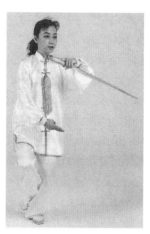

Fig. 4

1.3 Extend the Arms and T-Stance

Move the right foot to the right front (about 45 degrees), at the same time, swing the right sword-fingers to the upper front from below the left arm, bend the right arm slightly, with the wrist at shoulder height and the right palm inward; the left hand holds the sword and touches the inside of the right forearm (the handle of the sword is above the right forearm), the left palm downward. (Fig. 5)

Then, shift the body center to the right leg, the left foot pulls back to the inside of the right foot, with the ball of the left foot touching the ground. At the same time, extend the right sword-fingers to the right front, the palm slanted upward; bend the left elbow and draw the left hand holding

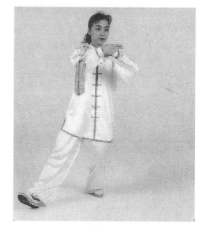

Fig. 5

the sword to the front of the right chest, with the left palm downward. Look in the direction in which the sword points. (Figs. 6, 7)

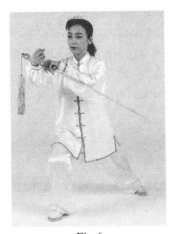
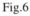

Fig.6

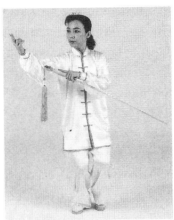

Fig. 7

1.4 Point Forward in Bow Stance

Shift the body center slightly to the left, draw the right toes inward, turn the body to the left (about 90 degrees), step the left foot to the left front, then shift the body center to the front to form a left bow stance; at the same time the left hand holding the sword strokes to the left past the front of the knee in an arc until it reaches the left hip, with the left arm slightly bent, the palm facing backward, the sword straight up and down with the tip of the sword pointed upward; bend the right elbow and move the right sword-fingers past the right ear and point them forward, with the right palm slanted forward, the finger-tips upward and the wrist at shoulder height. Look straight ahead. (Figs. 8, 9)

Important Points

- Coordinate all movements through shifting of the body center and turning the

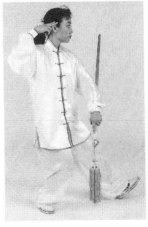

Fig. 8

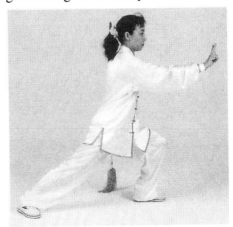

Fig. 9

waist. Keep the torso upright, steady and relaxed. Do not swing the body or let it lean. At the same time, relax and lower the shoulders. Let the arms be relaxed yet energized.

● When executing the bow stance and pointing the sword-fingers, turn the right foot to shift the body center a little in a steady movement. Do not swing the body; be agile and gentle in stepping with the left foot, heel touching the ground first before planting the whole foot as the body center shifts.

● Face South at the beginning, face Southwest when fixing the T-stance, and face due East in the left bow stance.

Common Mistakes

● The arms are stiff.

● The body sways, swings or leans

● The foot drops heavily on the ground when stepping,

● When holding the sword, the ball of the foot that is drawn in touches the ground.

● When the form is fixed, the sword is slanted instead of being held straight up and down.

2. Bìngbù Diǎnjiàn 并步点剑 (Stand with the Feet Together and Point the Sword)

2.1 Step Forward to Thread then Separate the Hands

Shift the body center forward, move the right foot past the inside of the left foot to the right front (about 45 degrees), then shift the body center forward, bend the right leg, lift and draw in the left foot to the inside of the right foot. At the same time, extend the left hand holding the sword past the front of the chest forward until it reaches above the right wrist (The handle of the sword touches the right wrist). Separate the hands to the left and right sides, swing them up, then pull the elbows back, moving the two hands in arcs to the sides of the hips, with the palms downward. Look straight ahead. (Figs. 10, 11, 12)

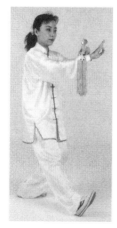 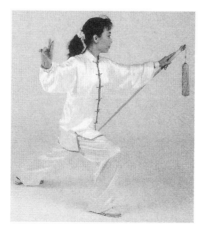 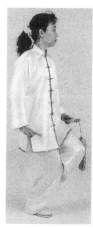

Fig. 10   Fig. 11   Fig. 12

2.2 Bow Stance and Take the Sword

Step the left foot to the left front (about 45 degrees), form a left bow stance with the shift of the body center; at the same time separate and swing the hands to both sides of the body a little higher than shoulder height, then move them in a curve and bring them together in front of the chest; the right palm faces outward, with the arms in an arc, the sword close to the left forearm and the tip of the sword slanted backward; the right hand is placed on the handle of the sword, ready to take the sword. Look straight ahead. (Figs. 13, 14)

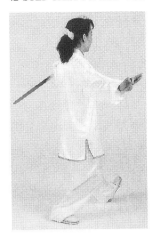

Fig. 13

2.3 Bring the Feet Together and Point the Sword

Shift the body center forward, move the right foot close to the left foot, and bend the knee into a half squat; at the same time the right hand holds the handle. Then using the right wrist as a pivot, raise the tip of the sword in a curve from the left rear of the body to the front. When the tip of the sword reaches the wrist and chest level, raise the right wrist and point down the tip of the sword to the lower front; change the left hand into sword-fingers and touch them to the inside of the right wrist. Look straight ahead. (Figs. 15, 16)

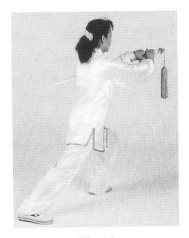

Fig. 14

Important Points

● Coordinate the movements of threading the sword (chuānjiàn 穿剑) with stepping forward; separating and swinging the hands while making a bow stance; and drawing the hands

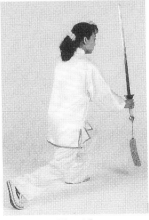

Fig. 15

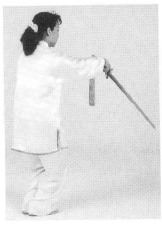

Fig. 16

inward while lifting the foot. Both arms should bend naturally. The sword held in the left hand touches the left forearm naturally from time to time.

- The right hand takes over the sword from the left hand with dexterity and without pause.

- When pointing the sword (diǎnjiàn 点剑), stretch the arm and raise the wrist, lower the shoulders and lift the head, straighten the torso, point the tip of the sword from upper to the lower front, and focus power in the sword tip.

- When moving the feet together, keep the feet parallel and close to each other; bend the legs and lower the hips. Face Northeast.

Common Mistakes

- The step forward is not in the correct direction; the first foot drops heavily and the other foot is drawn in too fast.

- The right hand takes over the sword in a movement that is too hurried, or which pauses.

- When standing with the feet together and pointing the sword, the back bends and the buttocks stick out, the shoulders are shrugged and the elbows raised; the sword is held too tightly, and the power does not focus on the tip of the sword when pointing the sword (diǎnjiàn 点剑) but forms instead a chopping sword (pījiàn 劈剑).

3. Gōngbù Xuējiàn 弓步削剑 (Bow Stance and Cut with the Sword)

3.1 Lower the Sword and Lift the Foot

Shift the body center to the left leg, raise the right heel. At the same time, with the right hand holding the sword, sink the right wrist and turn the right arm, with the palm upward so that the tip of the sword draws a small circle and points to the lower left corner; bend the left elbow and touch the left sword-fingers to the inside of the right forearm, with the left palm to the right and fingertips upward. Look in the direction the tip of the sword points. (Fig. 17)

3.2 Cut on the Diagonal in Bow Stance

Step back with the right foot behind to the right rear, with the heel landing on the ground, bend the right knee when shifting the body center to the right, move the left heel outward to form a right bow stance; turn the body to

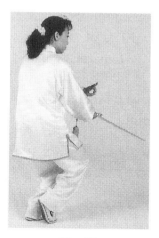

Fig. 17

the right (about 90 degrees); at the same time with the right hand holding the sword cut on the diagonal to the right upper corner, with the wrist at shoulder height and the palm slanted upward; swing the left sword-fingers to the left until they reach the side of the left hip, with the palm slanted downward and fingertips upward. Look in the direction to which the sword points. (Figs. 18, 19)

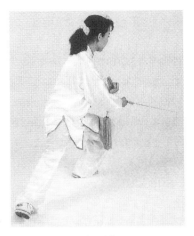

Fig. 18

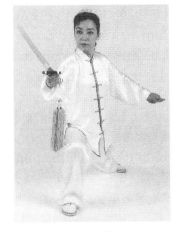

Fig. 19

Important Points

• Be gentle in lowering the sword. Circle the tip of the sword through the sinking of the wrist and the turning of the arm. Bring both hands together in front of the body.

• Stepping-back is a movement that occurs frequently in Taiji Sword and refers to moving one foot a half step directly back or back on the diagonal. For example, when standing with feet together, step one foot a half-step back, or move the front foot a half-step back, and so on. In Gōngbù Xuējiàn (Bow Stance and Cut with the Sword), when pulling back the right foot, land the heel on the ground first, and coordinate the movement with the turning of the waist and the extending of the hips. If beginners have difficulty doing this, they can land the ball of the foot first, then pivot on the heel to turn the foot due South.

• Coordinate the cutting with the turn of the waist, swing of the arm and bow stance. The waist directs the arm and the arm moves the sword, finally the right arm and the sword come to be on the same line, pointing to the upper right above the right leg.

• When cutting with the sword, keep the sword flat and cut from the lower left past the front of the chest to the upper right, with the palm slanted upward, and the sword tip slightly higher than the head. Concentrate the power of the sword along the upper edge of the blade from the handle area to the tip.

Common Mistakes

• Lowering the sword is too stiff, and the circular motion with the sword is too big.

• When stepping back and lowering the foot, the body center becomes unsteady.

• The cutting motion of the sword is not coordinated with the waist and legs. The torso leans forward; the legs move quickly while the hands move slowly; the waist is not coordinated with the movements of the hands; the right arm is not on the same line as the right leg when the sword cuts.

4. Tíxī Pījiàn 提膝劈剑 (Lift the Knee and Chop with the Sword)

4.1 Turn the Waist and Swing the Sword

Bend the left knee, shift the body center backward, and turn the torso slightly to the right, lift the ball of the right foot and turn the right foot outward; at the same time, bend the right elbow and the right hand holding the sword draws a curve backward to the right until it reaches behind the body on the right, with the right palm upward and the right wrist slightly higher than waist level; swing the left sword-fingers forward to the right until they reach the front of the right shoulder, with the left palm slanted downward. The eyes follow the tip of the sword. (Fig. 20)

4.2 Chop with the Sword in One-Leg Stance

Turn the body slightly to the left, shift the body center forward, plant the right foot firmly on the ground, and bend the left knee and raise the left leg to form a right one-leg stance; at the same time, the right hand chops (pījiàn 劈剑) forward with the sword, both the sword and the right arm straight and horizontal to the ground; swing the left sword-fingers in a curve from below to the left and raise them to shoulder height, with the left palm outward and fingertips forward. Look at the tip of the sword. (Fig. 21)

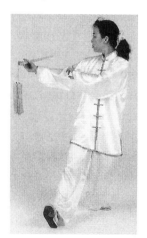

Fig. 20

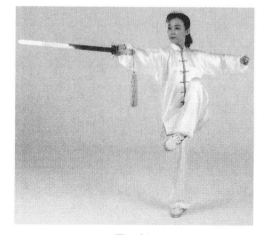

Fig. 21

Important Points

● Coordinate the movements of turning the waist and swinging the sword, of standing on one leg and cutting with the sword.

● When standing on one leg, keep the torso straight, lift the head and keep the lower back straight; bring the left knee up higher than the waist, straighten the ankle with the foot in front of the crotch; stand steadily on the right foot, press the right toes firmly on the ground.

● When cutting with the sword, have the edges of the sword on the vertical and extend the power through the bottom edge of the blade from the handle to the far end. Stretch the right arm straight, lift the left arm to the left side of the body, both arms are at shoulder height. In this movement, the sword chops to the Southwest.

Common Mistakes

● When standing on one leg, the body hunches and the supporting leg is bent, and the body center is unstable.

● The sword-fingers are raised too high or the arm is stretch too far back.

● The wrist is bent to point the sword, confusing the technique of chopping (pī 劈) with the technique of pointing (diǎn 点).

5. Zuǒ Gōngbù Lán 左弓步拦 (Left Bow Stance and Block)

5.1 Step Forward and Circle the Sword

Bend the right knee into a half squat, turn the torso slightly to the left, land the left foot on the ground to the left, with the left heel on the ground; at the same time, the tip of the sword draws a small arc clockwise in front of the body using the right wrist as the pivot; the left sword-fingers move in an arc to the right until they reach the inside of the right forearm, with the left palm downward. Look at the tip of the sword. (Fig. 22)

5.2 Block with the Sword in Bow Stance

Turn the body to the left (about 90 degrees); with the body center moving forward, plant the left foot firmly on the ground, push the right heel outward to form a left bow stance; at the same time, with the turning of the body, move the right hand with the sword up from below to the left front in an arc and block, the right palm is diagonally upward, and the right wrist is at chest level; the left sword-fingers draw a curve up from below to the left until they stop above and in front of the head, with the left arm curved and the left palm diagonally upward. Look at the tip of the sword. (Fig. 23)

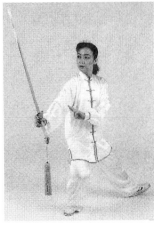
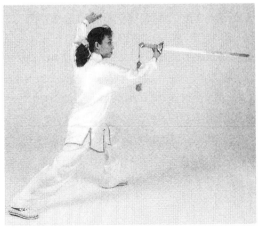

Fig. 22   Fig. 23

Important Points

• Coordinate lowering the foot and stepping forward with moving the sword in a circle; coordinate stepping into bow stance and blocking with the sword.

• Make the bow stance on the diagonal facing Northeast; block with the sword toward the East. Keep the torso relaxed and upright.

• When taking a left step forward, land the left heel on the ground first and keep the body center steady. Beginners who find this difficult can touch the ball of the left foot first, then turn the foot and body and bend the left leg to form a left bow stance.

• Blocking sword (lánjiàn 拦剑) means to block with the bottom edge of the blade forward from a lower position. Slant the blade toward the lower right front; do not bring the handle higher than the head or lower than the chest; do not bring the tip of the sword higher than the chest or lower than the waist. Focus power in the bottom edge of the sword.

Common Mistakes

• The left step forward lands heavily, and lacks balance; the circle made by the sword is too big.

• When blocking with the sword, the sword comes up higher than the head, thus making a lifting the sword (tuōjiàn 托剑); or the sword is flat, forming a slicing upward sword (liāojiàn 撩剑).

• The torso leans or bends forward.

• When the sword-fingers are raised, the left arm is too straight or too bent.

6. Zuǒ Xūbù Liāo 左虚步撩 (Left Empty Stance and Slice Upward)

6.1 Turn the Waist and Raise the Sword

Bend the right knee, shift the body center slightly backward, raise the left toes and turn them slightly outward, and turn the torso to the left. Move the sword upward in an arc. (Fig. 24)

6.2 Step Forward and Circle the Sword

With the body center shifting forward, plant the left foot firmly on the ground, turn the torso slightly to the right, step with the right foot forward to the right, with the right heel landing on the ground. At the same time, with the turning of the body bend the right elbow and move the right hand in an arc up-

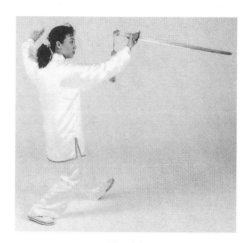

Fig. 24

ward to the left until it reaches the left hip side, the right palm turns inward and the tip of the sword is slanted to the upper rear; drop the left sword-fingers and touch them to the right wrist. Look at the tip of the sword. (Fig. 25)

6.3 Slice the Sword Upward in Empty Stance

Turn the body to the right, move the right toes outward and with the body center shifting forward plant the right foot, bend the right knee into a half squat; step the left foot forward to the left to form a left empty stance; at the same time, the right hand slices upward in a vertical circle with the sword to the left front until the right hand reaches the upper front side of the head, with the right arm slightly bent and the right palm outward and the tip of the sword slightly lower than the hand; touch the left sword-fingers to the right wrist. Look straight forward to the left. (Fig. 26)

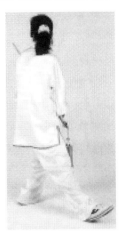

Fig. 25

Important Points

● Coordinate the circular motion of the sword with the turning of the body and the swinging of the arm; coordinate slicing the sword upward with stepping forward to the left. Move the sword in a vertical circle close to the body, and when fixing the form, face the Southeast. Move the body and sword in harmony; the whole sequence should flow.

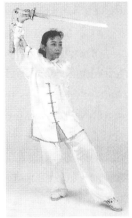

Fig. 26

● The slicing upward sword (liaojiàn 撩剑) is a reverse slice upward. Move the sword upward from below with the edges on the vertical. Focus the power along the bottom edge from the middle to the tip of the sword. If the right arm turns inward, slicing the sword upward is called normal slice upward. If the right arm turns outward, it is reverse slice upward.

Common Mistakes

● The circular motion of the sword is not coordinated with the turning of the body and the swinging of the arm, thus causing instead a swinging to the left and right or a "wrist flower" (extraneous turning of the wrist).

● The slicing upward with the sword is done faster than the movement of the feet.

● The fixed form faces due East.

● The focus of power is misplaced in slicing up the sword, resulting in raising the sword and blocking up.

7. Yòu Gōngbù Liao 右弓步撩 (Right Bow Stance and Slice Upward)

7.1 Step Forward and Circle the Sword

Turn the body slightly to the right, move the left foot to the left, with the left heel landing on the ground; at the same time, move the right hand holding the sword in an arc to the right until it reaches the right upper side of the body, with the right wrist slightly lower than the shoulder, the right arm slightly bent and the tip of the sword pointing upward to the right; bend the left elbow and lower the sword-fingers in front of the right shoulder, with the left palm diagonally downward. Look at the tip of the sword. (Fig. 27)

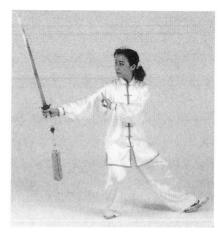

Fig. 27

7.2 Slice the Sword Upward in Bow Stance

Turn the body to the left, with the body center shifting to the left leg, turn the ball of the left foot outward and root it on the ground, then step forward with the right foot, forming a right bow stance as the body center shifts forward. At the same time, the right hand slices the sword with its edges on the vertical upward from below to the front, with the right wrist at shoulder height and the right palm slanted upward and the tip of the sword slightly slanted downward; the left sword-fingers draw a curve downward then upward to the left, with the left arm curved and raised at the upper side of the head, left palm slanted upward. Look at the tip of the sword. (Figs. 28, 29)

Important Points

• Move the circling sword in a vertical circle close to the body. Make a big swing of

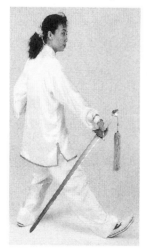

Fig. 28

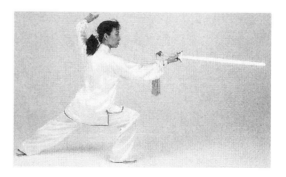

Fig. 29

the arm and turn of the waist, and let the mind and spirit (shén 神) flow with the movements.

● Be steady, agile and gentle in stepping forward. Make a clear difference between the empty and solid.

● Face due East when fixing the movement of slicing the sword upward, focus power on the lower edge of the blade from the middle to the tip.

Common Mistakes

● Moving the sword in a circle is not controlled and directed by the moving of the waist and arms. The vertical circle in which the sword is drawn does not come close enough to the body, and it is not big enough.

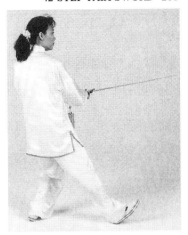

Fig. 30

● The sword moves faster than the leg.

● The slicing upward sword is over-slanted to form instead a blocking sword (lánjiàn 拦剑).

8. Tíxī Pongjiàn 提膝捧剑 (Lift the Knee and Hold the Sword)

8.1 Turn the Waist and Draw the Sword

Bend the left leg into a half squat, shift the body center backward, turn the body slightly to the left; at the same time, with the turning of the body, pull the right hand to the left with the blade flat, the right palm upward, the right wrist at the chest level and the tip of the sword forward to the right; bend the left elbow and drop the left sword-fingers to the right wrist, with the left palm downward. Look at the tip of the sword. (Fig. 30)

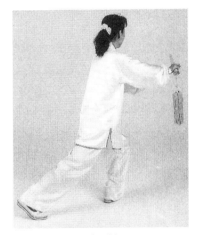

Fig. 31

8.2 Step Back and Draw the Sword

Turn the body slightly to the right, pull back the right foot. With shifting the body center back, form a left empty stance. At the same time with the turning of the body, the right hand holding the sword turns the palm downward. Pull the sword past the front of the body to the right with the blade flat until it reaches the side of the right hip, with the tip forward to the left; move the left sword-fingers downward to the left in an arc until it reaches the side of the hip at the left, with the left palm downward. Look straight ahead. (Figs. 31, 32)

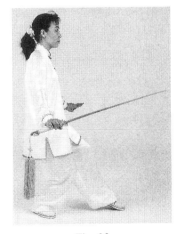

Fig. 32

8.3 Support the Sword in One-Leg Stance

Lift the left foot and then lower it, as the body center shifts forward. The left leg naturally straightens; raise the right knee to form a left one-leg stance; at the same time, turn the two palms upward, as the right knee raises, bring the hands from the sides of the body in front of the chest, place the left sword-fingers under the back of the right hand, at chest level; the tip of the sword points forward, slightly higher than the wrist. Look straight ahead. (Fig. 33)

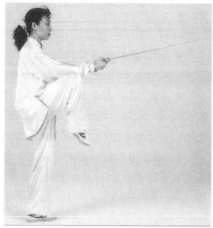

Fig. 33

Important Points

• Drive the arm with the waist and direct the sword with the arm when turning the body to the left or right and drawing the sword. Coordinate the movements of feet, waist, arms and sword. Swing the sword gently and continuously at a steady pace.

• Coordinate supporting the sword with lifting the knee and standing on one foot; lift the knee higher than waist level, and stand steady on one leg.

Common Mistakes

• When drawing the sword to the left, the wrist is twisted and the sword turned to form a "wrist flower" or extraneous turning of the wrist.

• When holding the sword, the sword fingers change into an open-palm hand or are clenched into a fist.

• When bending and lifting the right knee, the toes tilt up, the knee is not lifted high enough, the supporting foot is unsteady, and the torso bends and shrugs.

9. Dēngjiǎo Qiáncì 蹬脚前刺 (Kick and Stab Forward)

9.1 Support the Sword and Draw It Backward

Both hands support the sword and draw it slightly backward. (Fig. 34)

9.2 Kick the Right Foot and Stab Forward

The left leg straightens. Bend the right ankle and then kick the right foot forward with the power focused in the right heel. At the same time, hold the sword in both hands and stab forward with a flat sword. Look at the tip of the sword. (Fig. 35)

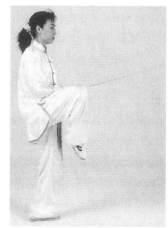

Fig. 34

Important Points

● Tuck in the hips, keep the lower back straight and the torso upright and stretched out when kicking with the right foot. Kick higher than horizontal.

● Draw the sword back to the abdomen; stab at shoulder height. Relax and drop the shoulders; when fixing the form, face due East.

● When stabbing, change the arm from bent to stretched out with the sword and the arm on the same straight line sending power to the tip of the sword. In the movement of stabbing with

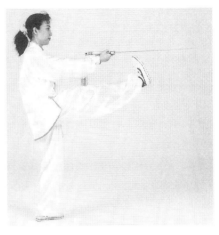

Fig. 35

the sword, the blade can be flat or on the vertical, the direction can be forward, backward, upward or downward.

Common Mistakes

● The torso bends forward or leans backward; the kicking foot is lower than the waist; the body center is unstable.

● When stabbing with the sword, the shoulders shrug to straighten the arm, the whole body is tense.

● The stabbing movement is unclear because the arms move in too small a range.

10. Tiàobù Píngcì 跳步平刺 (**Jump Step and Stab with a Flat Sword**)

10.1 Lower the Right Foot and Extend the Sword Forward

Lower the right foot forward to the ground, and with the body center shifting forward, let the left foot leave the ground. The hands support the sword as they extend forward to stab. (Fig. 36)

10.2 Jump Step and Draw Back the Sword

The right foot stomps the ground for a jump forward, swing the left foot forward and plant it firmly on the ground; with the left leg slightly bent; move the right foot quickly to the inside of the left foot just before the left foot almost touches the ground (Do not touch the right foot to the ground). At the same time, turn both hands inward

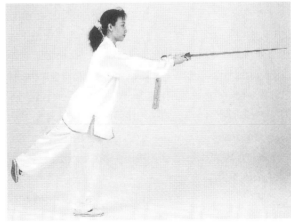

Fig. 36

and draw them back to the sides of the hips, with both palms downward. Look straight ahead. (Fig. 37)

10.3 Stab with the Sword in Bow Stance

Step the right foot forward to form a right bow stance; at the same time, the right hand stabs forward past the waist with the flat blade of the sword, with the right wrist at chest level, the right palm upward and the power focusing on the tip of the sword; the left sword-fingers draw an arc past the left side upward and forward, with the left arm curved and raised at the upper side of the head. The left palm is diagonally upward. Look at the tip of the sword. (Fig. 38)

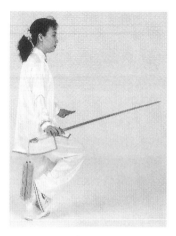

Fig. 37

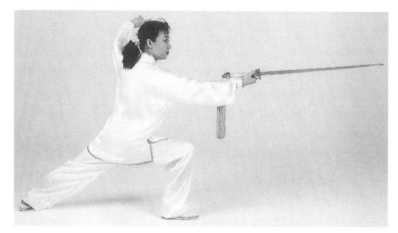

Fig. 38

Important Points

• When doing the jump step, there should be a moment when both feet leave the ground. Do not jump too high, but also don't walk.

• Lower the right foot to the ground a reasonable distance; when landing the left foot, land the ball of the foot first, then root the whole foot, and bend the left leg to buffer the reverse thrust. After drawing in the right foot to the inside of the left foot, stop the right foot for a very short moment, then step forward and stab with the flat sword.

Common Mistakes

• When doing the jump step, both feet fail to leave the ground, thus forming a walking step.

• The right foot lands too far out and too heavily. When the left foot lands, the knee does not bend as a buffer. The right foot is not drawn in and lifted tight enough and the body is unsteady.

• The movements of the hands and feet are not coordinated. The right arm does not stretch far enough when stabbing, or the sword handle does not come from the waist.

11. Zhuǎnshēn Xiàcì 转身下刺 (Turn the Body and Stab Downward)

11.1 Draw Back the Sword in Back Stance

Bend the left knee, shift the body center backward; the right leg is naturally straight, raise the ball of the right foot. At the same time, pull the right hand to the left and then to the right with the flat sword, bend the elbow and draw the sword back to the front of the chest, with the right palm upward; bend the left elbow and put the left sword-fingers in front of the chest, with the left palm downward; the blade is flat and touches under the left forearm, and the hands face each other on a slant. Look straight ahead. (Fig. 39)

11.2 Lift the Foot and Turn the Body

Turn the ball of the right foot inward and touch it to the ground, shift the body center to the right leg; taking the ball of the right foot as a pivot, spin the body around to the left rear (about 270 degrees); bend the left knee and raise it and draw the left foot to the inside of the right foot (Do not touch the left foot to the ground), both hands come together at the right side of the waist. Look straight ahead to the left. (Fig. 40)

11.3 Stab Downward in Bow Stance

Lower the left foot forward to the left to form a left bow stance. At the same time, the right hand stabs with the flat sword downward to the left front, with the right palm upward; move the left sword-fingers in an arc upward to the left above the front of the head, with the left arm curved and the left palm diagonally upward. Look at the tip of the sword. (Fig. 41)

Important Points

• When drawing back the sword, turn the waist, bend the arm and move the sword; after drawing the sword, turn to face due East.

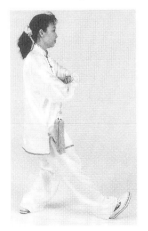 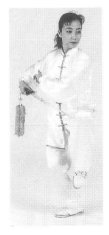 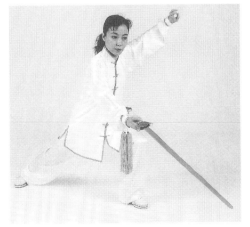

Fig. 39   Fig. 40   Fig. 41

• Lift the knee and turn the body in a steady and continuous way with agility, and keep the torso straight.

• When making the bow stance and stabbing with the sword, coordinate the movements of the hands and feet; when fixing the form, lean the torso slightly forward, to the Southeast.

Common Mistakes

• When turning the body, the torso bends forward or leans backward; the left lower leg relaxes and turns out.

• When executing the bow stance and stabbing with the sword, the stab does not come out from the waist.

Part II

12. Gōngbù Píngzhǎn 弓步平斩 (Bow Stance and Chop with the Flat Sword)

12.1 Draw In the Foot and Bring the Hands Together with the Sword

Shift the body center forward, raise and draw in the right foot to the inside of the left foot. (Do not touch the foot on the ground.) At the same time, sink the right wrist, and the right palm is diagonally upward; bend the left elbow and put the left sword-fingers over the right forearm. Look at the tip of the sword. (Fig. 42)

12.2 Cut with a Flat Sword in Side-Bow Stance

Step the right foot backward to the right, turn the left foot inward to form a right side-bow stance; turn the body to the right (about 90 degrees); at the same time the right hand stabs with a flat sword to the right; move the left sword-fingers to the left and raise them at the side of the body to a level slightly lower than the chest, with the left palm to the left and fingers forward. Look at the tip of the sword. (Fig. 43)

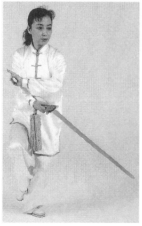

Fig. 42

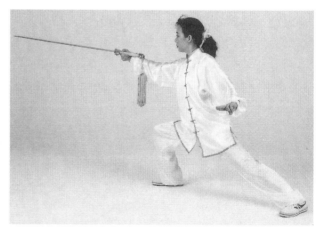

Fig. 43

Important Points

● A horizontal cut with the sword (zhǎnjiàn 斩剑) is made with the blade flat and moving to the left or right with power focused on the blade of the sword, at neck level. In this form, cut with the flat blade from left to right, with the right palm upward, pointing to the Southwest. The legs are in a side-bow stance (cègōngbù 侧弓步) (or hips sideways stance héngdangbù 横裆步).

● In the side-bow stance, have both feet parallel pointing forward or slightly in the Chinese character for "eight" (八) shape; pull the hips apart and turn the torso slightly. One leg is bent with the knee and the toes almost on the same line; the other leg is naturally straight.

Common Mistakes

● The chopping with a flat sword (píngzhǎn 平斩) is done in the manner of slicing on the diagonal (xuē 削) or snapping the sword flat (píngbēngjiàn 平崩剑).

● The horizontal cut in side-bow stance or hips sideways stance is done instead in a bow stance with the body turned toward the West.

● The left sword-fingers are raised too high.

13. Gōngbù Bēngjiàn 弓步崩剑 (Bow Stance and Snap the Sword)

13.1 Turn the Body and Swing the Sword

Shift the body center to the left, and turn the body to the left; with the turning of the body, bend the right elbow holding the sword and pull the sword to the left with the handle leading first until it reaches the front of the face, and palm faces backward; move the left sword-fingers in an arc to the left until they reaches the left hip side, with the left palm downward and fingertips forward. Look at the right hand. (Fig. 44)

13.2 Back Cross Step and Bring the Sword to the Right

Continue to shift the body to the right, extend the left foot past the back of the right foot to the right to form a cross stance (jiaochabù 交叉步); at the same time turn the right hand inward until the right palm faces downward after the right hand pulls the sword to the left, then the right hand pulls the sword back to the right, the right

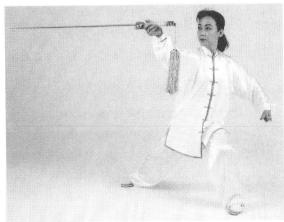

Fig. 44

wrist is at the chest level, the right arm is naturally straight, with the tip of the sword forward
at shoulder height; move the left sword-fingers
to the left and raise it to the head level, with the
left palm outward and fingertips forward. Look
at the right side. (Fig. 45)

13.3 Lift the Leg and Support the Sword

Shift the body center to the left leg, bend
the right knee and raise the right leg; at the
same time, move the two forearms inward in
curves and bring them together in front of the
abdomen, with the palms turned up and the tip
of the sword forward; the left sword-fingers are
placed under the back of the right hand. Look
straight ahead. (Fig. 46)

13.4 Snap the Sword in Bow Stance

Drop the right foot to the right to form a right
bow stance, and turn the torso slightly to the right;
at the same time, move the right hand to the right
and hold the sword flat (píngbēng 平崩), vibrate
the right wrist to exert power, sending the power
to the tip of the sword with the right wrist at shoulder height and the tip of the sword higher than the
right wrist. Keep the right arm slightly bent, with
the right palm upward; extend the left sword-fingers to the left and stop at the side of
the left hip with the left palm downward. Look at the tip of the sword.
(Fig. 47)

Important Points

● This movement originates from
Wudang Sword. The whole movement
requires continuity, agility and coordination of the waist, legs, arms and the
sword. It also involves exerting power
in the snapping of the sword (bēngjiàn
崩剑). To accomplish this, turn the

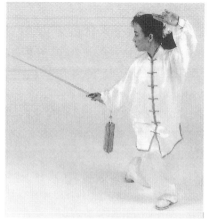

Fig. 45

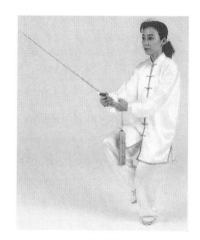

Fig. 46

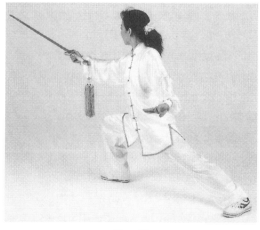

Fig. 47

waist, sink the hips, drop the elbow and snap the wrist to focus the movement on the tip of the sword in a burst of power.

• Steps move in a diagonal direction from the Southeast to Northwest. When fixing the form, face Northwest in the bow stance.

• Do not stop after extending the left foot past the back of the right foot to the right; when bending and raising the right leg and supporting the sword with both hands, do not stop so that it changes into standing on one leg.

• Snapping sword (bēngjiàn 崩剑) means to point and attack upward or to the right, focusing the power on the tip of the sword. When the tip points up, the technique is called snapping up; when the tip points to the right, it is called snapping flat.

Common Mistakes

• The movements are not continuous, but stop during the process.

• The body center rises and falls too much.

• The movements of the waist and the arms are not coordinated, the sword is pulled only with the arms, not with the turning of the waist.

• The effort to exert power is stiff and incomplete so that the power does not reach the tip of the sword.

14. Xiēbù Yājiàn 歇步压剑 (Resting Stance and Press the Sword)

14.1 Back Cross Step and Raise the Sword

Turn the body to the left, shift the body center to the left leg; extend the right foot to the back of the left foot, with the front ball of the right foot landing on the ground; at the same time move the right hand in an arc past the top to the left, and turn the right palm downward. Look straight ahead to the Southwest. (Fig. 48)

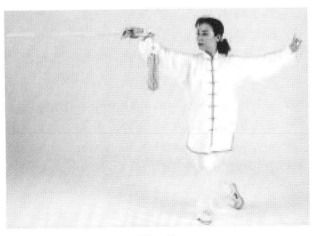

Fig. 48

14.2 Press the Sword in Resting Stance

Bend the two knees and crouch into a resting stance (xiēbù 歇步); at the same time, press the sword down with the right hand with the right arm slightly bent and the right wrist at the right knee level; move the left sword-fingers in an arc upward, with the left arm curved at the upper side of the

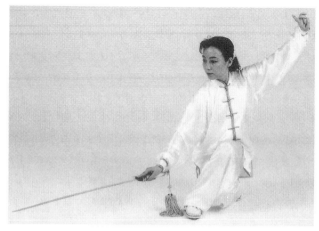

Fig. 49

head, left palm slanted upward. Look at the tip of the sword. (Fig. 49)

Important Points

• Pressing the sword involves pressing down on the opponent's attack by moving the flat sword from up to down with the power in the flat blade and with the tip of the sword forward. When doing resting stance and pressing the sword here, turn to Southwest with the blade about 4 inches or 10 centimeters away from the ground. Relax and lower the shoulders and elbows, lean the torso slightly forward.

• When stepping behind to the side (chābù 插步) and raising the sword, turn the left heel first inward, and extend the right foot to the left; at the same time, holding the sword in the right hand, draw a small curve upward from the right to the left, and rotate and raise the sword to the front of the head.

• In the resting stance, place the back knee to the outer side of the back of the front knee; keep the legs close to each other, sit the hips close to the rear heel.

Common Mistakes

• The stance is not steady, and the ball of the front foot is not turned outward.

• When pressing the sword, the sword is too far away from the body, the tip of the sword is diagonally downward, and the power is not on the blade.

15. Jìbù Jiǎojiàn 进步绞剑 (Step In and Circle to Entwine with the Sword)

15.1 Lift the Sword in Empty Stance

Turn the body slightly to the right, stretch out the legs with a heel stomp, bend the left knee, and step the right foot forward to form a right empty stance; at the same time, the right hand holds the sword with the "tiger's mouth" (hǔkǒu 虎口, the web between the thumb and the index finger) towards the upper front, raise the sword with the edges of the blade on the vertical, the right wrist at shoulder height and the tip of the sword slightly lower than the wrist; move the left sword-fingers in an arc forward and touch them to the inside of the right forearm, with the left palm downward. Look down to the front. (Fig. 50)

15.2 Step Forward to Entwine with the Sword

Move the right foot forward, with the whole foot landing on the ground; shift the body center forward; at the same time, the right hand makes a circle to entwine with the sword; move the left sword-fingers downward to the left in an arc and then raise them at the side of the body, with the left wrist slightly higher than the shoulder, the left palm outward, the left fingertips forward and the left arm curved. Look at the tip of the sword. (Fig. 51)

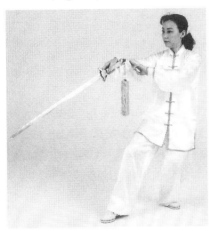

Fig. 50

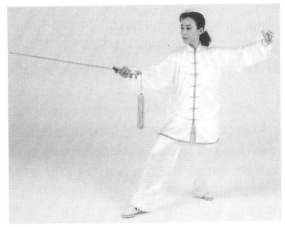

Fig. 51

15.3 Step Forward to Entwine with the Sword

Step the left foot forward, shift the body center forward; raise the right heel up; at the same time the right hand again makes a circle to entwine with the sword; keep the left sword-fingers in the same position. Look at the tip of the sword. (Fig. 52)

15.4 Entwine with the Sword in Bow Stance

Step the right foot forward to form a right bow stance; at the same time, the right hand continues to circle with the sword and push forward; raise the left sword-fingers forward and touch them to the right

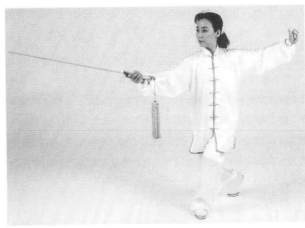

Fig. 52

forearm, with the left palm downward. Look at the tip of the sword. (Fig. 53)

Important Points

● Make the steps forward gentle, agile and steady. Do not let the body center go up and down. In this form, move forward continuously for three steps. With each step make one sword movement to entwine. The three continuous steps are

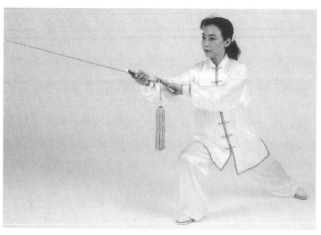

Fig. 53

all done in the direction of the Southwest. Coordinate stepping forward with circling to entwine with the sword.

● Circle to entwine with the sword (jiǎojiàn 绞剑) is to draw a counter-clock-wise circle in front of the chest with a flat sword, the palm upward, the tip of the sword forward, and the power placed on the front part of the blade. When entwining with the sword, keep the wrist relaxed and flexible so that the wrist, too, draws a circle.

Common Mistakes

● When stepping forward, the body center goes up and down in an unsteady motion.

● The entwining with the sword is very stiff with the sword grasped so tightly that the handle can't move in the palm. This makes the tip of the sword move too much.

● When doing the last entwining with the sword, a stabbing forward is added.

16. Tíxī Shàngcì 提膝上刺 (Lift the Knee and Stab Upward)

16.1 Turn the Waist and Draw In the Sword

Shift the body center backward, turn the torso slightly to the left, bend the left knee into a half squat, and bend the right knee slightly; at the same time, bend the right elbow and draw the sword back with the right hand to the left side of the abdomen, the right palm upward and the sword flat and straight, and the tip of the sword is forward; touch the left sword-fingers to the handle of the sword. Look straight ahead. (Fig. 54)

16.2 Stab Upward in One-Leg Stance

Shift the body center forward, turn the body slightly to the right, the right leg is naturally straight, bend the left knee and raise it to form a right one-leg stance; at the same time, the right hand holds the sword to stab upward to the front, with the right palm upward and left sword-fingers touching the inside of the right forearm. Look at the tip of the sword. (Fig. 55)

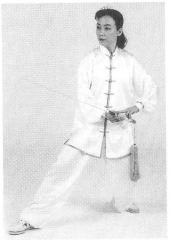

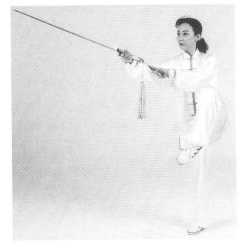

Fig. 54   Fig. 55

Important Points

● Point the direction of the stabbing sword (cìjiàn 刺剑) diagonally toward the upper corner, with the tip of the sword slightly higher than the head. Keep the torso upright and relaxed.

● When standing on one-leg, keep the body center stable, bend and raise the right knee to a level higher than the waist.

● When fixing the form, face Southwest.

Common Mistakes

● When turning the body and withdrawing the sword, the ball of the right foot lifts up, the torso turns too much. When withdrawing the sword, the sword moves in an arc to the left.

● When standing on one leg and stabbing upward, the body bends and shrugs, the body is tense and unstable.

17. Xūbù Xiàjié 虚步下截 (Empty Stance and Intercept Downward)

17.1 Land the Foot and Pull the Sword

Bend the right knee into a half squat; drop the left foot to the left, with the heel landing on the ground, and turn the torso slightly to the left; at the same time, with the turning of the body, bend the right elbow and turn the right hand outward and pull the sword to the upper left, with the right palm inward, the right wrist at the head level and the tip of the sword to the right; move the left sword-fingers in an arc downward to the left until it reaches the left hip side, with the left palm slanted downward. Look to the right. (Fig. 56)

17.2 Empty Stance and Intercept Downward

With the body center shifting to the left, plant the left foot firmly on the ground, bend the left knee into a half squat, and turn the torso to the right, move the right foot half a step to the left and touch the ball of the right foot to the ground to form a right empty stance; at the same time, with turning of the body the right hand pulls the sword slightly to the left then intercept with it to the right below until the sword reaches the right hip side, with the tip of the sword to the left at the right knee level, the power goes to the lower part of the blade; the left sword-fingers points upward, the left arm is bent into an arc at the upper side of the head and the left palm is diagonally upward. Look to the right side. (Fig. 57)

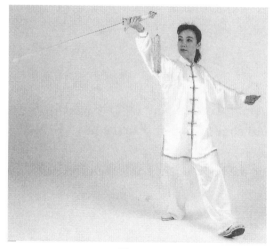 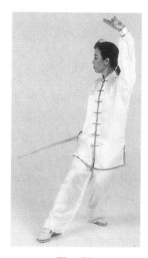

Fig. 56   Fig. 57

Important Points

• Lower the left foot in the direction of Southeast; fix the empty stance in the direction of Southwest, turn the head to the Northwest.

• Coordinate pulling the sword with the turning of the waist and lowering of the foot; coordinate intercepting with the sword with the movements of turning the waist and empty stance.

• Intercepting sword (jiéjiàn 截剑) is to use the blade to intercept the opponent's attack. The direction of intercepting can be upward, downward, forward or backward. The edges of the blade can be vertical or horizontal. The power goes to the lower blade.

Common Mistakes

● The direction is wrong in landing the foot and making the stance.

● When intercepting with the sword, the sword drops straight to become a chopping sword (pījiàn 劈剑).

● The intercepting with the sword is not coordinated with the empty stance. The feet move faster than the hands.

● When fixing the form, the torso leans to the right, the eyes look down.

18. Zuǒyòu Píngdài 左右平带 (Draw the Flat Sword Left and Right)

18.1 Lift the Knee and Extend the Sword Forward

Bend the left knee slightly, bend and raise the right knee, with the toes of the right foot dropping down; at the same time the right hand extends forward with the blade on the vertical, the right hand at the chest level, the right arm naturally straight and the sword tip slightly lower than the right hand; the left sword-fingers move forward from the top and touch the inside of the right forearm. Look at the tip of the sword. (Fig. 58)

18.2 Draw the Sword to the Right in Bow Stance

Move the right foot forward to the right, turn the torso slightly to the right to form a right bow stance. At the same time the right hand moves forward with the sword, turn the right palm downward, then bend the right elbow and pull the sword backward to the right until the sword reaches the front of the right ribs, with the tip of the sword slanted forward; the left sword-fingers still touch the inside of the right forearm. Look at the tip of the sword. (Fig. 59)

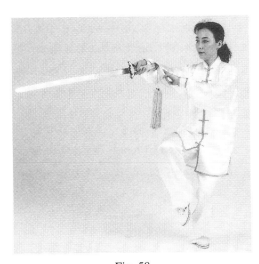

Fig. 58

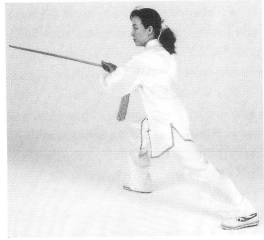

Fig. 59

18.3 Draw In the Foot and Extend the Sword Forward

With the body center shifting forward, withdraw the left foot to the inside of the right foot; at the same time, draw the sword back with the right hand. (Fig. 60)

18.4 Draw the Sword to the Left in Bow Stance

Then extend the sword forward; the left foot steps forward to the left, shift the body center forward to form a left bow stance; at the same time turn the forearm outward with the palm upward, and bend the right elbow and pull the sword backward to the left until it reaches the left ribs, with the sword tip slanted upward; move the left sword-fingers upward to the left from below until they reach the upper side of the head, with the left arm curved and the left palm slanted upward. Look straight ahead. (Fig. 61)

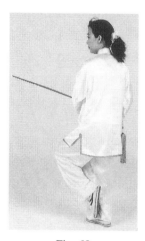

Fig. 60

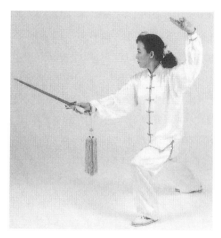

Fig. 61

Important Points

● Drawing sword (dàijiàn 带剑) refers to withdrawing and slashing with the flat sword from front to the diagonal rear. The power focus shifts from the back to the front along the edge of the blade. When pulling with the sword, the arm is stretched first, then bent, the wrist no higher than chest level, and the tip of the sword points forward diagonally. With the bending and bowing forward of the leg, pull back the sword to the right or left. Coordinate the movements of bow stance and pulling back the sword.

● The direction of the bow stance is on the diagonal toward front; draw the sword back slanted toward the rear. Keep the tip of the sword moving near the midline, do not swing the tip left and right too much.

Common Mistakes

● Pulling back the sword is not done correctly but rather is done in the manner of sweeping to the left or right (zuǒyòu sǎobǎi 左右扫摆), or pushing forward to the left or right (zuǒyòu qiántuī 左右前推).

- When fixing the form, the torso bends and the head is lowered.
- When extending the sword forward, the right hand turns too early.

19. Gōngbù Pījiàn 弓步劈劍 (Bow Stance and Chop with the Sword)

19.1 Turn the Torso and Intercept Downward

With the body center shifting forward, move the right foot forward, bend the right knee into a half squat; the left leg is naturally straight with the heel lifted; turn the torso to the right; at the same time, the right hand intercepts down to the right rear with the sword; bend the left elbow and put the left sword-fingers in front of the right shoulder, with the left palm slanted downward. Look at the tip of the sword. (Fig. 62 front and rear views)

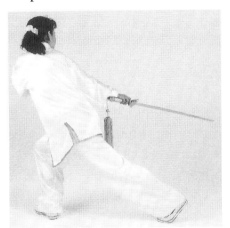 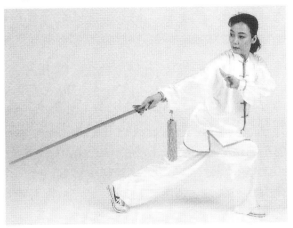

Fig. 62

19.2 Chop with the Sword in Bow Stance

Turn the torso to the left, move the left foot forward to make a left bow stance; at the same time bring the sword in the right hand over the top of the head and chop forward at shoulder height; move the left sword-fingers in an arc from below to the upper left until they are above the left side of the head, with the left arm curved and the palm slanted outward. Look forward. (Fig. 63)

Important Points

- When turning the body and intercepting down, move forward and turn the body to form a cross step. The sword moves in a hori-

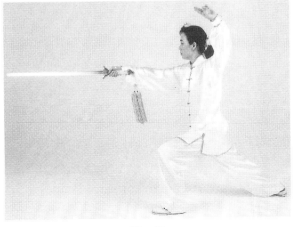

Fig. 63

zontal curve to the lower right rear, turn the palm downward with the right arm and the sword on the same diagonal line.

- Do the whole sequence without pause. Coordinate bow stance with chopping with the sword, facing due West.

Common Mistakes

- The movements of turning the body and intercepting down are done in a manner of back cross stance (chābù 叉步) and reverse slicing sword (fǎnliāo 反撩), the palm is turned backward, and the sword is moved in a vertical circle; or when doing the movements of cross stance and moving the foot, the waist is not turned enough, the torso leans forward and the head is lowered.

- There's a pause after doing intercepting down with sword.

- The chopping sword is not straight on the horizon, but is slanted downward.

20. Dīngbù Tuōjiàn 丁步托剑 (**T-Stance and Lift the Sword**)

20.1 Lift the Knee and Intercept to the Rear

With shifting the body center forward, bend the right knee and lift it up to form a one-leg stance; turn the torso to the right and lean slightly forward; at the same time the right hand intercepts down with the sword (jiéjiàn 截剑) to the right rear; bend the left elbow and move the left sword-fingers to the front of the right shoulder, with the left palm downward. Look at the tip of the sword. (Fig. 64 front and rear views)

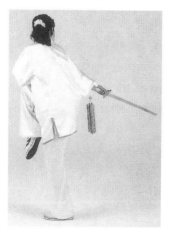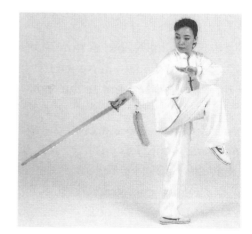

Fig. 64

20.2 Lift the Sword in T-Stance

Move the right foot forward, bend the right knee into a half squat, the left foot follows up to the inside of the right foot, and touch the left toes to the ground to form a left T-stance; at the same time bend the right elbow and lift the sword up, with the tip of the sword to the right; put the left sword-fingers at the inside of the right wrist, with the left palm forward. Look to the right. (Fig. 65)

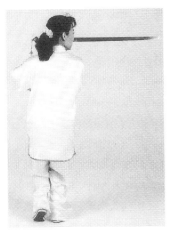

Important Points

● Lifting sword (tuōjiàn 托剑) means to lift the sword and block from the lower to the higher position with the edges of the blade on the vertical, the palm inward, the wrist at head level and the strength in the bottom edge of the blade

● Lean the torso forward slightly when raising the knee and intercepting (jiéjiàn 截剑) to the rear with the sword. Do all the movements without pause, and do not

Fig. 65

straighten the left supporting leg too much when lifting the right knee. Slant the intercepting sword down to the lower right, North by East.

● When fixing the lifting sword movement, face North. In the T-stance, bend the right knee into a half squat, and touch the ball of the left foot on the ground gently at the inside of the right foot.

Common Mistakes

● The movements of raising the knee and intercepting (jiéjiàn截剑) to the rear are done in a manner of slicing to the rear (hòuliáo 后撩) in a vertical circle.

● When raising the knee and intercepting to the rear, there is a pause in the process.

● When lifting the sword, the elbow is not bent and raised. Lifting the sword is done in the manner of pulling the sword from the rear to the left.

● Lifting the sword is not coordinated with the T-stance.

21. Fēnjiǎo Hòudiǎn 分脚后点 (Separate the Feet and Point Backward)

21.1 Turn In the Feet and Turn the Torso

Move the left foot forward to the left, with the ball of the left foot turned inward, bend the left knee slightly and turn the torso to the right (about 90 degrees). Taking the ball of the right foot as an axis, turn the right heel inward, bend the right knee slightly; move the tip of the sword in the right hand down in an arc downward to the right until the right wrist reaches shoulder height, with the palm slanted upward and tip of the sword slanted downward; the left sword-fingers are still on the right wrist. Look at the tip of the sword. (Fig. 66)

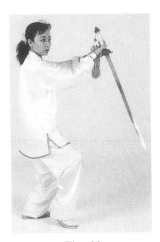

Fig. 66

21.2 Step Back and Thrust the Sword

Pull the right foot backward and straighten the right leg naturally, pivoting on the left heel, turn the ball of the left foot inward, bend the left knee into a half squat, and turn the body to the right (about 90 degrees); at the same time with the tip of the sword in the lead, the right hand thrusts (chuan 穿) the sword down to the rear in a curve until the right hand reaches the front of the abdomen, with the right palm outward, the tip of the sword to the right and slightly lower than the wrist; still with the left sword-fingers on the right wrist. Look at the tip of the sword. (Fig. 67)

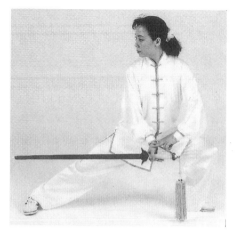

Fig. 67

21.3 Thrust the Sword in Bow Stance

As the body center shifts forward, bend the right knee to form a right bow stance; turn the torso slightly to the right; at the same time the right hand moves the sword forward along the inner edge of the right leg to stab (cì 刺) at shoulder height; the left sword-fingers move to the left rear in an arc until they reach shoulder height, with the palm outward. Look at the tip of the sword. (Fig. 68)

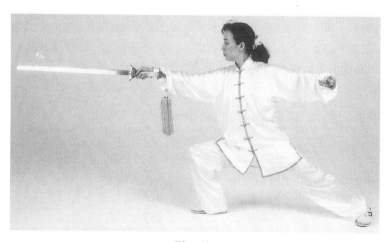

Fig. 68

21.4 Bring the Feet Together and Circle the Sword

While shifting the body center forward, move the left foot close to the right foot, bend both legs in a half squat, and turn the torso slightly to the left; at the same time, the right hand moves upward with the handle in the lead to the left in a curve until the right hand reaches the left side of the hip, with the palm inward and the tip of the sword to the upper left; the left sword-fingers move upward in a curve, after the left hand meets the right hand at the side of the head, bend the left elbow and lower the left sword-fingers and put them on the inside of the right wrist. Look to the left rear. (Fig. 69)

21.5 Lift the Knee and the Sword

Straighten the left leg naturally; bend the right knee and raise it, with the toes of the right foot dropping naturally; turn the torso to the right (about 90 degrees); at the same time the right hand moves the tip of the sword in a vertical circle at the left side of the body until it reaches the lower rear, then turn the right forearm inward, with the handle in the lead, pull the sword upward until the handle reaches above the front of the head,

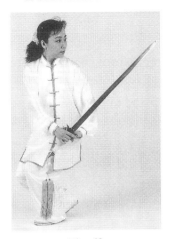

Fig. 69

with the palm to the right and the tip of the sword to the lower front; turn the left sword-fingers outward, extend them to the lower front until they reach the front of the inside of the right ankle, with the palm forward and upward. Look straight ahead. (Fig. 70)

21.6 Separate the Feet and Point Back with the Sword

Kick the right foot forward to separate the feet (fēnjiǎo 分脚) [a basic kicking technique of Taijiquan with power focused on the toes, see also movement 30 in 81-Step Taijiquan]; at the same time turn the torso to the right, with the turning of the body the right hand moves past the top of the head to the right rear and points with the sword (diǎnjiàn 点剑) with the wrist at shoulder height; move the left sword-fingers upward to the left, with the left arm curved above the side of the head, palm slanted upward. Look at the tip of the sword. (Fig. 71 front and rear views)

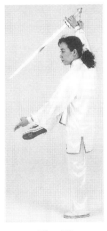

Fig. 70

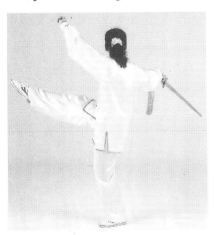
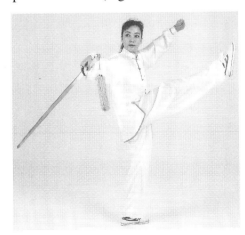

Fig. 71

Important Points

● Coordinate the bow stance with thrusting (chuan 穿) and stabbing (cì 刺) with the sword; coordinate the lifting of the knee with the pulling up of the sword; coordinate the separating of the feet with the pointing back with the sword. Pull and circle the sword up in a vertical circle. Be continuous and agile in pivoting on the heel, turning the body, pulling back the foot and bending the knee.

● Do all the movements with agility and without pause.

● When fixing the form, keep the torso upright, the separated foot is to the due West, the pointing sword is to the Northeast.

Common Mistakes

● Movements are stiff, with pauses in the shifts and without good balance.

● When thrusting and jabbing with the sword, the bow stance is done in a manner of crouch stance.

● When drawing one foot close to the other and moving the sword in a circle, the torso is not turned to the left, and the sword is not close to the body.

● When pulling the sword up, the sword-fingers are too close to the blade, forming a stroking sword (lǚjiàn 捋剑).

● When separating the feet and pointing with the sword, the body leans back with the hips thrust out, the sword-fingers are not held high but instead are stretched to the side of the body.

Part III

22. Pūbù Chuanjiàn 仆步穿剑 (Crouch Stance and Thread the Sword)

22.1 Bow Stance and Swing the Sword

Bend the left knee into a half squat, bend the right knee and move the right leg backward to form a left bow stance; at the same time turn the torso to the left, with the turning of the body the right hand moves the sword in an arc to the front of the body, with the wrist at the chest level, the palm upward, flat blade and tip of the sword forward; lower the left sword-fingers, bend the left elbow and touch the sword-fingers to the inside of the right forearm, with the palm downward. Look at the tip of the sword. (Fig. 72)

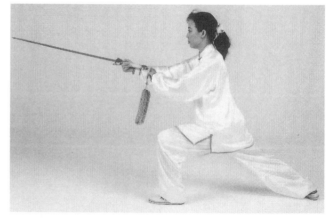

Fig. 72

22.2 Turn the Body and Cut with the Sword to the Right

Shifting the body center backward and pivoting on both feet, turn the body to the right (about 90 degrees) to form a right side-bow stance; at the same time the right hand cuts with the sword past the front of the chest to the right, bend the right arm slightly, with the palm upward and the tip of the sword slightly higher than the wrist; separate the left sword-fingers from the right forearm to stretch and raise them to waist level at the left side of the body, with the left arm slightly bent and palm outward. Look at the tip of the sword. (Fig. 73)

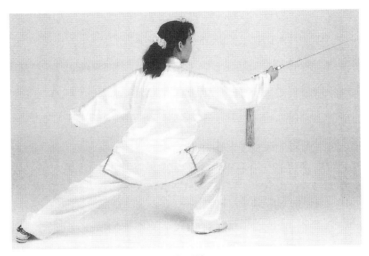

Fig. 73

22.3 Side-Bow Stance and Raise the Sword

Shift the body center to the left to form a left side-bow stance; turn the torso slightly to the left; at the same time bend the right arm and draw the sword back until the right hand reaches the upper front of the head, with the palm inward, blade flat and tip of the sword to the right; move the left sword-fingers up and touch them to the inside of the right wrist, with the left arm curved and the palm forward. Look at the tip of the sword. (Fig. 74)

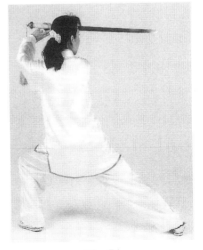

22.4 Crouch Stance and Thread the Sword

Bend the left knee into a squat to form a right crouch stance (pūbù 仆步), turn the torso slightly to the right; at the same time lower the right hand holding the sword until it reaches the front of the crotch,

Fig. 74

with the right palm outward, the blade on the vertical lowered at the inside of the right leg and the tip of the sword to the right; keep the left sword-fingers on the right wrist. Look to the right. (Fig. 75 front and rear views)

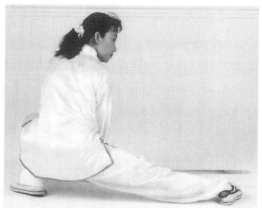 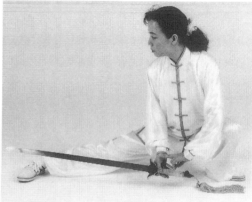

Fig. 75

22.5 Thread the Sword in Bow Stance

Shifting the body center to the right, turn the toes of the right foot outward, turn the toes of the left foot inward to form a right bow stance; at the same time turn the body to the right (about 90 degrees); as the body turns, thread the sword forward with the blade on the vertical along the inner edge of the right leg until the right wrist reaches chest level, with the arm naturally straight and palm to the left; the left sword-fingers still touch the inside of the right wrist. Look straight ahead. (Fig. 76)

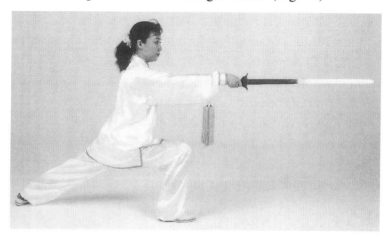

Fig. 76

Important Points

• Coordinate the sword's cutting to the right and its raising to the left with the body center's shifting left and right. Keep the body center balanced. Do not sway the torso.

- To thread the sword is to thrust the sword along the leg, arm or body in the direction in which the tip is pointing. Thrusting the sword is usually followed by stabbing to form an attacking movement, with the power focused on the tip of the sword. When fixing the form, face due East.

- To do the crouch stance, bend one leg into a squat, turn the toes of the foot and the knee slightly outward; the other leg is naturally straight out from the side of the body and close to the ground, with the toes of the foot turned inward. Plant both feet firmly on the ground, do not raise the ball or the heel of the foot. Lean the torso slightly forward.

Common Mistakes

- In the crouch stance, the waist is bent and the hips are raised, the ball or the heel of the foot is raised.

- The leg is moved backward slanted to the right, twisting and tensing the torso and making the direction of the fixed form slanted to the North.

23. Dēngjiǎo Jiàjiàn 蹬脚架剑 (Kick and Block Up with the Sword)

23.1 Turn the Waist and Draw the Sword

Turn the ball of the right foot outward, shift the body center forward, raise the left heel up and turn the body to the right; at the same time the right hand pulls the sword to the right rear until it reaches the upper front of the head (the wrist is about 4 inches or 10 centimeters away from the right forehead), with the right palm outward and the tip of the sword forward; bend the left elbow and touch the sword-fingers to the inside of the right forearm, with the left palm to the right. Look forward. (Fig. 77)

23.2 Lift the Knee and Draw the Sword

The right leg naturally stands straight. Move the left foot past the inside of the right ankle and raise it, with the ball of the foot dropping naturally; at the same time the right hand pulls the sword slightly to the right. Look straight ahead. (Fig. 78)

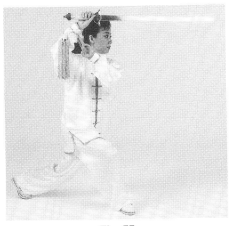

Fig. 77

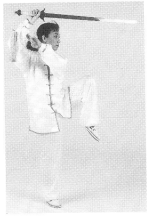

Fig. 78

23.3 Kick Forward and Block with the Sword

The left foot kicks forward with the power focused on the heel; at the same time the right hand blocks up with the sword, with the arm slightly bent; move the left sword-fingers forward and point, with the left arm naturally straight, the wrist at the shoulder height, the palm forward and the fingertips upward. Look forward. (Fig. 79)

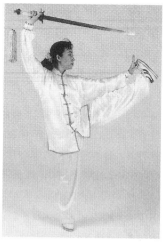

Fig. 79

Important Points

● Blocking up with the sword and lifting the sword are the same in that both are done with a vertical blade raised straight and horizontal above the head, the power focused in the middle part of the blade. The only difference is that the right palm faces outward in blocking up with the sword but faces inward in lifting the sword.

● When fixing the form, keep the tip of the sword, the sword-fingers and kicking foot in the same direction. The left arm and the left leg face each other. The sword-fingers and the tip of the sword face each other. Keep the torso upright, relaxed and steady.

● The kicking foot is higher than the horizontal level; the blocking sword is higher than the head; keep the blade level; point the sword-fingers out forward past the lower part of the chin.

● In this form, the sword is drawn backward with the blade on the vertical; the right arm changes from bent to straight.

Common Mistakes

● When kicking and blocking up with the sword, the torso leans backward with the abdomen thrust out, or the hips are thrust out.

● The sword fingers move along the edge of the blade to then separate in the manner of stroking sword.

● In the fixed form, the body center is unsteady; the torso sways and is tensed up.

24. Tíxī Diǎnjiàn 提膝点剑 (Lift the Knee and Point the Sword)

Bend the left knee to form a right one-leg stance, and turn the torso slightly to the right; at the same time the right hand points with the sword down from above the head to the lower right front, with the tip of the sword at the knee level; bend the left elbow and move the left sword-fingers to the right, and touch them to the inside of the right forearm, with the left palm downward. Look at the tip of the sword. (Fig. 80)

Important Points

● Coordinate bending the right knee, moving the ball of the foot inward and pointing.

● When fixing the form, stand steady on one leg. Bend the left knee and raise it up, draw in the calf and pull in the toes. Turn the torso to the Southwest and lean it slightly forward. The pointing sword is also towards the Southwest.

Common Mistakes

● When pointing with the sword, the left leg is not turned inward with the turning of the body, so the thighs are too far apart.

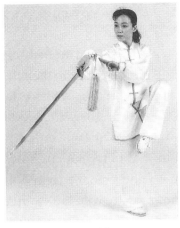

Fig. 80

● When pointing with the sword, the torso is not turned to the right, forming instead the movement of leaning the body and pointing back.

● When bending the leg, the back is hunched and the knee is not raised above waist height.

25. Pūbù Héngsǎo 仆步横扫 (Crouch Stance and Sweep to the Side)

25.1 Sweep with the Sword in Crouch Stance

Bend the right knee into a squat, move the left foot backward to the left to form a left crouch stance; turn the torso slightly to the left; at the same time, bend the left elbow and turn the left hand inward and extend the left sword-fingers backward past the left ribs until they reach the outer edge of the left leg, with the left palm backward; sink the right wrist and lower the right hand to the upper front of the right knee, with the palm upward. Look at the tip of the sword. (Fig. 81)

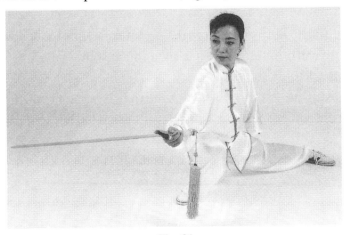

Fig. 81

25.2 Sweep with the Sword in Bow Stance

With shifting the body center to the left, turn the body to the left (about 90 degrees), bend the left knee, turn the toes of the left foot outward, pivot on the ball of the right foot and turn the right heel outward to form a left bow stance; at the same time the right hand sweeps horizontally with the sword to the left, with the right wrist at waist level and right palm upward, the right arm slightly

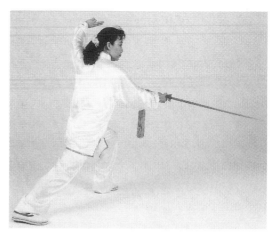

Fig. 82

bent and the tip of the sword slightly lower than the right wrist and facing to the lower front; move the left sword-fingers upward in a curve at the left side of the body until the left hand reaches over the head at the left side, with the left arm curved and palm slanted upward. Look at the tip of the sword. (Fig. 82)

Important Points

• Sweeping sword (sǎojiàn 扫剑) involves turning the waist and swinging the arm, sweeping with the flat sword in a curve from the back to the front and left, with power focused on the edge of the blade. The sword can be waist, leg or ankle height. In this form, sweep with sword as the crouch stance is shifted to bow stance, the height of the sword rises from the ankle level to waist level.

• When fixing the form, the bow stance faces on the diagonal to the Northeast with the tip of the sword due East.

• When doing crouch stance, pause a little bit to make the movement as accurate as possible.

• When shifting to bow stance, turn the hip joint, straighten the lower back, lower the hips. One also can turn the toes of the right foot inward.

Common Mistakes

• When moving the left foot backward, the right leg is not bent, the left foot is not extended along the ground, causing a mistake of raising the left foot and lowering it to the ground.

• The crouch stance does not meet the standard: The right leg is not fully bent into a squat, the lower back is bent and the hips are raised.

• When shifting the crouch stance to bow stance, the body leans forward and the hips are thrust out, the head is lowered and the lower back is bent.

26. Gōngbù Xiàjié 弓步下截 (Bow Stance and Intercept Downward)

26.1 Lift the Foot and Draw In the Sword

Shift the body center forward, withdraw the right foot to the inside of the left foot (do not touch the right foot to the ground); at the same time the right hand moves inward in a curve to sweep (bō 拨) to the right with the sword, with the right wrist at waist level, the right palm downward and the tip of the sword to the left lower front; bend the left elbow and lower the left sword-fingers and touch them to the inside of the right wrist, with the left palm downward. Look at the tip of the sword. (Fig. 83)

26.2 Intercept Downward in Right Bow Stance

Move the right foot forward to the right to form a right bow stance, turn the torso slightly to the right; at the same time as the right hand moves with the sword in a curve to the right front and intercept, bend the right arm slightly and turn it inward, with the right wrist at the chest level, the "tiger's mouth" (the web between the thumb and index finger) slanted downward, and the sword-fingers to the left lower front; keep the left sword-fingers on the right wrist. Look at the tip of the sword. (Fig. 84)

26.3 Lift the Foot and Draw In the Sword

Shift the body center to the right leg; withdraw the left foot to the inside of the right foot (do not touch the left foot to the ground), turn the torso to the left; at the same time, the right hand turns outward and sweeps in a curve to the left with the sword until the right hand reaches the right side of the hip, with the right palm upward and the tip of the sword to the right lower front; touch the left sword-fingers to the inside of the right wrist, with the palm downward. Look at the tip of the sword. (Fig. 85)

26.4 Intercept Downward in Left Bow Stance

Move the left foot forward to the left, shift the body center forward, turn the right heel outward to form a left bow stance, turn the torso to the left (about 45 degrees); at

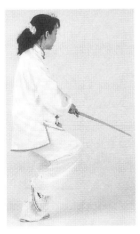

Fig. 83

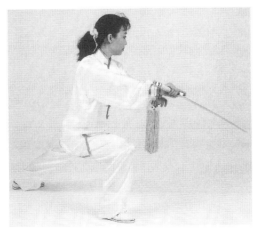

Fig. 84

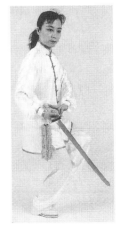

Fig. 85

the same time the right hand moves in a curve to the left with the sword and intercepts (jié 截) in front of the left part of the body, bend the right arm slightly and turn it outward, with the right wrist at the chest level and palm slanted upward; the tip of the sword points to the right lower front; move the left sword-fingers upward in an arc to the left, with the left arm curved above the front of the head and the left palm outward. Look at the tip of the sword. (Fig. 86)

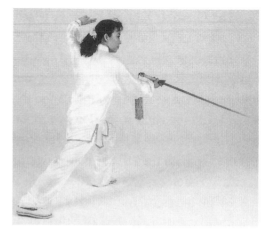

Fig. 86

Important Points
● When moving the sword in a curve to deflect (bō 拨), bend the arm and turn the wrist to draw a small arc with the tip of the sword. When intercepting with the sword (jiéjiàn 截剑), bend the leg and turn the waist in movements that are gentle and continuous. During the sequence, control the movements of the arms with the waist, control the movements of the sword with the arm. When turning the waist, turn the arm, bend or stretch the elbow. Draw a bigger arc with the handle of the sword than with the tip of the sword.

● When fixing the form, the right and left bow stances face Southeast and Northeast respectively, and the tip of the sword pauses near the midline.

● When intercepting with the sword, the power focuses on the bottom edge of the blade from middle to the tip, the intercepting sword is slanted to the left and right lower front.

Common Mistakes
● The sword is held too stiffly, and the tip of the sword moves around too much.

● The arm lacks agility in bending and stretching so that the movement becomes instead a sweeping sword (sǎojiàn 扫剑) made with a straight arm.

27. Gōngbù Xiàcì 弓步下刺 (Bow Stance and Stab Downward)
27.1 Stomp the Foot and Draw In the Sword

Shift the body center forward, the right foot stomps (zhèn震) at the back of the left foot, then bend the right knee to form a half squat, raise the left heel; turn the torso slightly to the right; at the same time bend the right elbow and draw the sword back to the front of the right ribs, with the right palm upward, the tip of the sword forward and slightly lower than the right hand; extend the left sword-fingers forward, then bend the left elbow, together with the right hand draw the left hand back and touch the sword-fingers to the inside of the right wrist, with the left palm downward. Look in the direction to which the tip of the sword points. (Fig. 87)

27.2 Stab Downward in Bow Stance

Move the left foot forward to the left, shift the body center forward to form a left bow stance; turn the torso to the left and exert power; at the same time the right hand stabs with the sword to the left lower front, with the right wrist at waist level and the palm upward; keep the left sword-fingers on the inside of the right wrist, with the left palm downward. Look at the tip of the sword. (Fig. 88)

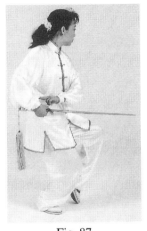
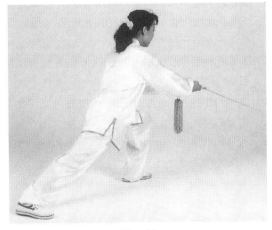

Fig. 87   Fig. 88

Important Points

• Stomping and stabbing with the sword here both involve exerting power, the second time this occurs. [The first occurs in 13. Gōngbù Bēngjiàn 弓步崩剑 (Bow Stance and Snap the Sword.)] When stomping, bend the left leg that supports the body, bend the right leg, stomp the ground with the sole of the right foot, solid and full of strength. Then shift the body center to the right leg, turn the torso to the right and bend the arms to bring the hands together, and draw the sword to the waist.

• When stabbing with the sword and exerting power, turn the waist and sink the hips, move the shoulder forward and extend the arm, send the power to the tip of the sword, stab quickly with agility with the sword forward down to the front.

• When fixing the form, face Northeast.

Common Mistakes

• Before stomping, the foot is raised too high, both feet jump into the air. After stomping, the whole left foot is raised and drawn to the inside of the right foot.

• The movements of stabbing sword and exerting power are not coordinated with the movements of turning the waist and kicking; before exerting power, the movements of bending the arm and drawing back the sword are added to the movements of the right hand.

28. Zuǒyòu Yúnmǒ 左右云抹 (Smear the Clouds Left and Right)

28.1 Lift the Foot and Bring the Hands Together with the Sword

Shifting the body center forward, pull the right foot back to the inside of the left foot (do not touch the foot to the ground), turn the body slightly to the left; at the same time sink the right wrist as the right hand draws the sword to the left, with the right wrist at waist level, the arm slightly bent, the palm upward and the tip of the sword slightly lower than the right hand; move the left sword-fingers slightly to the left, then move them in a curve to the right and bring them over the right arm, with the left palm to the right. Look at the tip of the sword. (Fig. 89)

28.2 Separate the Hands with the Sword in Side-Bow Stance

Step with the right foot to the right to form a right side-bow stance, turn the torso to the right; at the same time the right hand moves upward to the right in a curve and makes a slice (削 xiāo) with the sword, with the right arm slightly bent; the left sword-fingers move in a curve to the left and stop on the left front of the body at the chest level, with the left palm outward. Look at the tip of the sword. (Fig. 90)

28.3 Cross-Over Step and Circle with the Sword Like Clouds

Turn the torso slightly to the right, shift the body center to the right; then turn the torso slightly to the left, step the left foot crosswise over the right foot, with the knee slightly bent; kick the right foot down just as the left foot is about to land to lift the right foot and tuck it behind the left calf, with the toes of the right foot down (some 4 inches or 10 centimeters away from the ground); at the same time the right hand moves with the sword in an counter-clockwise circle like clouds until the right hand reaches the left side of the front of the body, with the right wrist at the chest level, the arm slightly bent, the palm downward and the tip of the sword to the left front; bring the left sword-fingers together with the right hand before the chest, and touch them to the inside of the right wrist, with the left palm down. Look at the tip of the sword. (Fig. 91)

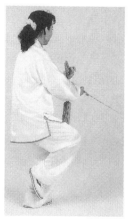
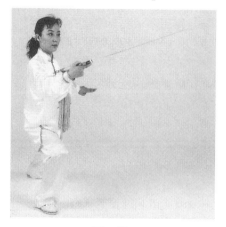
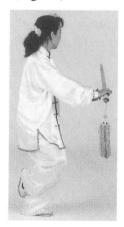

Fig. 89   Fig. 90   Fig. 91

28.4 Smear with the Sword in Bow Stance

Move the right foot to the right to form a right bow stance, and turn the torso to the right; at the same time the right hand smears with the sword to the right front, with the right palm downward; keep the left sword-fingers on the inside of the right wrist. Look at the tip of the sword. (Fig. 92)

28.5 Lift the Foot and Draw In the Sword

Shift the body center to the right, pull the left foot to the inside of the right foot (do not touch the left foot to the ground), turn the body slightly to the right; at the same time the right hand draws the sword to the right, with the right elbow bent and wrist at waist level and the tip of the sword to the left front; keep the left sword-fingers on the inside of the right wrist. Look straight ahead. (Fig. 93)

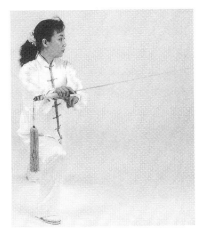

Fig. 92

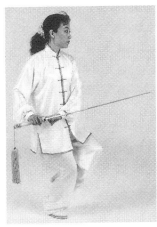

Fig. 93

28.6 Step Forward and Swing the Sword

Move the left foot to the left to form a left bow stance, turn the torso to the left; at the same time extend the right hand with the sword forward and then swing the right hand to the left, with the right wrist at chest level, the right palm downward and the tip of the sword forward; move the left sword-fingers in a curve past the front of the body to the left until they reach the left side of the body, with the left palm outward. Look at the tip of the sword. (Fig. 94)

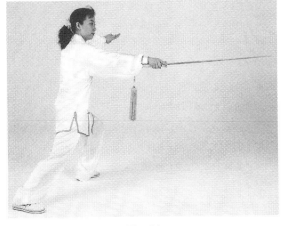

Fig. 94

28.7 Cross-Over Step and Circle with the Sword Like Clouds

Shift the body center to the left, the right foot crosses over the left foot; kick the ground with the left foot just before the right foot lands on the ground, raise the left foot to the back of the right calf, with the toes of the left foot down (about 4 inches or 10 centimeters away from the ground); turn the torso slightly to the right; at the same time the right hand moves the sword in a clockwise circle like clouds until the right hand reaches the right side of the front of the body, with the right wrist at chest level, the right palm upward and the tip of the sword to the right front; when moving the sword, bring the left sword-fingers to the right close to the right hand and touch it to the inside of the right wrist, with the left palm downward. Look at the tip of the sword. (Fig. 95)

28.8 Smear with the Sword in Bow Stance

Move the left foot to the left to form a left bow stance, turn the torso slightly to the left; at the same time the right hand smears to the left with the sword, with the right palm upward; move the left sword-fingers in an arc to the left, with the left arm in a curve above the side of the head. Look at the tip of the sword. (Fig. 96)

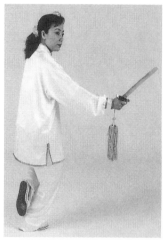
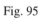
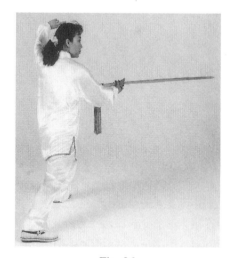

Fig. 95   Fig. 96

Important Points

● In moving the sword like clouds (yúnjiàn 云剑), taking the wrist as the axis, bend the wrist and turn it to move the sword in a horizontal circle in front of the head or above the head to deflect an opponent's attack to the side.

● In smearing sword (mǒjiàn 抹剑), move the sword in a curve with a flat blade from the left to the right or from the right to the left. The handle leads the sword, the focus of the power slips along the sword edge from the back to the tip.

● Cross-over stance (gàibù 盖步) involves one foot stepping crosswise in front of the supporting foot. In this form, just before landing the left foot in its cross-over step, kick the right leg down to get a lift in the right knee so that the right foot tucks, toes down, behind the left calf. In this brief jump and change of feet, keep the movements agile, smooth and gentle. Step crosswise with the left foot landing slightly ahead of the right foot in a line that forms a "Z" or Chinese-character 之 shape to help keep the body relaxed, upright and steady.

● The bow stances in their fixed forms face due South and due North respectively.

C

●

head,

●

maki

●

feet

ing s

●

forw

(Do

the r

from

abdo

right

the s

hip l

the

fore

at th

rear

Star

to fc

slightly to the right; at the same time the

sword is raised higher than the
ing something around the head.
o far away from the other foot,
d and body center unstable.
ifting and jumping between the
ement instead becomes a walk-

ight and the tip of the sword is

d Chop with the Sword)

back to the inside of the left foot
body to the left; at the same time
blade leading forward in a curve
hand reaches the left front of the

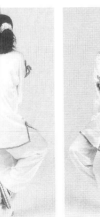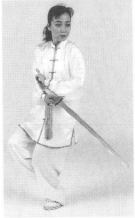

Fig. 97

right hand moves the sword forward in a curve and chops with the sword, with the right wrist at the chest level and the sword and the arm on the same line; the left sword-fingers draw an arc from a lower position to the left, with the left arm curved and held above the left side of the head, left palm outward. Look at the tip of the sword. (Fig. 98)

Important Points

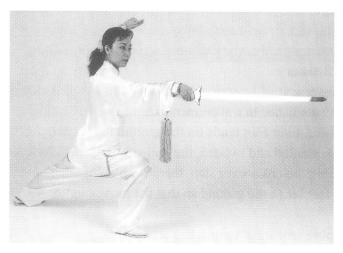

Fig. 98

- Coordinate the movements of swinging the sword with withdrawing the foot, lifting the sword and stepping forward; and chopping the sword with bow stance. All the movements are continuous and coordinated.

- When fixing the form, the right arm and the right leg are aligned; the direction of the chopping sword and the bow stance is Southeast.

Common Mistakes

- When swinging the sword (lūnjiàn 抡剑), the waist and the head are not turned, and the sword lacks harmony with the spirit.

- When chopping with the sword, the torso leans and twists, the movement of the right arm is not coordinated with that of the right leg.

- The bow stance is not coordinated with the chopping sword in that the leg moves faster than the hand.

30. Hòu Jǔtuǐ Jiàjiàn 后举腿架剑 (Lift the Leg Behind and Block Up with the Sword)

30.1 Hook Out Step and Hook the Sword

Shift the body center forward, hook the left foot out, bend the left knee into a half squat; lift the right heel up, and turn the torso to the left; at the same time the right hand moves the sword to the left in a hooking motion, with the right wrist at waist level, the tip of the sword to the left; bend the left elbow and lower the left sword-fingers and touch them to the right forearm, with the left palm outward. Look down to the left. (Fig. 99)

30.2 Raise the Leg Backward and Block Up with the Sword

Stand on the left leg, bend the right knee to lift up the lower leg until the top of the of the foot is horizontal to the ground at hip level; turn the torso slightly to the left; at the same time raise the sword with the right hand (about 4 inches or 10 centimeters away from the head); point the tip of the sword to the left; move the left sword-fingers to the left past the front of the face, with the left arm slightly curved and the fingertips upward. Look at the sword-fingers. (Fig. 100 front and rear views)

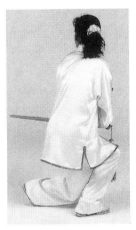
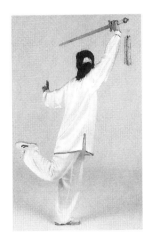
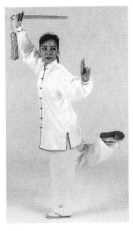

Fig. 99   Fig. 100

Important Points

• This form contains a set of balanced movements. Be steady in supporting the body on one leg; keep the torso upright and turn it to the left rear.

• The sword-fingers, the tip of the sword, the raised rear leg and the eyes all face the same direction, Northwest.

• When blocking up with the sword (jiàjiàn 架剑), bend the arm first and then stretch it; raise the sword above the head, keep the blade horizontal to the ground.

• Coordinate raising the sword, lifting the leg backward and the sword-fingers.

Common Mistakes

• The tip of the sword, the sword-fingers, the raised rear leg and the eyes are not in alignment.

• When fixing the form, the torso leans forward, the waist is bent, the head is lowered and stance is unsteady.

• When lifting the leg behind the body, the leg is not bent or tight enough, and the bottom of the foot is not stretched out flat.

31. Dīngbù Diǎnjiàn 丁步点剑 (**T-Stance and Point the Sword**)

31.1 Step Forward and Raise the Sword

Bend the left knee, and turn the body slightly to the right; move the right foot to the right and land it to the ground, with the right heel touching the ground and the right leg naturally straight; at the same time the right hand raises the sword slightly to the right to make the tip of the sword slanted upward and higher than the right wrist. Look to the left front. (Fig. 101)

31.2 Point the Sword in T-Stance

Shift the body center to the right, turn the body to the right, plant the right foot firmly on the ground, bend the right knee into a half squat, step the left foot to the inside of the right foot, with the toes of the left foot touching the ground to form a left T-stance; at the same time the right hand points with the sword to the lower front, with the right wrist at the chest level; the left sword-fingers move in a curve to the right past the front of the body, bend the left elbow and touch the sword-fingers to the inside of the right wrist. Look forward. (Fig. 102)

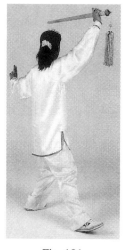
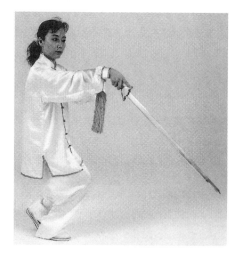

Fig. 101   Fig. 102

Important Points

● Coordinate T-stance (dīngbù 丁步) with pointing the sword.

● When fixing the form, face Southeast.

Common Mistakes

● Lack of coordination in making the T-stance and pointing the sword, one faster than the other.

● When pointing the sword, the right arm is not straight; the sword is grasped too hard, the wrist is not bent and raised enough.

32. Mǎbù Tuījiàn 马步推剑 (Horse Stance and Push the Sword)

32.1 Step Back and Draw In the Sword

Draw back the left foot to the left rear, bend the left leg; shift the body center back, bring the right foot half a step back, with the ball of the right foot moving along the ground and the right heel raised with the right leg slightly bent, turn the torso to the right; at the same time, bend the right elbow and draw the right hand to the side of the right ribs with the "tiger's mouth" (the web between the thumb and the index finger) up, the blade of the sword upright and the tip of the sword up; put the left sword-fingers on the right wrist, with the left palm down. Look at the sword to the right. (Fig. 103)

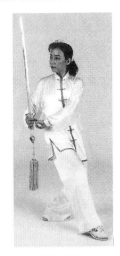

Fig. 103

32.2 Push with the Sword Forward in Horse Stance

Stomp the ground with the left foot, shifting the body center forward, move the right foot to the right front, with the toes of the right foot turned inward, the left foot slides towards the right foot as the knees half bend into a horse stance; turn the torso to the left; at the same time, the right hand push with the sword to the right front with force, the right wrist is at the chest level, the tip of the sword points up and the power goes through the blade of the sword; push the left sword-fingers to the left past the front of the chest, with the left palm outward and the fingertips forward, at shoulder height. Look at the sword to the right. (Fig. 104)

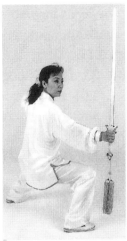

Fig. 104

Important Points

• Pushing with the sword in this movement is the third and last sword technique that involves exerting power.[The other two are 13. Gōngbù Bēngjiàn 弓步崩剑 (Bow Stance and Snap the Sword) and 27. Gōngbù Xiàcì 弓步下刺 (Bow Stance and Stab Downward.)] First, store power by withdrawing the foot and turning the waist. Then in an explosive release of power turn the waist, bend the legs, lower the hips and push with the sword with strength in horse stance.

• Pushing sword (tuījiàn 推剑) involves pushing and blocking or pushing and attacking outward with the blade on the vertical (from a position close to the body to a position far away from the body). Focus power on edge of the blade near the handle, keep the blade upright.

- When drawing the right foot back or following-in with the left foot, the feet should slide without leaving the ground. Be flexible in controlling the distance of the slide, according to needs.

- In horse stance, the feet are parallel, some three-feet width distance apart, toes forward; bend the legs into a half squat, lower the hips and tuck in the buttocks, lift the head and straighten the lower back, and keep the torso upright. In this form, the toes of the feet and the chest in horse stance face Northeast.

Common Mistakes

- The sword is not firmly withdrawn, the torso is not turned, and the stored power is not strong.

- When pushing with the sword, the right foot moves too short a distance; the exertion of power lacks coordination with the movements of the turning waist and thrusting leg.

- In horse stance, the toes of the feet are turned outward, the hips are open; the torso leans forward, the hips are thrust out and the waist is bent.

Part IV

33. Dúlì Shàngtuō 独立上托 (Stand on One Foot and Lift Up)

33.1 Back Cross Step and Pull the Sword

Shift the body center to the left, cross the right foot back to the left, turn the body to the right; at the same time, taking the right wrist as an axis, turn the right hand with the sword outward, moving the tip of the sword backward and downward and then upward to make a vertical circle at the right side of the body until the tip of the sword reaches the right side of the head, with the tip of the sword pointing up to the right, the "tiger's mouth" (the web between the thumb and the index finger) upward, and the right wrist at the chest level; raise the left sword-fingers slightly forward. Look forward to the right. (Fig. 105)

33.2 Turn the Body and Swing the Sword

With shifting the body center backward, bend the knees and squat, pivot on the left heel and the right sole, turn the body to the right rear (about 180 degrees); at the same time turn the right forearm inward, move the sword to the lower right rear with the handle leading forward in a curve until the handle reaches the front top of the right knee, with the tip of the sword forward; bend the left elbow and move the left sword-fingers to the right and touch them to the inside of the right wrist, with the left palm downward. Look at the tip of the sword. (Fig. 106)

33.3 Hold the Sword Up in One-Leg Stance

Turn the torso slightly to the right, the right leg is naturally straight, stand on the right leg, bend the left knee and raise it to form a right one-leg stance; at the same time turn the right arm inward and lift the sword up until the right hand is above the right side of the forehead (about 4 inches or 10 centimeters away from the head). The blade of the sword is horizontal to the ground, the tip of the sword points forward; bend the left elbow and touch the left sword-fingers to the inside of the right forearm, with the left palm outward. Look to the left. (Fig. 107)

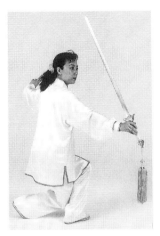
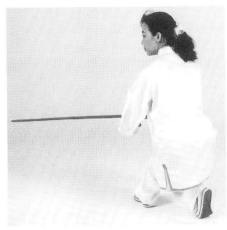
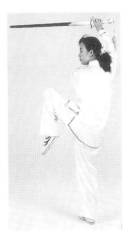

Fig. 105   Fig. 106   Fig. 107

Important Points

● When moving the sword in a circle with the wrist as axis, use the power of the wrist and the fingers to wield the sword. Do not hold the sword so tightly that the handle cannot easily move around in the hand.

● When pivoting on the foot and turning the body, bend the leg and turn the hips, keep the torso upright.

● When lifting the sword, turn the right arm inward, bend the arm first and then stretch it, lift the sword to a position higher than the head, and coordinate this movement with lifting the knee and standing on one leg.

● When fixing the form, keep the body balanced and stable, straighten the lower back and hold the head high, sink the shoulders and relax the arms. Face due West.

Common Mistakes

● When turning on the feet and turning the body, the waist is bent and buttocks stick out.

● The arm is straight when it moves to raise the sword.

● The one-leg stance is unsteady; the torso is hunched, not extended.

34. Jìnbù Guàdiǎn 进步挂点 (Forward Step, Hook, and Point)

34.1 Hook Out the Foot and Hook the Sword to the Left

Lower the left foot and hook it out; shifting the body center forward, raise the right heel up, turn the torso to the left; at the same time the right hand moves the sword in a curve to the lower left and hooks, with the right palm inward; bend the left elbow and touch the left sword-fingers to the inside of the right upper arm, with the left palm outward. Look at the tip of the sword. (Fig. 108)

34.2 Hook Out the Foot and Raise the Sword

With shifting the body center forward, hook the right foot out forward, turn the torso slightly to the right; at the same time the right hand moves the sword forward in a curve past a higher position, turn the right forearm outward, with the right palm upward, the tip of the sword forward and lower than the right wrist;

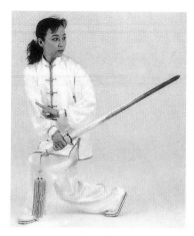

Fig. 108

keep the left sword-fingers on the inside of the right forearm, with the left palm to the right. Look at the tip of the sword. (Fig. 109)

34.3 Turn the Torso and Hook the Sword to the Right

Shifting the body center forward, plant the right foot firmly on the ground, raise the left heel, and turn the torso to the right; at the same time the right hand moves the sword in a curve to the right in a hooking motion, with the right palm outward; the left sword-fingers point upward, hold the left arm in a curve above the head, with the left palm to the left. Look in the direction in which the tip of the sword points. (Fig. 110)

34.4 Step Forward and Raise the Sword

Shifting the body center forward, hook the left foot outward and move it forward, with the left heel touching the ground; turn the body slightly to the left; at the same time the right hand raises the sword up, with the right palm upward, the wrist at head level,

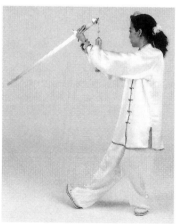

Fig. 109

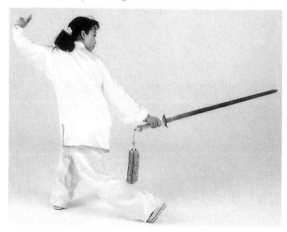

Fig. 110

the tip of the sword to the lower rear; lower the left sword-fingers to shoulder height, with the left palm outward. Look forward. (Fig. 111)

34.5 Point the Sword in Empty Stance

Again shifting the body center forward, plant the left foot firmly on the ground, bend the left knee into a half squat, move the right foot to the right front to form a right empty stance; turn the torso to the left (about 90 degrees); at the same time the right hand points with the sword, moving above head to the lower right front; move the left sword-fingers past a lower position to the left in an arc, with the left arm curved above the left side of the head and the left palm outward. Look at the tip of the sword. (Fig. 112)

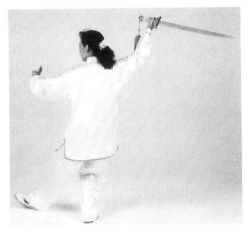 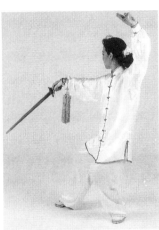

Fig. 111   Fig. 112

Important Points

• Hooking sword (guàjiàn 挂剑) involves hooking back with the blade on the vertical. Draw a vertical circle with the sword tip close to the body from the front to the back in a hooking motion to defend against an attack. Focus the power in the front part of the sword. When hooking the sword, turn the waist, turn the arm and bend the wrist. Synchronize the movements of the body and sword. Do the whole sequence in one continuous motion.

• In this form, when hooking the sword on the left and right, hook out the foot and step forward to the West; the direction of the empty stance and the pointing of the sword is about 30 degrees West by North.

Common Mistakes

• When hooking the sword, the sword is too far away from the body, or the wrist is not bent enough, the sword and the right arm are on the same straight line to form a circling sword (lūnjiàn 抡剑).

● The body is not turned enough. The hooking sword is slanted to the South or North.

● When doing the movements of empty stance and pointing sword, the hands and the feet are not coordinated; the direction of the empty stance and pointing sword is not on the diagonal to the Northwest.

35. Xiēbù Bēngjiàn 歇步崩剑 (Resting Stance and Snap the Sword)

35.1 Turn the Torso and Lower the Sword

Turn the right heel inward and root the right foot on the ground, and bend the right knee into a half squat; raise the left heel up and shift the body center forward; turn the torso to the right; at the same time sink the right wrist as the right hand draws the sword to the right side of the hips, with the right palm inward and the tip of the sword to the upper left; bend the left elbow and lower the left sword-fingers and touch them to the right wrist, with the left palm downward. Look to the right front. (Fig. 113)

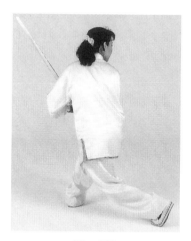

Fig. 113

35.2 Turn the Torso and Slice the Sword Upward

Bend the right knee; move the left foot to the left front and turn it in to form a right side-bow stance, and turn the torso to the right rear; at the same time the right hand slices the sword in a reverse slice down and up to the right, with the right wrist at the chest level, the right palm backward and the tip of the sword to the right; move the left sword-fingers down and up to the left in a curve until the sword-fingers reach shoulder height. Look at the tip of the sword. (Fig. 114)

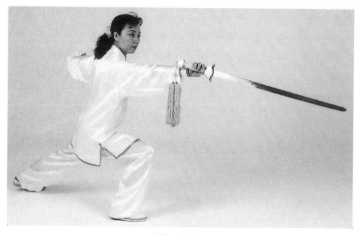

Fig. 114

35.3 Resting Stance and Snap the Sword

Shift the body center backward, cross the right foot to the back of the left foot to form a resting stance; turn the body to the right; at the same time turn the right hand outward until the "tiger's mouth" (the web between the thumb and index finger) turns up, then sink the right wrist and point up with the sword, with the right wrist at waist level; the left sword-

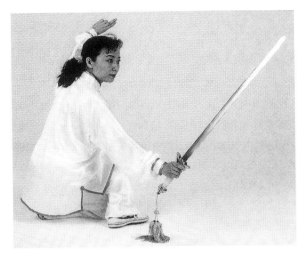

Fig. 115

fingers point upward, with the left arm curved above the left side of the head, left palm slanted upward. Look to the right front. (Fig. 115)

Important Points

• In this form, the footwork includes pivoting on the foot, turning in the foot, back cross stepping, bending and squatting. There is also a turning of the body to the rear. Be agile and make the movements flow without pause.

• Move the foot forward in a diagonal line of West by North. When fixing the form, that is resting stance, look East by South.

• Pointing up the sword is to sink the wrist and point up with the sword, the blade is slanted to the upper front, the tip of the sword is slightly higher than the head.

Common Mistakes

• The movement pauses midway.

• Turning on the feet in empty stance becomes instead a lift-foot step with the right leg.

• After snapping the sword, the blade becomes vertical or turned inward.

• The feet move and the form is fixed in the direction of East-West.

36. Gōngbù Fǎncì 弓步反刺 (Bow Stance and Reverse Stab)

36.1 Lift the Knee and Raise the Sword

With the right foot rooted on the ground, straighten the right leg and stand on it, bend the left knee and raise it up, with the toes of the left foot dropping; lean the torso slightly to the left; at the same time bend the right elbow and raise it at the side of the body, with the right wrist lower than the chest, hold the blade of the sword slanted at the top of the right shoulder, with the right palm forward and the tip of the sword to the upper left; lower the left sword-fingers to shoulder height. Look to the right front. (Fig. 116)

36.2 Bow Stance and Stab Upward

Lower the left foot and land it to the left to form a left bow stance, turn the torso slightly to the left; at the same time lean the body forward and the right hand stabs with the sword to the upper front; move the left sword-fingers to the right and bring them together with the right arm in front of the body, and put the left sword-fingers to the inside of the right forearm. Look at the tip of the sword. (Fig. 117 front and rear views)

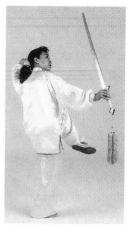

Fig. 116

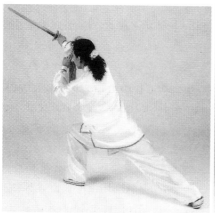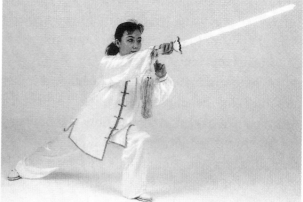

Fig. 117

Important Points

• Reverse stabbing sword (fǎncìjiàn 反刺剑) means to turn the right arm inward, with the "tiger's mouth" (the web between the thumb and the index finger) downward, reverse the hand and stab forward with the blade of the sword on the vertical. In this form, lean the torso forward, turn slightly to the left. The right arm and the sword are on the same straight line. Stab to the upper front.

• When fixing the form, face 30 degrees West by North.

Common Mistakes

• The left foot is landed on the ground too heavily, the bow stance and the stabbing sword are not coordinated.

• The torso is not leaned forward and to the side.

• The head is lowered and looks down.

37. Zhuǎnshēn Xiàcì 转身下刺 (**Turn the Body and Stab Downward**)

37.1 Turn the Foot In and Draw In the Sword

Shifting the body center backward, turn the body to the right, turn the ball of the left foot in; at the same time bend the right elbow while the right hand draws the sword back until the right hand reaches the front of the left shoulder, with the right palm inward and the tip of the sword to the right; put the left sword-fingers on the inside of the right wrist, with the left palm outward. Look to the right. (Fig. 118)

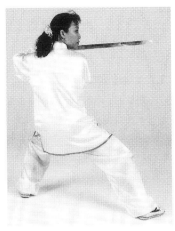

Fig. 118

37.2 Lift the Foot and Turn the Body

Shift the body center to the left, bend the right knee and lift the foot, with the toes of the right foot dropping down; pivot on the ball of the left foot, turn the body to the right back; at the same time the right hand moves the sword to the right past the right shoulder and lowers it to the waist, the tip of the sword moves downward in a curve until it reaches the outer side of the right knee, with the right palm upward and the tip of the sword slanted downward; keep the left sword-fingers on the right wrist. Look at the tip of the sword. (Fig. 119)

37.3 Bow Stance and Stab Downward

With turning the body to the right back (about 180 degrees), lower the right foot to the right rear to form a right bow stance; at the same time the right hand stabs down forward with the sword, with the right wrist at waist level and the right palm upward; put the left sword-fingers on the right wrist, with the left palm downward. Look at the tip of the sword. (Fig. 120)

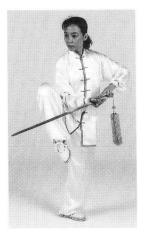

Fig. 119

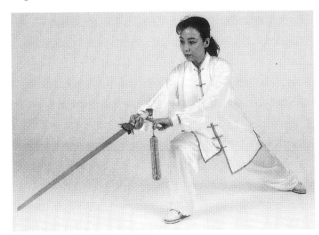

Fig. 120

Important Points

• Turn the right arm outward first when turning in the foot and drawing back the sword, then bend the right elbow and the right wrist to draw the hand back to the front of the left shoulder.

• Lift the foot and turn the body in a smooth movement and without pausing.

• Coordinate the bow stance with the stabbing down. When fixing the form, lean the torso slightly forward, face Southwest.

Common Mistakes

• When drawing back the sword, the sword is raised and smeared in the manner of moving the sword like clouds horizontally or wrapping something around the head.

• The body is not turned enough, the right foot is stepped backward and landed on the ground.

38. Tíxī Tíjiàn 提膝提劍 (Lift the Knee and the Sword)

38.1 Draw the Sword and Circle to the Left

Shift the body center backward, turn the torso to the left; turn the toes of the left foot outward, bend the left knee into a half squat, and straighten the right leg naturally; at the same time bend the right arm and turn it outward and the right hand draws the sword with the handle leading forward to the upper left (about 8 inches or 20 centimeters away from the head), with the right palm inward and the tip of the sword to the right; put the left sword-fingers on the inside of the right forearm, with the left palm outward. Look at the tip of the sword. (Fig. 121)

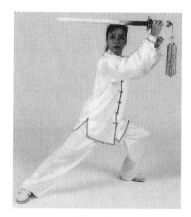

Fig. 121

38.2 Draw the Sword and Circle to the Right

Shift the body center to the right, bend the right knee, straighten the left leg naturally, turn the left heel outward, and turn the torso slightly to the right; at the same time turn the right forearm inward and the right hand moves the sword with the handle leading forward past the front of the abdomen until the right hand reaches the front of the right chest (about 12 inches or 30 centimeters away from the chest), draw the tip of the sword in a curve upward to the right front, with the tip of the sword lower than the right wrist; touch the left sword-fingers to the inside of the right wrist, with the left palm outward. Look at the tip of the sword. (Fig. 122)

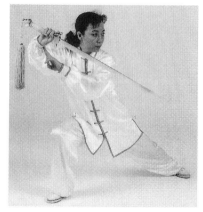

Fig. 122

38.3 One-Leg Stance and Raise the Sword

Bend the left knee and lift the left leg to form a right one-leg stance; turn the torso slightly to the right and lean it slightly forward; at the same time the right hand leads with the handle to raise the sword upward in a curve to the right, hold the right arm in an arc at the right front, with the right wrist at the level of the forehead and the right palm outward, the "tiger's mouth" is slanted downward and the tip of the sword is at the outer side of the left knee; move the left sword-fingers in a curve past the front of the abdomen to the left and hold them at waist level, with the left palm outward. Look to the left front. (Fig. 123)

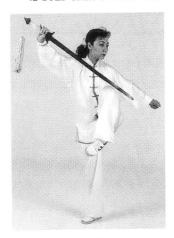

Fig. 123

Important Points

● Drawing the sword to the left or right entails drawing a vertical circle in front of the body. Coordinate drawing the sword with shifting the body center and turning the waist. Make an agile, flowing movement without stopping.

● Relax and stretch the torso when lifting the knee and raising the sword. Turn the torso slightly to the left and lean it forward; hold the arms so they are symmetrical, keep the body center steady. Look to the Southeast.

● When raising the sword, turn the right arm inward, move the sword-fingers along the blade away from the right hand.

Common Mistakes

● In the fixed form, the torso does not turn to the left; the body is out of balance; the knee is not raised higher than the waist, and the left foot is not close enough to the crotch.

● Drawing the sword in circles is not coordinated with shifting the body center as the arm is not driven by the waist and the sword is not directed by the arm, which results in swinging the sword.

● When lifting the sword, the right arm fails to turn inward, the left sword fingers move along the edge of the blade and then move away in the manner of stroking sword.

39. Xíngbù Chuānjiàn 行步穿剑 (Walking Step and Thread the Sword)

39.1 Land the Foot and Thread the Sword

Bend the right knee, lower the left foot to the left and land it with the left heel touching the ground, and turn the torso to the left; at the same time turn the right palm up and thread the sword with the tip leading forward past the front of the left ribs and under the left arm to the left front, the right wrist is at waist level and the tip of the sword points forward; move the left sword-fingers in a curve to the right upper front until they reach the front of the right shoulder, with the left palm downward. Look at the tip of the sword. (Fig. 124)

39.2 Walking Step and Thread the Sword

With shifting the body center forward, plant the left foot, bend the knee slightly, hook out the right foot to the right front, turn the torso to the right; at the same time, with the tip of the sword leading forward, the right hand threads the sword in a curve to the right front, with the right wrist at the chest level and tip of the sword to the right;

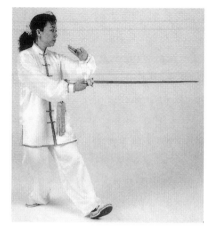

Fig. 124

move the left sword-fingers to the left past the front of the chest and hold them at the side of the body, with the left arm curved and the left palm outward. Look at the tip of the sword. (Fig. 125)

39.3 Walking Step and Thread the Sword

With shifting the body center forward, move the left foot to the right and turn it in, and turn the torso slightly to the right; keep both hands unchanged. Look at the tip of the sword. (Fig. 126)

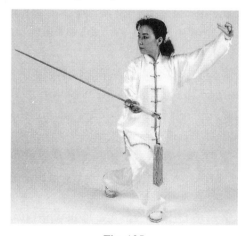

Fig. 125

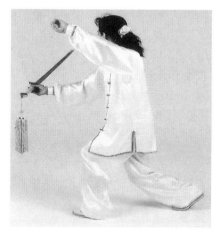

Fig. 126

39.4 Walking Step and Thread the Sword

With shifting the body center forward, hook out the right foot to the right, turn the torso slightly to the right; keep both hands unchanged. Look at the tip of the sword. (Fig. 127)

39.5 Walking Step and Thread the Sword

With shifting the body center forward, move the left foot to the right and turn it in, and turn the torso slightly to the right; hold the hands in the same position. Look at the tip of the sword. (Fig. 128)

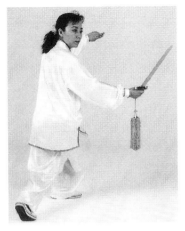
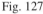

Fig. 127

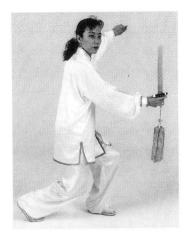

Fig. 128

Important Points

● Walking step (xíngbù 行步) includes five steps, in a circular track. When walking, keep the body center balanced; step the left foot forward and turn it in, step the right foot forward and turn it outward; sink the hips and twist the waist, turn the torso to the right. Look at the tip of the sword.

● In the last step, turn the left foot to the Southeast, and also turn the torso to the Southeast.

● When threading the sword, thrust the tip of the sword to the left first, then move it in a curve and thread it to the right.

Common Mistakes

● Walking steps are floating, the body center rises and falls.

● When walking, the waist is not turned enough, the radius of the track is too wide, and the five walking steps do not reach the designated place.

● When threading the sword, the edge of the sword touches the body.

40. Bǎituǐ Jiàjiàn 摆腿架剑 (Swing Out the Leg and Block Up with the Sword)

40.1 Swing Out the Leg and Join the Hands with the Sword

The right hand holds the sword, turn the right forearm inward and move the tip of the sword in a counter-clockwise curve in front of the head, bend the right elbow and move the right hand to the left until it reaches the front of the left ribs, with the tip of the sword to the upper left; when the right hand moves to the front of the face, hook out the right leg, then lower it until it reaches a position horizontal to the ground, bend the right leg and pull it back; point the left sword-fingers upward, bring them close to the right hand, bend the left elbow and touch the left sword-fingers to the inside of the right wrist, with the left palm downward. Look forward. (Figs. 129, 130)

40.2 Step Forward and Smear with the Sword

Bend the left knee, lower the right foot to the right front, turn the body slightly to the right; at the same time the right hand smears with the sword in a curve past the front of the body to the right, with the right wrist at the chest level, the right palm downward and the tip of the sword to the left; touch the left sword-fingers to the inside of the right forearm, with the left palm downward. Look at the front part of the blade. (Fig. 131)

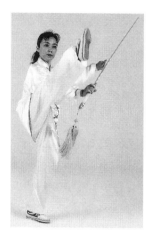
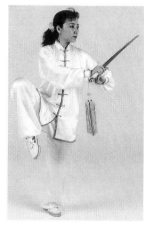
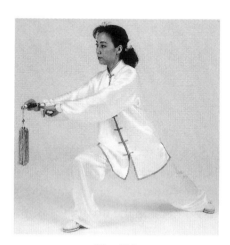

Fig. 129   Fig. 130   Fig. 131

40.3 Block Up the Sword in Bow Stance

Bend the right knee and bow forward, push the left heel outward to form a right bow stance, turn the torso slightly to the left; at the same time the right hand raises the

sword to block up, with the tip of the sword to the left front; raise the left sword-fingers together with the right hand, then point with the sword-fingers to the left front past the front of the face, with the fingertips upward at the nose level. Look in the direction the sword points. (Fig. 132)

Important Points

● When swinging out the leg (wàibǎituǐ 外摆腿), bend the left leg slightly and stand steady; starting from the left side, the right leg hooks out in a fan-shaped arc past the front of the chest to the right, straighten the ankle with the foot no lower than the shoulder. At the

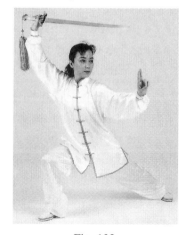

Fig. 132

same time, coordinate hooking out the leg with the moving of the sword and turning of the forearm from right to left.

● When moving the sword to the left, turn the arm inward, move the blade of the sword in front of the head in a fan-shaped arc.

● When the right hand smears (mǒ 抹) with the sword, as soon as the right hand reaches over the right knee, bend the right arm and withdraw and raise the sword to block up, do the movements smoothly. Coordinate blocking up with the sword and pointing forward with the bow stance.

● When fixing the form, the bow stance faces Southwest, the direction of the tip of the sword, the sword-fingers and the eyes is Southeast.

Common Mistakes

● The hooking out leg is too low; the leg is hooked out in a too short distance; the hips are tense; after hooking out the leg, the body is unbalanced.

● The sword is raised too high, the arm is thrown out and the hand is held up.

● The smearing sword is overdone, the movements of raising the sword and blocking up are done in a manner of reverse stabbing.

● When fixing the form, the hips are turned to form a side-bow stance.

● The sword-fingers are moved along the edge of the blade to point forward, forming by mistake a stroking sword (lǚjiàn 捋剑).

● When fixing the form, the leg moves faster than the hand. The bow stance is not coordinated with raising the sword and blocking up.

41. Gōngbù Zhícì 弓步直刺 (Bow Stance and Stab Straight)

41.1 Draw In the Foot and Sword

Shift the body center to the right leg, raise and withdraw the left foot to the inside of the right foot (do not touch the left foot to the ground); at the same time the right hand moves the sword downward past the right side of the body until the right hand reaches the side of the right hips, with the "tiger's mouth" forward and the tip of the sword forward; move the left sword-fingers downward past the left side of the body and withdraw them to the side of the left hips, with the left palm downward and fingertips forward. Look to the right front. (Fig. 133)

41.2 Stab Forward in Bow Stance

Move the left foot forward to form a left bow stance; turn the torso slightly to the left; at the same time the right hand stabs forward with the blade of the sword on the vertical; bring the left sword-fingers close to the right hand before the chest,

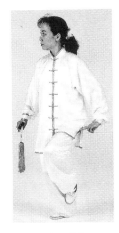

Fig. 133

and touch them to the inside of the right wrist, then extend both hands forward, with the left palm slanted downward. Look forward. (Fig. 134)

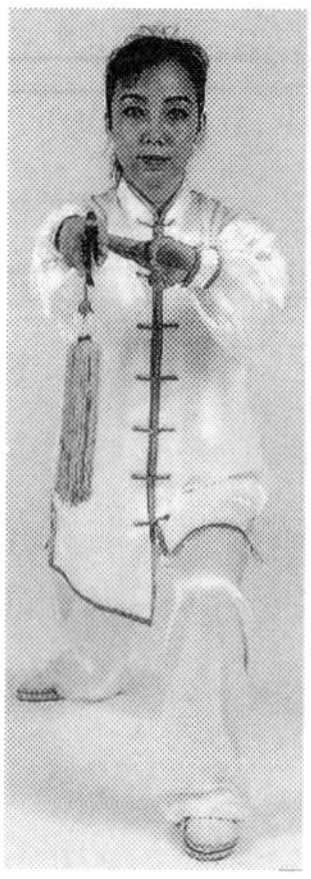

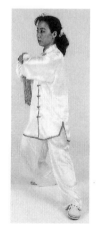

Important Points

● When pulling back the sword and foot, turn the torso to the right, lower the hands in curves.

● Stab with the blade vertical and as high as the shoulder. The direction of the stabbing sword and the bow stance is the same as in the beginning posture.

Common Mistakes

● When stabbing with the sword, the foot moves faster than the hand, the torso and the lower body are not coordinated.

Fig. 134

● When pulling back the sword, the torso is not turned, the movement does not flow.

● When fixing the form, the torso leans forward or backward.

42. Shōushì 收势 (Finish)

42.1 Turn the Waist to Take Over the Sword

Shift the body center backward, bend the right knee, and turn the torso to the right; at the same time bend the right elbow while the right hand draws the sword to the right until the right hand reaches the front of the right chest; the left sword-fingers are still on the right wrist and move to the right with the right hand, the palms face each other (ready to take over the sword), the blade slightly touches the outer side of the left forearm. Look forward. (Fig. 135)

42.2 Follow-Up Step and Draw In the Sword

Turn the torso to the left, shift the body center forward, move the right foot half a step forward to form a standing parallel feet-apart stance; at the same time, change the left sword-fingers into an open-palm hand to take over the sword (reverse holding), then move the sword in the left hand past the front of the lower abdo-

Fig. 135

men to the left until the left hand reaches the left side of the body, with the left palm facing backward, the blade of the sword upright and the tip upward. Meanwhile, change the right hand into sword-fingers and move the right hand in a curve past the lower position to the right rear, then bend the right elbow and raise the right hand to the side of the right ear, with the palm inward, the fingertips pointing up at head level. Look forward. (Figs. 136, 137)

42.3 Stand Straight with the Arms Hanging Naturally

The legs stand naturally straight; at the same time lower the right sword-fingers past the front of the chest to the right side of the body. Look forward. (Fig. 138)

42.4 Bring the Feet Together and Return to the Beginning Position

Move the left foot close to the right foot, stand naturally, with the hands naturally at the sides of the body. Look forward. (Fig. 139)

Important Points

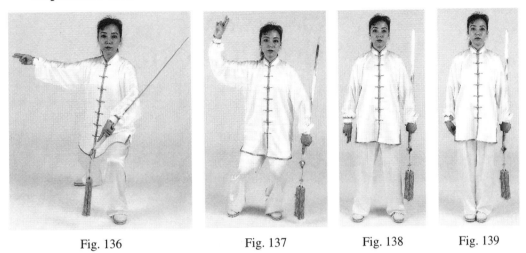

| Fig. 136 | Fig. 137 | Fig. 138 | Fig. 139 |

- Make a smooth exchange of the sword between the hands.
- Make the whole sequence a continuous one, flowing, gentle and steady.
- After bringing the feet together, keep the torso relaxed and upright, and pause for a moment before relaxing and walking away.

Common Mistakes

- On the exchange of the sword between the hands, there is a pause.
- The ending is done in a rush. After bringing the feet together and standing, the body immediately loses its attention.
- In holding the sword backhand in the left hand at the end, the blade of the sword is not upright.

CHAPTER IX
32-STEP TAIJI SWORD
Sānshí'èr Shì Tàijíjiàn 三十二式太极剑

Introduction

The first instructional material on 32-Step Taiji Sword was published by China's State Physical Culture and Sports Commission under editor-in-chief Li Tianji in 1957 in the form of a wall chart. This was followed by book editions that now have reached a circulation of over one million — an indication of how much this sword form has contributed to promoting the popularity of Taiji Sword. With basic material, a clear routine, precise sword techniques and traditional movements, 32-Step Taiji Sword is simple to learn and to remember. It is suitable for practice by individuals or in a group, and it takes about three minutes to complete which makes it convenient to practice on a regular basis.

Adapted from the Yang-style Taiji Sword, 32-Step Taiji Sword preserves the style and features of traditional Taiji Sword, but also provides a breakthrough in the routine by eliminating complications to provide an easy method for group instruction and for beginners who want to learn the basic form and techniques of Taiji Sword.

The 32-Step Taiji Sword includes 32 representative movements divided into four parts, with eight movements in each part. From start to finish, the entire routine goes back and forth on its axis (or line of movement) just twice. The 32-Step Taiji Sword includes 13 sword techniques: point (diǎn 点), stab (cì 刺), sweep (sǎo 扫), draw (dài 带), chop (pī 劈), pull back (chōu 抽), slice upward (liāo 撩), block (lán 拦), hook (guà 挂), intercept (jié 截), lift (tuō 托), strike (jī 击), and smear (mǒ 抹).

The 32-Step Taiji Sword also includes seven stances (bùxíng 步型): Front bow stance, empty stance, crouch stance, one-leg stance, feet-together stance, T-stance, and side-bow stance; and over 10 footwork techniques (bùfǎ 步法): Step in, step back, forward step, draw-in step, follow-up step, jumping step, stabbing step, standing upright with feet together step, toes-out step, toes-in step, and step with the pivot on the ball or heel of the foot; and self-defense techniques of moving the body (shēnfǎ 身法) such as shift (zhuǎn 转), rotate (xuán 旋), contract or draw back (suō 缩), and turn around (fǎn 反).

Names of the Movements of 32-StepTaiji Sword

Yùbèishi 预备势 (Ready Position)
Qǐshì 起势 (Beginning Position)
Also known as Sanhuán Tàoyuè 三环套月 (Three Rings Envelop the Moon)

Part I

1. Bìngbù Diǎnjiàn 并步点剑 (Stand with the Feet Together and Point)
   Also known as Qīngtíng Diǎnshuǐ 蜻蜓点水 (Dragonfly Skims over the Water)
2. Dúlì Fǎncì 独立反刺 (One-leg Stance and Reverse Stab)
   Also known as Dàkuíxīng Shì 大魁星势 (Big Dipper)
3. Pūbù Héngsǎo 仆步横扫 (Crouch Stance and Sweep to the Side)
   Also known as Yànzi Chaoshuǐ 燕子抄水 (Swallow Brushes the Water)
4. Xiàngyòu Píngdài 向右平带 (Horizontal Draw to the Right)
   Also known as Yòu Lánsǎo 右拦扫 (Right Block and Sweep)
5. Xiàngzuǒ Píngdài 向左平带 (Horizontal Draw to the Left)
   Also known as Zuǒ Lánsǎo 左拦扫 (Left Block and Sweep)
6. Dúlì Lūnpī 独立抡劈 (One-leg Stance, Circle and Chop Down)
   Also known as Tànhǎi Shì 探海势 (Probe the Sea Position)
7. Tuìbù Huíchōu 退步回抽 (Step Back and Draw the Sword Back)
   Also known as Huáizhōng Bàoyuè 怀中抱月 (Embrace the Moon)
8. Dúlì Shàngcì 独立上刺 (One-leg Stance and Stab Up)
   Also known as Sùniǎo Teulín 宿鸟投林 (Birds Fly into the Woods)

Part II

9. Xūbù Xiàjié 虚步下截 (Empty Stance and Intercept Downward)
   Also known as Wūleng Bǎiwoi 乌龙摆尾 (Black Dragon Waves Its Tail)
10. Zuǒgōngbù Cì 左弓步刺 (Left Bow Stance and Stab)
    Also known as Qīngleng Chūshuǐ 青龙出水 (Blue Dragon Emerges from Water)
11. Zhuǎnshēn Xiédài 转身斜带 (Turn the Body and Draw on a Slant)
    Also known as Fēngjuǎn Héyè 风卷荷叶 (Wind Curls Lotus Leaves)

12. Suōshēn Xiédài 缩身斜带 (Contract the Body and Draw on the Diagonal)

    Also known as Shīzi Yáoteu 狮子摇头 (Lion Nods Its Head)

13. Tíxī Pongjiàn 提膝捧剑 (Raise the Knee and Hold the Sword)

    Also known as Hǔbàoteu 虎抱头 (Tiger Covers Its Head)

14. Tiàobù Píngcì 跳步平刺 (Jump Step and Stab with a Flat Sword)

    Also known as Yomǎ Tiàojiàn 野马跳涧 (Wild Horse Leaps over Ravine)

15. Zuǒ Xūbù Liao 左虚步撩 (Left Empty Stance and Slice Upward)

    Also known as Xiǎokuíxīng Shì 小魁星势 (Little Dipper)

16. Yòu Gōngbù Liao 右弓步撩 (Right Bow Stance and Slice Upward)

    Also known as Hǎidǐ Laoyuè 海底捞月 (Dredge for the Moon in the Sea)

Part III

17. Zhuǎnshēn Huíchōu 转身回抽 (Turn the Body and Pull Back)

    Also known as Shèyàn Shì 射雁势 (Shoot at the Wild Goose)

18. Bìngbù Píngcì 并步平刺 (Stand Upright with Feet Together and Stab with a Flat Sword)

    Also known as Báiyuán Xiànguǒ 白猿献果 (White Ape Offers Fruit)

19. Zuǒ Gōngbù Lán 左弓步拦 (Left Bow Stance and Block)

    Also known as Yíngfēng Dǎnchén 迎风掸尘 (Wind Flicks the Dust)

20. Yòu Gōngbù Lán 右弓步拦 (Right Bow Stance and Block)

    Also known as Yíngfēng Dǎnchén 迎风掸尘 (Wind Flicks the Dust)

21. Zuǒ Gōngbù Lán 左弓步拦 (Left Bow Stance and Block)

    Also known as Yíngfēng Dǎnchén 迎风掸尘 (Wind Flicks the Dust)

22. Jìnbù Fǎncì 进步反刺 (Step In and Stab Backhand)

    Also known as Shùnshuǐ Tuīzhōu 顺水推舟 (Push the Boat Along with the Current)

23. Fǎnshēn Huípī 反身回劈 (Reverse Body and Chop Behind)

    Also known as Liúxīng Gǎnyuè 流星赶月 (Meteor Chases the Moon)

24. Xūbù Diǎnjiàn 虚步点剑 (Empty Stance and Point the Sword)

    Also known as Tianmǎ Xíngkōng 天马行空 (Celestial Horse Transverses the Void)

Part IV

25. Dúlì Píngtuō 独立平托 (One-leg Stance and Lift Horizontally)

    Also known as Tiǎolián Shì 挑帘势 (Lift the Curtain)

26. Gōngbù Guàpī 弓步挂劈 (Bow Stance, Hook and Chop)

    Also known as Zuǒ Chēlúnjiàn 左车轮剑 (Wheel the Sword to the Left)

27. Xūbù Lūnpī 虚步抡劈 (Empty Stance, Circle Sword and Chop)

    Also known as Yòu Chēlenjiàn 右车轮剑 (Wheel the Sword to the Right)

28. Chèbù Fǎnjī 撤步反击 (Back Step and Strike Backhand)

Also known as Dàpéng Zhǎnchì 大鹏展翅 (Great Eagle Spreads Its Wings)

29. Jìnbù Píngcì 进步平刺 (Step In and Stab with a Flat Sword)

Also known as Huángfēng Rùdòng 黄蜂入洞 (Yellow Bee Enters the Cave)

30. Dīngbù Huíchōu 丁步回抽 (T-Stance and Pull Back)

Also known as Huáizhōng Bàoyuè 怀中抱月 (Embrace the Moon)

31. Xuánzhuǎn Píngmǒ 旋转平抹 (Turn Around and Smear Horizontally)

Also known as Fēngsǎo Méihuā 风扫梅花 (Wind Sweeps the Plum Blossoms)

32. Gōngbù Zhícì 弓步直刺 (Bow Stance and Stab Straight)

Also known as Zhǐnánzhēn 指南针 (Compass Points South)

Shōushì 收势 (Closing Position)

Movements and Illustrations of 32-Step Taiji Sword

Yùbèishi 预备势 (Ready Position)

Stand with the feet together and the body upright. Assume the direction faced is South. Let the arms hang naturally at the sides of the body, hold the handle of the sword in the left hand with the tip of the sword pointing upward, while the right hand makes "sword-fingers" with the index and middle fingers held straight down and the palm in. Look straight ahead. (Fig. 1)

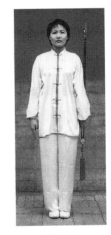

Fig. 1

Important Points

● Keep the neck straight, the chin slightly drawn in. Concentrate.

● Relax the torso. Do not intentionally stick out the chest or hold in the abdomen.

● Relax and lower the shoulders, bend the elbows slightly; keep the sword against the back of the left forearm without the sword edge touching the body.

Common Mistakes

● The body is strained, the shoulders are shrugged and the chest is stuck out.

● The sword is not held correctly in the left hand so that the sword touches the body.

Qǐshì 起势 (Beginning Position)

Also known as Sanhuán Tàoyuè 三环套月 (Three Rings Envelop the Moon)

1. Step with the Left Foot

Move the left foot half a step to the left until the feet are shoulder-width apart, parallel with each other. Turn the right sword-fingers inward, and turn the palm to the back. (Fig. 2)

2. Raise the Arms

Raise the arms slowly forward to shoulder height, palms down. Look straight ahead. (Fig. 3)

Important Points

● When raising the arms, relax and keep the shoulders naturally low; do not shrug the shoulders.

● Keep the sword against the lower part of the left forearm, point the handle of sword straight ahead with the tip of the sword slightly lowered.

Common Mistakes

The body strains to apply strength, the shoulders shrug and the arms straighten.

3. Turn the Body and Swing the Arm

Turn the torso slightly to the right. Shift the body center onto the right leg, bend the knee to a squat, and then lift the left foot and draw it in to the inside of the right ankle. (Do not touch the toes to the ground.) At the same time, turn and lower the right sword-fingers, then lift them up to the right past the abdomen, right palm facing up. Hold the sword in the left hand while bending the elbow until the left hand reaches in front of the right shoulder passing the face, palm down, and then hold the sword with the blade flat in front of the chest. Look at the right sword-fingers. (Figs. 4, 5)

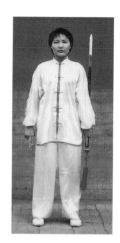

Fig. 2

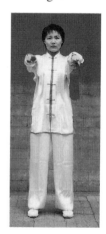

Fig. 3

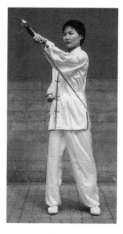

Fig. 4

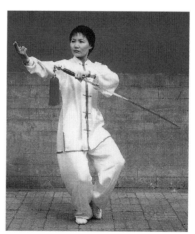

Fig. 5

Important Points

- Shift the body center onto the right leg and keep it steady; then draw in the left foot and bend the left leg.
- When holding the sword in the left hand and drawing an arc in the air, do not shrug the shoulders and do not let the body lean.

Common Mistakes

- When holding the sword in the left arm to draw an arc in the air, the shoulders are shrugged and the body leans.
- The arm is swung and the head turned without coordination through the turning of the waist.

4. Bow Stance and Point Forward

Turn the body to the left. Step forward with the left leg (toward the East) to form a left bow stance. At the same time, holding the sword in the left hand, brush the left hand toward the lower left, passing the sword in front of the body until it reaches the side of the left hip. Then, hold the sword straight up and down along the back of the left forearm, with the sword tip pointing upward. Bend the right arm, pass the sword-fingers by the ear, and then point the sword-fingers forward while turning the body, fingertips pointing naturally upward at the same level with eyes. Look at the right sword-fingers. (Figs. 6, 7)

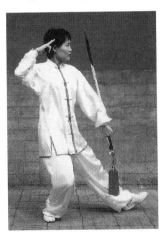

Fig. 6

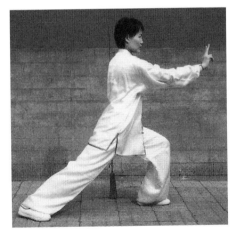

Fig. 7

Important Points

- While stepping forward, shift the body center onto the right leg and keep it steady before stepping forward with the left foot. Put the heel on the ground first, then bend the left knee forward, and shift the body center gradually forward with the left foot slowly becoming solid on the ground. The left toes face forward, and the knee does not go beyond the toes. Naturally straighten the right leg, and push the right heel back on the ground in bow stance. While making the bow stance, try to avoid moving the body center forward immediately with your forward step, which is known as "rushing the step." As for the bow stance in its fixed form, land the left foot at a suitable point so that the width between the feet is about 12 inches or 30 centimeters.

• Be soft and coordinated in turning the body, stepping forward, bowing the leg, and moving the arms. Complete these movements all at the same time.

• Be continuous in the second, third and fourth movements.

Common Mistakes

• When stepping forward into a bow stance, the body center is shifted forward too early, and the ball of the foot hits the ground hard.

• The width between the feet is too short, and the body center is not stable. For instance, the feet are in a straight line as in "tightrope walking." Or the legs cross like a "fried dough twist," which causes stiff movements and a strained body.

• The heel of the rear foot is not pushed down and backward, causing the knee and hip to turn outward, not coordinated with the torso.

5. Cross the Legs and Spread the Arms

Turn the body to the right. Bend the left elbow, hold the sword in the left hand, and thread the sword through above the right hand in front of the chest. Turn over the right sword-fingers and slowly lower them, passing by the waist, palm upward, to the right side of the body. The left and right arms spread out to the sides. At the same time, lift the right leg and step forward with the toes pointing out, the legs crossing, and the knees overlapping in the front and at the back. Then raise the left heel, slightly lower the body center, forming a half-sitting posture with legs crossed. Look at the right sword-fingers. (Figs. 8, 9)

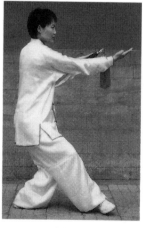

Fig. 8

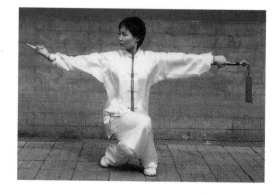

Fig. 9

Important Points

• When crossing the hands in front of the body, hold the sword in the left hand and thread (chuɑn 穿) the sword straight forward in front of the body. Do not bend the elbow and push the sword horizontally forward.

• When stepping forward with the right foot, be light in landing the right foot as it steps across, and be stable when moving the body. Try to avoid "rushing the step," that is, try to avoid a heavy landing of the foot accompanied by a sudden shifting of the body center forward.

• Draw back the right hand while lowering it, drawing an arc along the front of the abdomen. Do not draw back in a straight line. Take care to coordinate the movement with the turning of the body to the right.

• After threading the sword held in the left hand, turn the left forearm in and keep the sword close to the back of the left arm.

Common Mistakes

• The right foot lands too far as it steps across forward; the knees are not placed against each other; the body center is mostly on the front leg and thus the half-sitting posture (bànzuòpán 半坐盘) is changed into a cross-legged stance (jiɑochɑbù 交叉步).

• The right toes are not pointed out, and the torso is not turned to the right, and the half-sitting posture is changed into a kneeling stance in which the knees do not cross.

6. Bow Stance and Take Over the Sword

Holding the sword in the left hand, rotate the blade slightly out, turn the palm downward, with the tip of the blade slightly lowered. Step forward with the left foot forming a left bow stance. At the same time, turn the body to the left, move the right sword-fingers forward past the side of the head and place them on the sword handle, ready to take over the sword. Look straight ahead. (Figs. 10, 11)

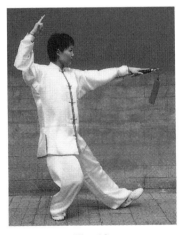

Fig. 10

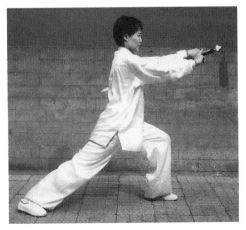

Fig. 11

Important Points

• When lifting the leg and stepping forward, raise the right arm upward. And then bend the knee to form a bow stance, lower the right arm in front. Slightly bend the elbows and relax the shoulders; keep the torso naturally upright.

• Maintain the width between the feet in bow stance at about 12 inches or 30 centimeters apart.

Common Mistakes

• The front foot of the bow stance points to the Northeast (It should be pointing due East); and the heel of the rear foot is not pushed down and backward (The back foot should be slanted toward the Southeast).

• The distance between the feet of the bow stance is not wide enough, leading to a strained torso and unstable body center.

Part I

1. Bìngbù Diǎnjiàn 并步点剑 (Stand with the Feet Together and Point)

Also known as Qīngtíng Diǎnshuǐ 蜻蜓点水 (Dragonfly Skims over the Water)

Loosen the right sword-fingers, with the web between the thumb and the index finger facing the sword handle. Grasp the sword handle with the right hand, then bend the right wrist, lower and draw it back, with the wrist circling and drawing a circle perpendicular to the ground from the left of the body. Stretch out the arm, lift the wrist, and point forward, sending the strength to the tip of the sword in front of the body. Meanwhile, the left hand assumes the sword-fingers position with the middle and index fingers straight, placed on the right wrist. At the same time, move the right foot to the left foot to form a standing stance with feet together and half-squat over the heels. Look at the sword tip. (Fig. 12)

Important Points

• When using the wrist to turn the sword blade in a vertical circular motion from the left to the front, do not lift the arms upward.

• To point (diǎn 点) means to point and pierce with the sword tip downward by bending the wrist and focusing power on the sword tip. When pointing, hold the sword firmly with the thumb, ring finger and little finger, and lightly grasp with the other two fingers. Hold the sword loosely with flexibility, and point

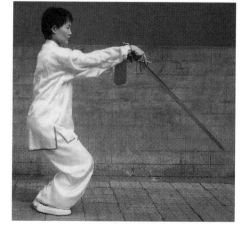

Fig. 12

the sword downward to the front mainly through the action of the wrist, with the sword slanted downward and the right arm naturally straight.

● When standing straight with feet together, do not place the feet too close together, and stand with the soles of the feet completely on the ground. Squat slightly and shift the body center mainly onto the left leg. Do not form a T-stance with the ball of the right foot on the ground; do not distribute the body center weight onto both legs. Keep the body straight.

Common Mistakes

● When pointing, the power does not reach the sword tip, the arm and the sword are in the same line, and the wrist is not bent and raised sufficiently.

● When standing upright with feet together, empty is not differentiated from solid; the right heel comes off the ground.

● The torso leans forward too much.

2. Dúlì Fǎncì 独立反刺 (One-Leg Stance and Reverse Stab)
Also known as Dàkuíxīng Shì 大魁星势 (Big Dipper)

2.1 Draw Back the Foot and the Sword

Draw back the right foot to the right, and at the same time shift the body center back. Draw back the sword in the right hand to the front of the abdomen, the sword tip slightly elevated. Place the left sword-fingers on the right wrist, so that the left hand stays with the right hand when it draws back the sword. Look at the sword tip. (Figs. 13, 14)

Important Points

● When drawing back the right foot, land the ball of the foot first, and then bend the right leg and shift the body center back. The landing point of the withdrawing right foot is slightly to the right rear. Land the right foot with the toes pointing 60 degrees out.

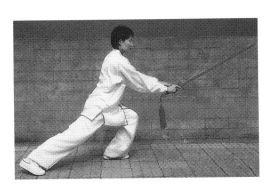

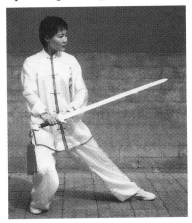

Fig. 13   Fig. 14

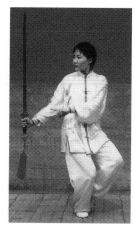

Fig. 15

- When drawing back the sword with the right hand, drop the right arm and lower the right wrist, with the sword tip naturally lifted.

Common Mistakes

- The right foot is withdrawn to the West (It should be Southwest), or the toes point out at too big an angle.

- The foot drops heavily, and the body center shifts backward too fast.

2.2 Draw In the Foot and Spear Up the Sword

Turn the body to the right rear (Southwest). Then draw in the left foot to the inside of the right foot, with the toes touching the ground. At the same time, hold the sword in the right hand, and continue to draw back and slice up (liao 撩) backhand to the right rear. And then turn the right arm outward and lower the right wrist, turning up the sword tip until the blade is up on a slant on the right side of the body. Draw the left sword-fingers back with the sword to the inside of the right forearm. Look at the sword tip. (Fig. 15)

Important Points

- Do not let the right foot move around.

- Be continuous, smooth and natural when turning and lowering the wrist, and then turning up the sword. Try to avoid leaning the torso to the left or raising the right shoulder and the right elbow.

- When turning up the sword, bend the wrist and hold the sword lightly.

Common Mistakes

- The sword is held too tightly in the right hand; the torso is twisted when drawing back and slicing upward; the shoulders are shrugged and elbows raised.

- When the right hand slices the sword upward, it moves around, so the track of the sword is not circular.

2.3 Lift the Knee and Reverse Stab (Fǎncì 反刺)

Turn the torso to the left. Raise the left knee into a one-leg stance. At the same time, hold the sword in the right hand and lift it above and past the right side of the head before jabbing it straight forward backhand with a vertical blade, sending power to the tip of the sword, the thumb of the right hand downward, the palm facing out. Pass the left sword-fingers under the chin and point the left hand to the front, the fingertips naturally upward and at the eye level. Look at the sword-fingers. (Fig. 16)

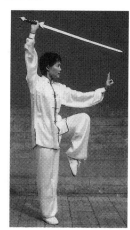

Fig. 16

Important Points

● Stand with the right leg naturally straight, try to lift the left knee as high as possible, let the left toes drop, stretch the left foot, and pull the sole of the left foot and the left calf slightly inside to protect the groin. Keep the torso straight, head and neck upright, and the chin slightly drawn in. Do not bend forward or backward.

● The left knee should be directly in front, just below the left elbow. Do not lean to the right. If in the previous movement, the right foot was positioned in the right direction, the right foot will help stabilize the body when raising the left knee to stand on one leg.

● To stab (cì 刺) the sword means to deliver the power to the sword tip by stretching the arm and swinging. Be careful not to raise the sword blade on the horizontal straight up from below.

Common Mistakes

● The direction in which the knee is lifted is not directly to the front (due East), but to the Southeast; the left elbow and the left knee are not in line with each other.

● The right toes point due South, which affects the stability when lifting the knee and standing on one leg.

● The technique of stabbing is executed as blocking up with the sword (shàngjià jiàn 上架剑).

3. Pūbù Héngsǎo 仆步横扫 (Crouch Stance and Sweep to the Side)

Also known as Yànzi Chāoshuǐ 燕子抄水 (Swallow Brushes the Water)

3.1 Draw the Foot Back and Chop

Turn the torso to the right rear. Cut down with the edge of the sword at the right rear while turning the body until the right arm is level with the ground and in line with the sword, and place the left sword-fingers on the right wrist. While turning the body, bend the right leg, step with the left foot back to the left rear (Northeast), and straighten the left knee. Look at the sword tip. (Fig. 17)

Important Points

● When stepping with the left foot to the left rear, do not change the direction of the right foot.

● Cut down with the sword in the direction opposite to that in which left leg stepped back.

Common Mistake

The sword tip is dropped and is not in a straight line with the right arm.

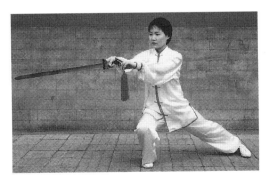

Fig. 17

3.2 Crouch Stance and Sweep

Turn the body to the left. The left sword-fingers point toward the rear as they pass in front of the body along the left ribs. They then draw up in a semi-circle to the upper left with the palm slanted upward. Hold the sword in the right hand and turn the palm upward, bring the sword down from the right rear, and then sweep it in a horizontal curve to the left front. Bend the right leg in a crouch stance, and shift the body center gradually to the left; form the left bow stance with the left toes out, the left leg bent, the right toes in and the right leg naturally straight. When fixing this form, hold the sword at chest level. Look at the sword tip. (Figs. 18, 19)

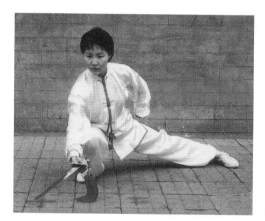

Fig. 18

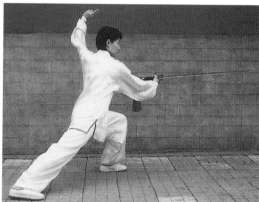

Fig. 19

Important Points

• While turning the body and shifting the body center to the left, try to turn the left toes out rather than facing straight, and then form the left bow stance with the right toes turned in. During the shift, the stance can be either a deep full crouching stance or a half-crouching stance. Keep the body upright.

• To sweep (sǎojiàn 扫剑) is to hold the sword with the flat side up and draw the blade edge to the left or to the right, with the strength on the edge of the sword. In this movement, hold the sword steady, start the sweep downward and then on the horizontal to the left front, in an arc from a higher position to the low (at the same level as the knee or the ankle) and then up again; do not sweep horizontally at waist level. When fixing the form, settle the right hand in front of the left ribs, and place the sword in front of the body in the same direction as the right arm at the chest level.

• When fixing the form, extend the left arm in an arc; do not bend or stretch it too much.

Common Mistakes

• The crouch stance is not deep enough, or it is done as a bow stance.

● The left sword-fingers do not point backward.

● In crouch stance, the waist is bent and buttocks stick out, or the sole of the foot is not fully on the ground and the heel is raised.

● The tip of the sword points on a slant to the Southeast.

4. Xiàngyòu Píngdài 向右平带 (Horizontal Draw to the Right)

Also known as Yòu Lánsǎo 右拦扫 (Right Block and Sweep)

4.1 Draw In the Foot and the Sword

Draw in the right foot to the inside of the left foot without the toes touching the ground. At the same time, hold the sword in the right hand, and draw it in slightly with the left sword-fingers placed on the right wrist. Look at the sword tip. (Fig. 20)

Important Point

When drawing back the sword in the right hand by bending the arm, raise the sword tip slightly, and keep the tip near the central line in front of the body; do not swing the sword tip to the left.

Common Mistake

The sword tip is swung away from the central line.

4.2 Step Forward and Send Out the Sword

Stride one step to the right front, and land the heel. At the same time, hold the sword in the right hand, and extend it slightly forward. Place the left sword-fingers on the right wrist. Look at the sword tip. (Fig. 21)

Important Point

Step forward in a direction about 30 degrees to the right of the central line.

Common Mistake

Stepping forward too far to the side or too far straight ahead, thus facing almost due South or due East.

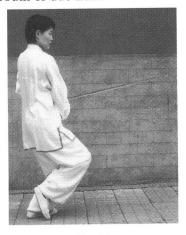

Fig. 20

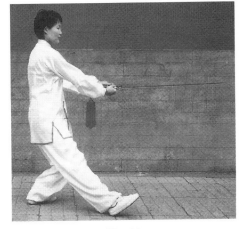

Fig. 21

4.3 Bow Stance and Draw to the Right

Shift the body center forward and land the right foot firmly in a right bow stance. Hold the sword in the right hand with the palm turned downward, and draw back the sword to the right rear. Keep the left sword-fingers on the right wrist. Look at the sword tip. (Fig. 22)

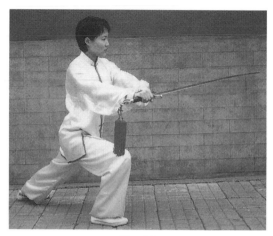

Fig. 22

Important Points

• To draw the sword is to hold the sword horizontally and draw back in an arc from the front to the rear on a slant gently, slowly and steadily, with the strength in the blade edge. In this movement, when drawing the sword horizontally, turn the sword while drawing it back on a slant. Swing the handle to the left or the right in a wide range, while continuously keeping the sword tip around the central line in front of the body, not swinging the tip too much. Coordinate drawing back the sword and making a bow stance, and at the same time, turn the torso slightly to the right, so that the movement can be coordinated and complete.

• Coordinate the drawing of the sword with bow stance with the upper and lower limbs working together in harmony.

• Draw the sword from front to back; do not push (tuī 推) it or make a sweeping (sǎo 扫) motion.

Common Mistakes

• The movements are unnatural and sudden; the hand does not turn over at the same time as the sword is drawn.

• The sword is drawn after the bow stance has been completed; the feet are quicker than the hands.

• The technique of drawing is executed as pushing or sweeping.

5. Xiàngzuǒ Píngdài 向左平带 (Horizontal Draw to the Left)

Also known as Zuǒ Lánsǎo 左拦扫 (Left Block and Sweep)

5.1 Draw In the Foot and the Sword

Holding the sword in the right hand, bend the right arm and draw back. At the same time, lift the left foot to the

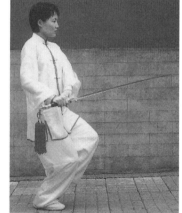

Fig. 23

inside of the right foot with the toes not touching the ground. Look at the sword tip. (Fig. 23)

Important Points

The same points apply here as in the first movement of Horizontal Draw to the Right, but in the opposite direction.

Common Mistakes

The same points apply here as in Horizontal Draw to the Right.

5.2 Step Forward and Send Out the Sword

Step to the left front with the heel first. Hold the sword in the right hand and extend the sword forward. Turn the left sword-fingers and pull back to the side of the waist. Look at the sword tip. (Fig. 24)

Important Points

The same points apply here as in the second movement of Horizontal Draw to the Right, but in the opposite direction.

Common Mistakes

The same points apply here as in 4.2 of Horizontal Draw to the Right, only in the opposite direction.

5.3 Bow Stance and Draw to the Left

Turn over the right hand and draw the sword horizontally in an arc to the left rear, the right hand pausing before the left ribs and the strength focused on the edge of the blade. Continue to draw an arc with the left sword-fingers until they are to the left above the head, the palm slanted upward. At the same time, bend the left leg. Shift the body center forward, and form a left bow stance. Look at the sword tip. (Fig. 25)

Important Points

Except for the movement of raising the left sword-fingers in an arc, the points that apply here are the same as 4.3 Bow Stance and Draw to the Right, but in the opposite direction.

Common Mistakes

The same points apply here as 4.3 Bow Stance and Draw to the Right.

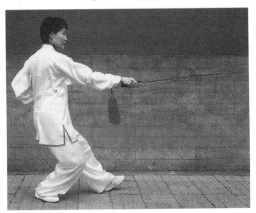 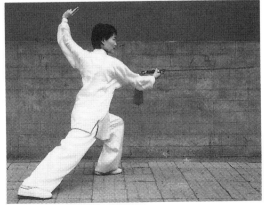

Fig. 24 Fig. 25

6. Dúlì Lūnpī 独立抢劈 (One-Leg Stance, Circle and Chop Down)

Also known as Tànhǎi Shì 探海势 (Probe the Sea Position)

6.1 Turn the Body and Circle the Sword

Turn the body to the left, draw in the right foot to the inside of the left foot, and land the toes. Turn the body to the left, hold the sword in the right hand, draw an arc from the front downward and back, and then hold the sword with vertical blade on the diagonal to the lower left of the body. Lower the left sword-fingers and cross both hands in front of the abdomen. Look back to the left. (Fig. 26 front and rear views)

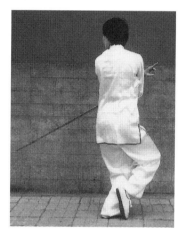
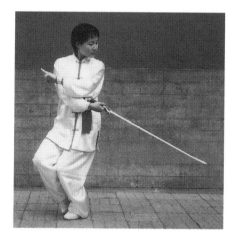

Fig. 26

Important Points

● When circling the sword in the right hand, keep the right palm slanted out and the left palm slanted downward.

● When turning the body to the left, keep the body straight and do not bend forward.

Common Mistakes

● When circling the sword, the body is not turned enough, and the eyes do not follow the sword tip to look to the lower left.

● When circling, the right palm turns down, and the sword tip points back, to form a hooking sword (guàjiàn 挂剑).

6.2 Step Forward and Raise the Sword

Step forward with the heel of the right foot. Turn the right hand in and raise it while lifting the sword in an arc above the head. Turn the sword-fingers and pull them in beside the waist. (Fig. 27)

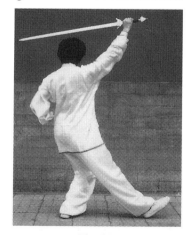

Fig. 27

Important Points

Join together the circling and the raising of the sword when drawing a vertical circle in one continuous motion, which should be coordinated with the turning of the waist and the arm.

Common Mistakes

● The sword is grasped too tightly; the sword tip is raised.

● The foot lands heavily in the step forward, and the body center shifts onto the right leg.

6.3 One-Leg Stance and Chop

Shift the body center forward, firmly landing the entire right foot, and bend and lift the left leg to form a right one-leg stance. At the same time, turn the torso to the right and slightly bend the body forward. Hold the sword in the right hand; while turning the body to the right, hold the sword with the edge of the blade upright and then chop to the lower front, with the power in the blade edge and with the right arm on the same diagonal line as the sword. Point the left sword-fingers back, and draw an arc upward until they are extended to the upper left, palm slanted upward. Look at the lower front. (Fig. 28 front and rear views)

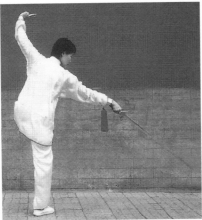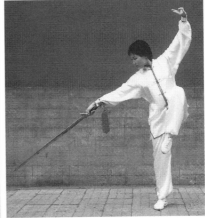

Fig. 28

Important Points

● To chop (pījiàn 劈剑) involves holding the sword with the blade edges vertical and chopping downward, with the power in the blade edge. In this movement, swing the sword with the right hand in a vertical circle downward, back, and then upward on the left side of the body. Then swing the chop from above down to the lower front, with the sword tip stopping a bit higher than knee level. When swinging the sword, take the shoulder as the axis, and stretch the arm naturally straight. When chopping, do not raise the wrist as in the technique of pointing (diǎn 点).

- Coordinate the left sword-fingers with the right hand that holds the sword. When lifting the sword with the right hand, draw an arc crosswise with the left sword-fingers downward and back. When chopping to the lower front with the sword in the right hand, draw an arc with the left sword-fingers upward until they are above the head. The hands cross as they draw vertical circles symmetrically, from up to down, and from front to back.

- Be continuous in the whole movement without pausing.

Common Mistakes

- The arm is not in a straight line with the sword, and the power is not on the edge of the sword, but rather the movement is done like the movement of raising the knee and pointing the sword.

- When circling the arm and the sword, the direction points Southeast (It should be pointing due East).

7. Tuìbù Huíchōu 退步回抽 (Step Back and Draw the Sword Back)

Also known as Huáizhōng Bàoyuè 怀中抱月 (Embrace the Moon)

7.1   Step Back and Raise the Sword

Land the foot at the back. Hold the sword in the right hand, turn it out and lift it. (Fig. 29)

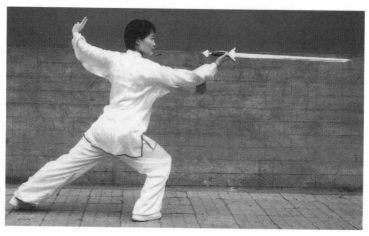

Fig. 29

7.2   Empty Stance and Draw Back the Sword

Shift the body center back, draw back the right foot half a step, and touch the ground with the ball of the left foot, forming a right empty stance. At the same time, pull back the sword in the right hand, and draw the handle beside the left ribs, the palm in and the sword tip slanted upward. Place the left sword-fingers on the handle. Look at the sword tip. (Fig. 30 front and rear views)

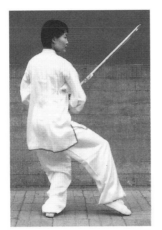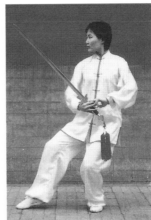

Fig. 30

Important Points

● To draw back the sword (chōujiàn 抽剑) is to draw the sword back in a circular motion with the blade edge vertical, the focus of power sliding along the blade edge. When drawing the sword upward in this form, first turn the right hand with palm up, lift the sword slightly, and then draw an arc in front of the body and pull it back beside the left ribs. Try not to draw the sword back in a straight line.

● The distance should not be too narrow when stepping back with the left foot. Be bold in shifting the body center forward or back. And make a clear distinction in the legs between empty or solid.

● When fixing the movement, extend the arms as if embracing a circle, and turn the torso to the left, with the sword tip pointing to the upper right. At the same time, turn the head to the right, relax and lower the shoulders, and keep the sword handle about 4 inches or 10 centimeters away from the left ribs.

Common Mistakes

● The difference between empty and solid is not distinct in the legs, and the body center shifts too fast.

● The sword is held with too much tension, the handle is grasped too tightly, the sword is vertical; the hands are too close to the body, clamping the elbows and closing the armpits.

8. Dúlì Shàngcì 独立上刺 (One-Leg Stance and Stab Up)

Also known as Sùniǎo Teulín 宿鸟投林 (Birds Fly into the Woods)

8.1 Turn the Body and Move the Feet

Turn the body slightly to the right, facing the front, and move the right foot slightly forward. At the same time, move the right hand in front of the abdomen, with palm up, and the sword tip slanted upward. Place the left sword-fingers on the right wrist. Look at the sword tip. (Fig. 31)

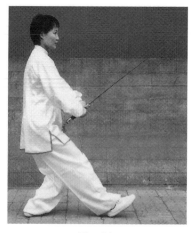

Fig. 31

Important Points

Turn with the body upright. And when taking a half-step forward, do not step farther than one foot's length.

Common Mistakes

The half-step forward is too long, the body center shifts onto the front leg.

8.2 Raise the Knee and Stab Upward

Shift the body center forward, bend the left leg and lift it. At the same time, hold the sword in the right hand, and stab to the upper front, sending power to the sword tip at head level. Keep the left sword-fingers on the right wrist. Look at the sword tip. (Fig. 32)

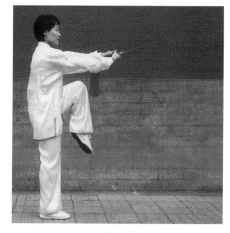

Important Points

• When stabbing upward, keep the hands at shoulder height with the arms slightly bent.

• With the motion of stabbing upward, lean the torso slightly forward, do not shrug the shoulders or hunch the back. Lift the left knee in front of the body.

Fig. 32

Common Mistakes

• The arms straighten.

• The one-leg stance is unstable, and the left thigh is not lifted to the horizontal level.

Part II

9. Xūbù Xiàjié 虚步下截 (Empty Stance and Intercept Downward)

Also known as Wūleng Bǎiwoi 乌龙摆尾 (Black Dragon Waves Its Tail)

9.1 Turn the Body and Swing the Sword

Put the left foot down to the left rear, then shift the body center to the left, and turn the body to the left. At the same time, hold the sword in the right hand, and swing the sword horizontally to the left with the turn of the body. Turn over the sword-fingers and drop them next to the waist on the left. Look at the sword tip. (Fig. 33 front and rear views)

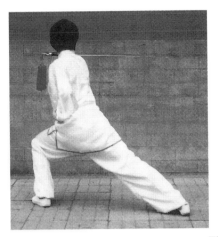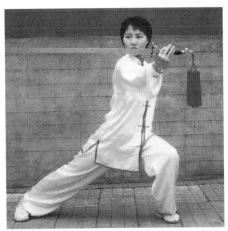

Fig. 33

Important Points

• Do not move the left foot back in a straight line, but leave a distance of about 4 to 8 inches or 10 to 20 centimeters between the feet.

• When turning the body to the left, bend the left leg, push the right heel down and outward, and naturally straighten the right leg into a left side-bow stance. With the turn of the body, hold the sword in the right hand and swing it flat to the front of the body at head level, with the palm up, the sword tip pointing to the right.

Common Mistakes

• The sword is swung to the left and upwards in an arc.

• The right heel is not pushed down and extended, and the turn of the body to the left does not reach the correct position (due South).

9.2 Empty Stance and Intercept Downward

Turn the torso to the right, and pull the right foot slightly in with the toes touching the ground, forming a right empty stance. At the same time, with the turn of the body, hold the sword in the right hand and turn the arm and the wrist (palm down) to intercept and push down to the right, passing before the body, with the sword tip hanging slightly down at knee level. Circle the left sword-fingers up to the left (the palm slanted upward). Look forward to the right. (Fig. 34)

Important Points

• To intercept with the sword (jiéjiàn 截剑) means to cut with the middle to the far end of the blade edge to stop the opponent, mostly used as a crosscut in a side attack, with the power in the edge

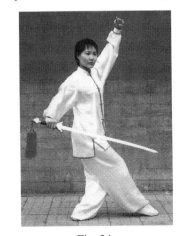

Fig. 34

of blade. When intercepting in this movement, drive the sword to intercept on the lower right mainly by turning the body and swinging the arm. Be coordinated and continuous in the movement of the body, sword, hand and feet. When fixing the form, bend the right arm a little and pull back, the sword placed to the right of the body.

- The direction of the right empty stance is 30 degrees facing East by North. The direction in which to turn the head to look is about 45 degrees to the Southeast. In the empty stance, the width between the feet is about 4 inches or 10 centimeters; try to avoid too short a width, or even a crossing of the feet.

Common Mistakes

- The movement of Empty Stance and Intercept Downward does not make full use of the turn of the body to swing the arm and intercept with the sword. It is often done in a movement of tucking in the sword, that is, using a swing of the wrist to push the sword down.

- The width between the feet in the right empty stance is too short, and the feet are even crossed.

- When turning the body to the right, the body does not reach the correct position (The direction should be Southeast).

10. Zuǒ Gōngbù Cì 左弓步刺 (Left Bow Stance and Stab)
Also known as Qīnglěng Chūshuǐ 青龙出水 (Black Dragon Emerges from Water)

10.1 Step Back and Lift the Sword

Hold the sword in the right hand and raise it in front of the body at chest level, the sword tip pointing 30 degrees to the left front. Drop the left sword-fingers on the

right wrist. At the same time, move back one step with the right foot. Look at the sword tip. (Fig. 35)

Important Points

Hold and lift the sword with the right hand; do not stab the sword.

Common Mistake

The sword is held in the right hand and lifted without being extended forward.

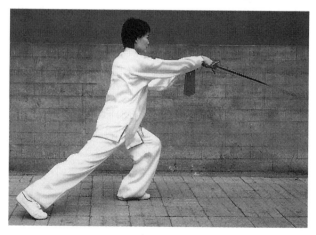

Fig. 35

10.2 Turn the Body and Draw the Sword

Shift the body center to the right and turn the body to the right. At the same time, holding the sword in the right hand, pull the sword back passing in front of the head, and turn the palm out. Draw the sword back with the left sword-fingers on the right wrist. Look at the sword tip. (Fig. 36)

Important Points

● When holding the sword in the right hand to draw back, turn the forearm in and the palm out. At the same time, control the sword tip so that it does not swing out.

● Kick and turn the right heel out, shift most of the body center onto the right leg, and keep the torso straight.

Common Mistake

The sword in the right hand is drawn back directly without being drawn in an arc passing in front of the head.

10.3 Draw In the Foot and the Sword

Turn the body to the left. Draw in the left foot to the inside of the right foot (with the toes not touching the ground). At the same time, hold the sword in the right hand, roll the sword downward and pull it in to the right side of the waist. Turn and draw back the left sword-fingers in front of the abdomen. Turn the eyes to look to the left front. (Fig. 37)

Important Points

When holding the sword in the right hand to roll downward and draw back, turn the forearm out with the palm facing up. At the same time, control the sword by pointing the tip in the direction that you will stab.

Common Mistake

The sword makes a circle; the sword tip is circled upward and backward.

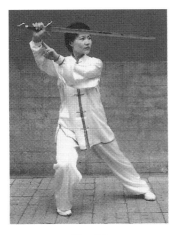

Fig. 36

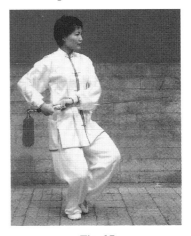

Fig. 37

10.4 Bow Stance and Stab Horizontally

Move the left foot to the left front, heel first, and shift the body center forward, forming a left bow stance. At the same time, turn the torso to the left. Hold the sword in the right hand, stab past the right side of the waist to the left front, palm up and the power going into the sword tip. Circle the left sword-fingers up and to the left, the palm slanted up and the arm rounded. Look at the sword tip. (Fig. 38)

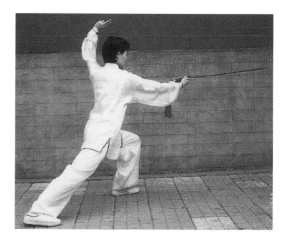

Fig. 38

Important Points

• The direction of the bow stance is about 30 degrees left of the center line (that is, facing Northeast). Be careful not to rush the step into bow stance, and keep the width between the feet at about 12 inches or 30 centimeters. Keep the torso straight and relax the waist and hips.

• When stabbing, keep the sword tip at chest level on the same line as the arm.

• Make all the movements flexible, consistent and natural, driven by the turning of the waist.

Common Mistake

The sword points due East, not in the same direction as the bow stance.

11. Zhuǎnshēn Xiédài 转身斜带 (Turn the Body and Draw on a Slant)

Also known as Fēngjuǎn Héyè 风卷荷叶 (Wind Curls Lotus Leaves)

11.1 Turn the Left Toes In and Draw Back the Sword

Shift the body center back, turn the left toes in, and turn the torso to the right. At the same time, holding the sword in the right hand, bend the arm and pull back to place the sword horizontal to the ground in front of the chest, palm up. Place the left sword-fingers on the right wrist. Look at the sword tip. (Fig. 39)

Important Points

Try to turn the left toes in as far as you can. Relax and keep the shoulders down, and draw the hands to

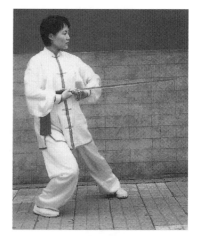

Fig. 39

the front of the right chest.

11.2 Lift the Foot and Turn the Body

Shift the body center again onto the left leg. Lift the right foot to the inside of the left calf. Extend the sword to the left front. Look at the sword tip. (Fig. 40)

Important Point

When lifting the right foot, bring it next to the calf and not up to the knee as in the one-leg stance.

11.3 Bow Stance and Draw to the Right

Turn the body to the right rear. Move the right foot to the right front (facing Northwest) in a right bow stance. At the same time, hold the sword in the right hand, turn it in with palm down, and make a horizontal draw to the right (with the sword tip a little higher than the handle) with the power in the edge of the sword. Keep the left sword-fingers attached to the right wrist. Look at the sword tip. (Fig. 41)

Important Points

● The direction of the bow stance is about 30 degrees to the right of the center line, toward the Northwest. That is, turn the body about 240 degrees from the "left bow stance" in the previous movement to the "right bow stance" in this movement.

● To draw on a diagonal refers to the route of the sword. The key points for movements are the same as those for "horizontal draw."

Common Mistakes

● The left toes are not turned in enough, the movement of turning the body to the right does not reach the correct position, and the right bow stance is not done with ease, agility and precision.

● For common mistakes of drawing the sword, the same points apply here as in Step 4: Horizontal Draw to the Right.

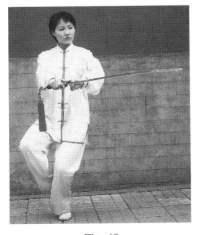

Fig. 40

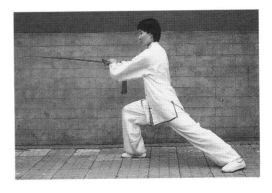

Fig. 41

12. Suōshēn Xiédài 缩身斜带 (Contract the Body and Draw on the Diagonal)

Also known as Shīzi Yáoteu 狮子摇头 (Lion Nods Its Head)

12.1 Lift the Foot and Pull Back the Sword

Lift the left foot and draw it to the inside of the right foot, with the left toes not touching the ground. At the same time, hold the sword in the right hand and slightly pull back. Keep the left sword-fingers on the right wrist. Look straight ahead. (Fig. 42)

12.2 Move the Foot Back and Send Out the Sword

Move the left foot back to its original place. Holding

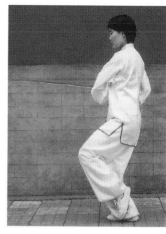

Fig. 42

the sword in the right hand, send the sword out forward (to the Northwest). Pull the left sword-fingers past the left ribs backhand with the left wrist bent, and thread the sword-fingers to the back. Look at the sword tip. (Fig. 43)

Important Points

Stretch the torso forward slightly and send out the sword in the same direction as that of the bow stance.

Common Mistakes

● The direction of the bow stance and the extended sword is West (It should be Northwest).

● The sword-fingers are pulled back to the left side, not threaded backhand to the rear.

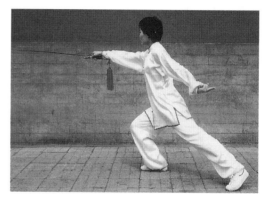

Fig. 43

12.3 T-Stance and Draw to the Left

Shift the body center onto the left leg, then draw the right foot to the inside of the left foot, and touch the ground with the right toes, forming a T-stance. At the same time, turn over the right hand with the palm upward, draw the sword horizontally to the left (the sword tip a bit higher than the handle) with the power going into the edge of the sword. Circle and draw an arc with the left sword-fingers upward and forward, and place the sword-fingers on the right wrist. Look at the sword tip. (Fig. 44)

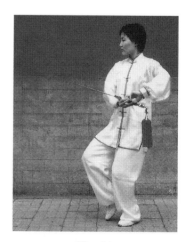

Fig. 44

Important Points

When moving the foot back and drawing the sword, turn the body to the left, with the body center on the left leg. Keep the torso upright, relax the waist and hips, and do not let the buttocks stick out.

Common Mistakes

● The sword is held with the edges of the blade vertical, the palm inward, the same as in drawing back the sword [See Step 7: Step Back and Draw the Sword Back].

● The stance is done as an empty stance.

13. Tíxī Pongjiàn 提膝捧剑 (**Raise the Knee and Hold the Sword**)

Also known as Hǔbàoteu 虎抱头 (Tiger Covers Its Head)

13.1 Empty Stance, Separate the Sword and Sword-Fingers

Step back one step with the right leg, shift the body center back, draw the left foot slightly back, and touch the ground with the left toes to form an empty stance. At the same time, extend the hands forward, and then bring them back to the sides of the body with both palms downward, and place the sword on an upward angle at the right of the body, with the tip pointing forward. Look straight ahead. (Fig. 45)

Important Points

● For the front view of this movement, see Fig.102. After separating the hands to the left and the right sides of the body, still keep the sword tip near the body center in front, with the tip of the sword a bit raised.

● Step slightly back to the right rear with the right foot, and turn the torso to the front.

Common Mistakes

● The right foot steps back to the East (It should step to 30 degrees East by North); the sword extends due West (It should extend to 30 degrees West by South).

● The sword tip swings to the right, far off the middle line.

13.2 Lift the Knee and Hold the Sword in Both Hands

Move a little forward with the left foot, lift the right knee forward into a one-leg stance. At the same time, holding the sword in the right hand, turn it outward, draw and swing the sword up in an arc in front of the body. Change the left sword-fingers into an open-palm hand and swing the left hand in front of the body, and hold and lift the sword under the

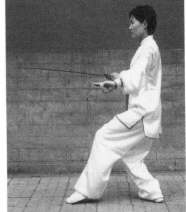

Fig. 45

back of the right palm. Slightly bend both arms, and send out the sword straight forward, the tip slightly raised. Look straight ahead. (Fig. 46)

Important Points

When swinging the hands to the front of the body, do it in an arc: First move the hands slightly out, then in, and finally clasped in front of the chest. When holding the sword, slightly bend the arms with the handle at chest level.

Common Mistakes

● When holding the sword with both hands, the movement goes from a lower level to a higher level.

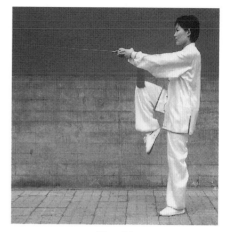

Fig. 46

● In the one-leg stance, the right knee is too low, the toes point up, or the right knee lifts to the side of the body.

14. Tiàobù Píngcì 跳步平刺 (Jump Step and Stab with a Flat Sword)

Also known as Yomǎ Tiàojiàn 野马跳涧 (Wild Horse Leaps over Ravine)

14.1 Land the Foot and Draw Back the Sword

Land the right foot in front, with the heel on the ground. Carry the sword in both hands, and draw back slightly downward and back until the hands are in front of the abdomen. Look straight ahead. (Fig. 47)

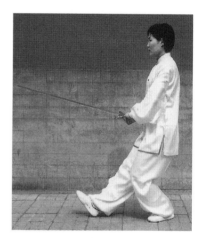

Fig. 47

Important Points

Do not land the right foot too far in front, and do not bend the torso forward.

14.2 Hold the Sword and Stab It Forward

Shift the body center onto the right leg, stretch out the right leg and drive the hips forward, and lift the left foot in the rear off the ground. At the same time, carry the sword in both hands and extend and send it out to the front. Look straight ahead. (Fig. 48)

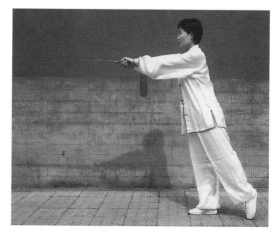

Fig. 48

Important Point

When stabbing, hold the sword at the chest level with the tip a bit raised.

14.3 Jump and Draw In the Sword

Push off the right foot, jump-stride one step forward with the left foot, and then as the left foot is about to land, pull the right foot forward rapidly to the inside of the left calf. At the same time, separate the hands and withdraw them to the sides of the body, palms downward, and change the left hand into sword-fingers. Look straight ahead. (Fig. 49)

Important Points

● Jump forward far, but not too high, and be light, nimble and gentle in the movements.

● When landing the left foot, turn the toes slightly out, bend the knee as a buffer, and keep the body center steady on the left leg.

Common Mistakes

● The jump is too high and too far, and the movement is rapid and strong.

● The torso sways, and the landing of the foot is not steady.

● The jumping step is done as a walk, the feet do not leave the ground.

14.4 Bow Stance and Stab with Flat Sword

Move the right foot forward, and shift the body center forward, forming a right bow stance. At the same time, holding the sword in the right hand, stab with a flat sword to the front, palm up. Circle and hold high the left sword-fingers above the left forehead, the palm slanted up. Look at the sword tip. (Fig. 50)

Important Points

The bow stance faces in the same direction as the arm and sword. Relax the waist and lower shoulders, and do not twist the waist or turn the hip.

Common Mistakes

In Bow Stance and Stab with Flat Sword, the body leans to one side too much, the front foot turns in, and the bow stance becomes a side-bow stance.

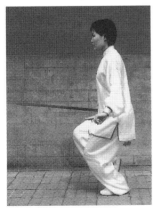

Fig. 49

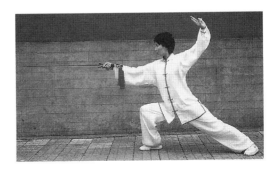

Fig. 50

15. Zuǒ Xūbù Liao 左虚步撩 (Left Empty Stance and Slice Upward)

Also known as Xiǎokuíxīng Shì 小魁星势 (Little Dipper)

15. 1 Draw In the Foot and Circle the Sword

Shift the body center back, turn the torso to the left, and draw in the right foot to the front of the left foot, right toes touching the ground. At the same time, hold the sword in the right hand, draw an arc upward and back with the turn of the body, drop the handle to the left side of the waist, the sword tip slanted upward. Lower the left sword-fingers onto the right wrist. Look to the left. (Fig. 51)

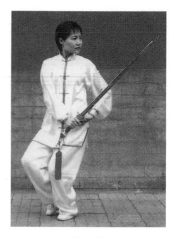

Fig. 51

Important Points

• When circling the sword back, make a full turn with the body, with the eyes turning to the left with the body.

• When circling the sword, hold it close to the body and draw a vertical circle, and at the same time, turn the right forearm in, the palm in.

Common Mistakes

• The sword is held too tightly, and the movement is not gentle.

• The turn of the waist and the swing of the arm are not full enough, and the sword circles far away from the body.

15.2 Step Forward and Circle the Sword

Turn the torso slightly to the right, step forward with the right foot, the toes turned out. At the same time, holding the sword in the right hand, circle downward to the front of the abdomen, and place the blade of the sword on an inclined plane to the left of the body. The left sword-fingers are on the right wrist and turn with the wrist. Look straight ahead. (Fig. 52)

Important Points

Keep the sword close to the body, and point the sword tip to the upper rear.

Common Mistakes

• The sword is held too tightly; the sword tip touches the ground.

• The torso leans forward.

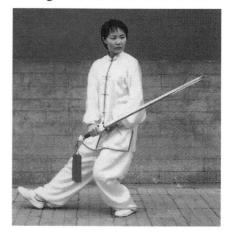

Fig. 52

15.3 Empty Stance and Slice the Sword Upward to the Left

Continue to turn the torso to the right. Shift the body center forward onto the right leg, step forward with the left foot into a left empty stance. At the same time, holding the sword in the right hand with the edges of the sword on the vertical, slice the sword upward to the front with the palm turned out, and then stop in front of the right side of the forehead, with the sword tip slightly lowered. Keep the left sword-fingers on the right wrist. Look at the sword tip. (Fig. 53)

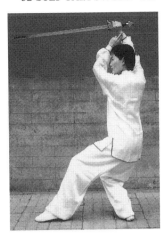

Fig. 53

Important Points

● To slice up (liao 撩) the sword means to hold the sword backhand with the edges of the blade of the sword vertical and then pull forward and upward, with the power in the far end of the blade edge. When pulling up the sword to the left in this movement, first make a vertical circle with the sword on the left side of the body, then pull up the sword to the upper front. Keep the path of the sword close to the body and also in a vertical circle. At the same time, turn the right forearm in, the right palm out, the web of the hand between the thumb and index finger downward, holding the handle loosely with the power focused on the far end of the blade.

● Complete all this movement of slicing up the sword through the drive of the turn of the body. Make a coordinated and integrated movement. And do not touch the ground with the sword tip.

● Do not lift the sword in a block.

16. Yòu Gōngbù Liao 右弓步撩 (Right Bow Stance and Slice Upward)

Also known as Hǎidǐ Laoyuè 海底捞月 (Dredge for the Moon in the Sea)

16.1 Turn the Body and Circle the Sword

Turn the body to the right. Move the left foot forward, with the left toes pointing out. At the same time, hold the sword in the right hand, draw a circle and wind back, hold the sword straight up and down to the right of the body, the palm out. The left sword-fingers circle with the sword, and pull back in front of the right chest. Look at the sword tip. (Fig. 54)

Important Points

When circling the sword back, turn the body

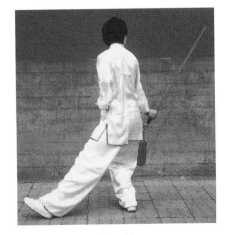

Fig. 54

to the right and look to the northeast, and
turn the body fully.

Common Mistakes

• The swing of the arm and the turn
of the body are not full enough, and the
sword is too far away from the body.

• The back and the head are bent.

16.2 Bow Stance and Slice Upward
to the Right

Turn the body to the left. Move the right

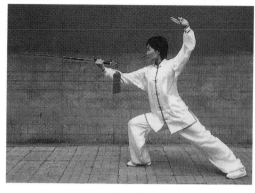

Fig. 55

foot a step forward, and shift the body center forward, forming a right bow stance. At the
same time, holding the sword in the right hand, slice the sword upward backhand in a
downward and then forward motion with the edges of the blade vertical, the palm facing out
at shoulder height, the sword tip slightly lowered. Circle the left sword-fingers upward until
they are above the left side of the head, the palm slanted up. Look straight ahead. (Fig. 55)

Important Points

• Hold the sword handle loosely and do not let the sword tip touch the ground.

• The rest is the same as that of Empty Stance and Slice the Sword Upward to the
Left in 15.3.

Common Mistakes

• The bow stance and the slicing up of the sword are not completed at the same
time. Usually the feet are faster than the sword or the sword is faster than the feet.

• When slicing up the sword, the sword tip is too low, as in blocking (lánjàn拦剑).

Part III

17. Zhuǎnshēn Huíchōu 转身回抽 (Turn the Body and Pull Back)

Also known as Shèyàn Shì 射雁势
(Shoot at the Wild Goose)

17.1 Turn the Body and Draw the Sword

Turn the body to the left, bend the left leg, and
shift the body center onto the left leg, with the right
toes slightly in. At the same time, bend the right arm
and draw the sword in front of the body at shoulder
height, with the sword horizontally straight and the
tip pointing to the right. Place the left sword-fingers
on the right wrist. Look at the sword tip. (Fig. 56)

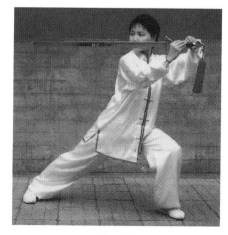

Fig. 56

Important Points

When drawing the sword, hold the sword mainly with the thumb, index finger and the web between them, the other three fingers loosely holding the sword, so that the sword can be straight horizontal to the ground.

Common Mistakes

The sword tip is raised, and the sword circles to the rear.

17.2 Bow Stance and Chop

Continue to turn the body to the left. With the left toes out, straighten the right leg to form a bow stance. At the same time, hold the sword in the right hand and slice down to the left front. Look at the sword tip. (Fig. 57)

Important Point

The direction of the bow stance and slicing down is at about a 30-degree angle to the right from the central line, that is, toward the Southeast.

Common Mistake

The sword and the right arm are not in a straight line.

17.3 Sit Back and Draw Back the Sword

Shift the body center onto the right leg, and bend the right leg. At the same time, holding the sword in the right hand, draw the sword back beside the right hip, pulling back the left sword-fingers with the right hand. Look to the lower right. (Fig. 58)

Important Point

While pulling back the sword, turn the body to the right.

Common Mistakes

The sword is pulled back in a straight line, and there is a pause at the waist.

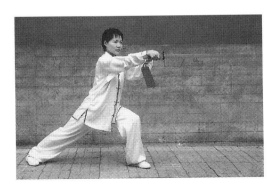

Fig. 57

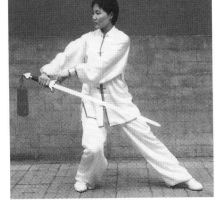

Fig. 58

17.4 Empty Stance and Point Forward

Turn the torso a little to the left, and draw the left foot half a step back into a left empty stance. At the same time, draw the right hand back behind the hip, place the sword to the right side of the body, with the sword tip a bit lowered. Point the left sword-fingers forward, passing the chin at eye level. Look at the sword-fingers. (Fig. 59)

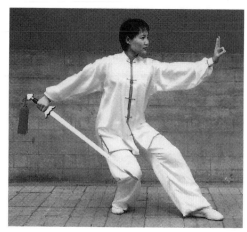

Fig. 59

Important Points

• When pointing forward with the sword-fingers, coordinate the hand movement with the movements of touching the ground with the left foot in an empty stance, and turning the torso to the left.

• The direction of the empty stance and the sword-fingers is about 30 degrees to the right of the front center, that is, toward the Southeast.

• When drawing the sword downward in this movement, draw it downward and back along an arc with the blade edges vertical and with the power in the far end edge of the sword. When fixing the movement, place the sword to the right of the body, draw the handle behind the hip, and bend the right arm slightly.

Common Mistake

The sword handle stops beside the body, not behind the hip.

18. Bìngbù Píngcì 并步平刺 (Stand Upright with Feet Together and Stab with a Flat Sword)

Also known as Báiyuán Xiànguǒ 白猿献果 (White Ape Offers Fruit)

18.1 Turn the Body and Move the Foot

Move the left foot slightly to the left, and turn the body to the left. At the same time, turn the left sword-fingers in and draw an arc to the left. Look ahead. (Fig. 60)

Important Point

When moving the left foot, turn the toes to the front.

18.2 Stand Upright with Feet Together and Stab with Flat Sword

Move the right foot next to the left foot. At the

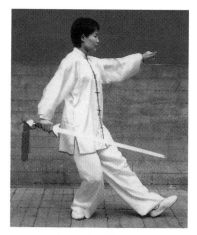

Fig. 60

same time hold the sword in the right hand, turn the hand out and jab forward with a flat sword from the waist. Pull back the left sword-fingers, turn the hand over and change it into an open-palm hand passing the waist to hold it under the right hand, both palms facing upward. Look straight ahead. (Fig. 61)

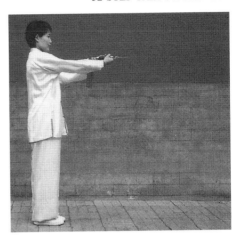

Important Points

● When holding the sword, keep the left hand in the form of sword fingers.

● Be coordinated and consistent in

Fig. 61

stabbing and standing upright with feet together. After stabbing out the sword, bend the arms slightly, and relax and lower the shoulders.

Common Mistakes

● When stabbing, the sword is not stabbed from the waist, but rather is swung in an arc from the side of the body to the front, as in holding the sword with both hands (pongjiàn 捧剑).

● The body is stiff, the chest is intentionally thrust out, the abdomen is drawn in or the torso leans forward.

● The right hand is not turned up, and the sword is held on the vertical to stab.

19. Zuǒ Gōngbù Lán 左弓步拦 (Left Bow Stance and Block)

Also known as Yíngfēng Dǎnchén 迎风掸尘 (Wind Flicks the Dust)

19.1 Turn the Body and Make a Circle with the Sword

Turn the right toes out, turn and lift the left heel out, turn the body to the right and bend both legs. Hold the sword in the right hand, turn the palm out and circle upward and rightward from the front with the turn of the body. Change the left hand to sword-fingers and place them on the right wrist so that they circle along with the right hand. Look to the right rear. (Fig. 62)

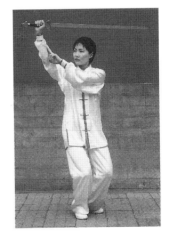

Important Point

When turning the body, lift the left heel after shifting the body center onto the right leg.

19.2 Step Forward and Circle the Sword

Move the left foot forward to the left front, heel first. Hold the sword in the right hand and continue to circle

Fig. 62

back. Turn the left sword-fingers and pull back before the abdomen. Look to the right rear. (Fig. 63)

Important Points

When circling the sword, the sword handle goes first, then the waist turns, the arm swings, and the sword is held close to the body as it makes a vertical circle.

Common Mistakes

● The left foot steps directly forward (It should be 30 degrees toward the Northeast).

● The head and the waist bend.

● When circling the sword, the sword is too far away from the body, or the sword tip touches the ground.

19.3 Bow Stance and Block

Turn the body to the left, shift the body center forward, forming a left bow stance. At the same time, hold the sword in the right hand, block and intercept from the right rear downward then to the upper left front, with the strength in the edge of the sword which is held at head level, the tip slightly lower. Turn the right arm outward with the palm slanted in. At the same time, circle the left sword-fingers to the upper left and hold them above the left forehead. Look at the sword tip. (Fig. 64)

Important Points

● To block (lán 拦) means to block upward with the bottom edge of the sword held backhand from below to the upper front, with the power in the blade edge. When blocking in this movement, turn the body to the left or the right with the sword close to the right side of the body drawing a complete vertical circle. Be careful not to touch the ground with the sword tip and also do not have the sword too far away from the body.

● At the end of the block, the right hand is in front of the left forehead, with the sword tip near the central line.

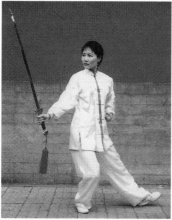
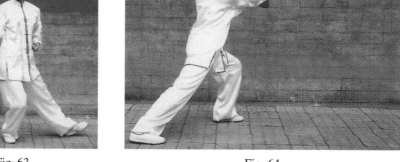

Fig. 63   Fig. 64

Common Mistakes

● The direction of the bow stance is not correct; the width between the two feet is too narrow.

● The torso is not upright, the body leans to one side, and the hips are twisted. The body is not extended, relaxed or agile.

● Blocking up with the sword in the right hand, circling the left sword-fingers, and bending the left leg forward are not coordinated in a synchronized movement.

20. Yòu Gōngbù Lán 右弓步拦 (Right Bow Stance and Block)

Also known as Yíngfēng Dǎnchén 迎风掸尘 (Wind Flicks the Dust)

20.1 Turn the Toes Out and Make a Circle with the Sword

Shift the body center slightly back, turn the left toes out and turn the body slightly to the left. At the same time, hold the sword up in the right hand, and circle to the left rear. Look at the right hand. (Fig. 65)

20.2 Draw In the Foot and Make a Circle

Continue to turn the body to the left, and draw the right foot in to the inside of the left foot (the toes not touching the ground). At the same time, holding the sword in the right hand, draw a vertical circle at the left side of the body upward, back and downward to the front of the left ribs, with the sword close to the body. Place the left sword-fingers on the right wrist. Look to the left rear in the same direction as the sword. (Fig. 66)

20.3 Bow Stance and Block

Turn the body to the right, move the right foot one step forward to the right front, and shift the body center forward into the right bow stance. At the same time, hold the sword in the right hand, draw an arc from below upward and block to the upper front, the palm out at head level, the tip slightly lowered and the sword blade

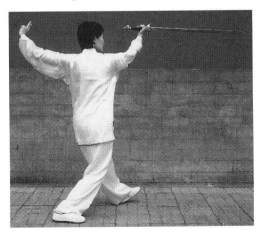

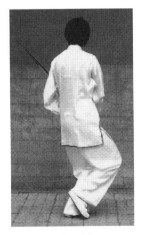

Fig. 65   Fig. 66

on a slant inward. Place the left sword-fingers on the right wrist. Look ahead. (Figs. 67, 68)

Important Points

The same points apply as in the previous movement, but in the opposite direction. And the direction of the bow stance is about 30 degrees toward the Southeast.

Common Mistakes

See previous Movement: Left Bow Stance and Block.

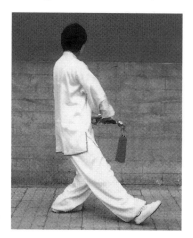

Fig. 67

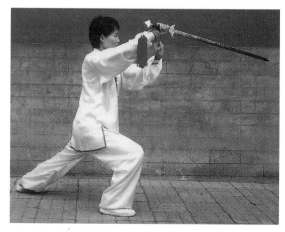

Fig. 68

21. Zuǒ Gōngbù Lán 左弓步拦 (Left Bow Stance and Block)

Also known as Yíngfēng Dǎnchén 迎风掸尘 (Wind Flicks the Dust)

21.1 Turn the Toes Out and Circle the Sword

Shift the body center slightly back, turn the right toes out, and turn the body slightly to the right. At the same time hold the sword up in the right hand, and start to make a circle with the sword to the right rear. Keep the left sword-fingers on the right wrist. Look straight ahead. (Fig. 69)

21.2 Step Forward and Circle the Sword

Continue to turn the body to the right. Draw in the left foot to the inside of the right foot. (Do not touch the left toes on the ground.) At the same time, holding the sword in the right hand, draw a vertical circle up, back and down at the side of the right hip, the sword on a slant at the right side of the body.

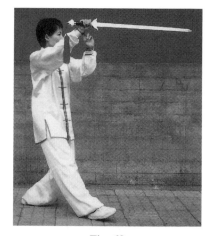

Fig. 69

The left sword-fingers circle to the front of the abdomen. The eyes move with the movement of the sword. Turn and look to the right rear. (Fig. 70)

21.3 Bow Stance and Block

Turn the body to the left, move the left foot one step forward to the left, and shift the body center forward into a left bow stance. At the same time, holding the sword in the right hand, swing the arm to draw an arc and block to the upper front, the palm on a slant inward at head level, the sword tip slightly lowered and the sword blade slanted inward. Draw an arc with the left sword-fingers leftward and upward passing the waist and stop above the left forehead, the palm obliquely upward. Look straight ahead. (Fig. 71)

Important Points & Common Mistakes

See Step 19: Left Bow Stance and Block.

22. Jìnbù Fǎncì 进步反刺 (Step In and Reverse Stab)

Also known as Shùnshuǐ Tuīzhōu 顺水推舟 (Push the Boat Along with the Current)

22.1 Step Forward and Draw Back the Sword

Move the right foot forward with the toes out, and turn the torso slightly to the right. At the same time, draw back the sword with the right palm downward and the wrist bent, drop the sword handle in front of the chest and turn the sword tip downward. Place the left sword-fingers on the right wrist. Look at the sword tip. (Fig. 72)

Important Points

● When stepping forward, keep the body center on the left leg.

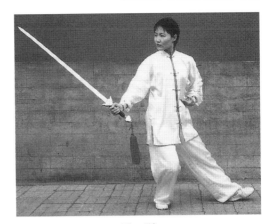

Fig. 70

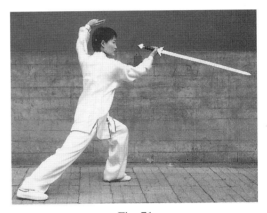

Fig. 71

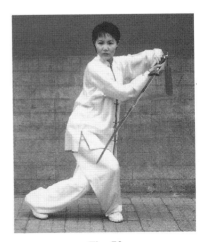

Fig. 72

• When drawing back the sword in the right hand and lowering it in front of the chest, bend the wrist and drop the elbow with the palm slanted out and the thumb side of the hand slanted downward; hold the sword loosely, with the sword tip pointing to the lower rear, and the sword blade placed on a slant at the right side of the body.

Common Mistake

The sword is held too tightly so that the sword tip cannot turn down.

22.2 Turn the Body and Stab Behind

Continue to turn the body to the right. Cross the legs, bend the knees into a half squat, with the body center more on the front leg and the left heel off the ground, forming a half-sitting posture with legs crossed (bànzuòpán 半坐盘). Hold the sword

with its edges up and down in the right hand, and stab to the back with the sword horizontal to the ground, palm facing the front (the same direction as the starting form, South). Point with the left sword-fingers straight, palm down and then straighten both arms. Look at the sword tip. (Fig. 73)

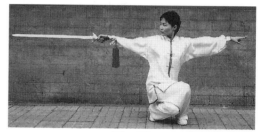
Fig. 73

Important Points

• When executing the half squat, turn the body and bend the knee, place the right foot crosswise (foot points South) with the whole bottom of the foot on the ground. Raise the left heel, and keep the left knee close to the back of the right knee. Keep the torso upright.

• When jabbing back, stab horizontal to the ground to the rear with the sword close to the body passing beside the right side of waist, with the sword and the right arm in a straight line. At the same time, point the left sword-fingers forward and stretch out the arms level to the front and back.

Common Mistakes

The step forward is too far, the knees do not touch each other, and the body center is mostly on the front leg, forming a cross-legged stance.

22.3 Bow Stance and Reverse Stab

Flick the sword tip up and back, turn the torso to the left, move the left foot one step forward into a left bow stance. At the same time, bend and draw the right arm back, hold the sword with the edges of the blade vertical and stab backhand to the front passing the side of the head, palm out at head level and the sword tip slightly lowered. Pull the left sword-fingers back onto the right wrist. Look at the sword tip. (Figs. 74, 75, 76)

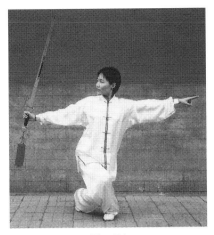

Fig. 74

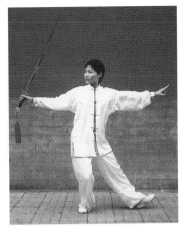

Fig. 75

Important Points

• When doing a reverse stab, bend the right arm first and then straighten it, so as to stab the sword from the rear to the front, the power reaching the tip. Keep the right hand in front of the head slightly inclined to the right and the sword tip on the middle line at face level. The arm and the sword form a broken line.

• When fixing the bow stance, face due East with the feet about 12 inches or

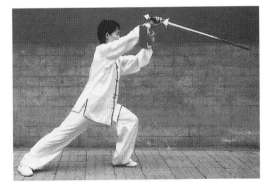

Fig. 76

30 centimeters apart. Relax the waist and hips, and keep the torso upright. Do not make a side-bow stance.

Common Mistakes

• The right arm and the sword are in a straight line, pointing forward or to the upper front.

• The torso is turned to one side and leans forward to make a forward-leaning stabbing movement.

23. Fǎnshēn Huípī 反身回劈 (Reverse Body and Chop Behind)

Also known as Liúxīng Gǎnyuè 流星赶月 (Meteor Chases the Moon)

23.1 Turn the Body and Draw Back the Sword

Bend the right knee, turn the left toes in, and turn the torso to the right. At the same time, draw back the sword to the upper front of the head, with the left sword-fingers still on the right wrist. Look at the sword tip. (Fig. 77)

Important Point

Try to turn your left toes in as much as you can to prepare for the next movement.

Common Mistake

The sword is drawn back and held high above the head.

23.2 Lift the Foot and Hold the Sword High

Continue to turn the torso to the right. Shift the body center again onto the left leg, lift the right foot and pull it to the inside of the left calf. At the same time, raise the sword with the right hand. Lower the left sword-fingers to the abdomen. Look to the left front, that is, the Northwest direction. (Fig. 78)

Important Point

Do not form a one-leg stance when lifting the right foot and withdrawing it.

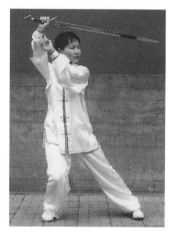

Fig. 77

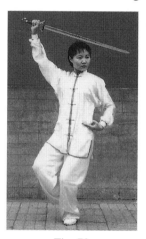

Fig. 78

23.3 Bow Stance and Chop

Move the right foot to the right front, and shift the body center forward to form a right bow stance. At the same time, hold the sword in the right hand, and chop to the right front as the body turns. The left sword-fingers circle to the upper left of the forehead, with the palm slanted up. Look at the sword tip. (Fig. 79)

Important Points

● The direction of the bow stance and the chop is about 30 degrees to the right of the center line, in the direction of North by West.

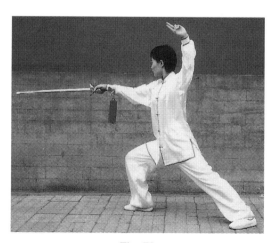

Fig. 79

● Chop the sword to a position horizontal to the ground, keeping the sword and the arm in a straight line, applying power to the middle of the sword blade.

● Coordinate the chopping and the movement into bow stance, completing them both at the same time.

Common Mistakes

● The movement of Bow Stance and Chop is made to the West. Or the bow stance faces West, the chop is in the direction of North by West, so the right arm and the right leg are not in alignment.

● The chopping and the bow stance are not coordinated: the bow stance is done first, followed by the chop.

24. Xūbù Diǎnjiàn 虚步点剑 (Empty Stance and Point the Sword)

Also known as Tianmǎ Xíngkōng 天马行空 (Celestial Horse Transverses the Void)

24.1 Lower the Fingers and Draw In the Foot

Draw the left foot in to the inside of the right foot (the toes not touching the ground). At the same time, drop the sword-fingers to the inside of the right arm. Look at the sword tip. (Fig. 80)

Important Point

Do not change the direction of the sword.

24.2 Turn the Body and Hold the Sword

Turn the torso to the left. Move the left foot in the same direction as the beginning

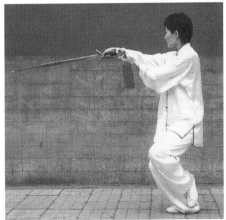

Fig. 80

form, toes out. At the same time, turn the right arm out, draw an arc and lift the sword, with the sword tip pointing behind the body. Lower the left sword-fingers to the front of the abdomen passing in front of the body, with the palm facing up. Look in the same direction as the beginning position. (Fig. 81)

Important Point

When raising the sword, keep the right hand slightly higher than the head and the sword slanted down backward, with the blade not touching the body.

Common Mistake

When turning the body and stepping forward, the body center is unstable.

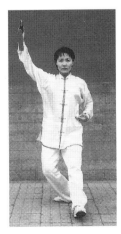

Fig. 81

24.3 Empty Stance and Point

Move the right foot forward in front of the left foot, toes touching the ground, and form a right empty stance. At the same time, hold the sword in the right hand and point to the lower front, with the arm stretched, the wrist lifted and the power focused into the sword tip. Move the left sword-fingers up in a curve from the left side of the body to join with the right hand in front of the body, with the left sword-fingers placed on the right wrist. Look at the sword tip. (Fig. 82)

Important Points

• The direction of the empty stance and the pointing is the same as that of the beginning position, South.

• When pointing, hold the sword handle loosely, and raise the wrist. In this movement, first sink and drop the right arm to point, then stretch the arm and raise the wrist to shoulder height. Be coordinated and consistent in pointing and landing the right foot. Keep the body upright.

Common Mistakes

First the sword is pointed, then the empty stance is assumed — the hands are fast while the feet are slow.

Part IV

25. Dúlì Píngtuō 独立平托 (One-Leg Stance and Lift Horizontally)

Also known as Tiǎolián Shì 挑帘势 (Lift the Curtain)

25.1 Back-Cross Step and Make a Circle with the Sword

Step back to the left with the right foot crossing behind the left foot, land the ball of the foot, and bend both legs into a half squat. At the same time, turn the right hand holding the sword out, make a circle in front of the body from the right upward and to the left, lower the handle to the left side of the waist, palm in, and place the sword to the left of the body with the tip pointing on a slant to the upper left. Place the left sword-fingers on the right wrist so that they circle along with the right hand. Look at the sword tip. (Fig. 83)

Important Points

Make the circle with the sword while executing a back-cross step to the left. Keep the torso upright, and turn it slightly to the left.

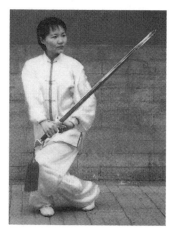

Fig. 83

Common Mistakes

When circling the sword, the right arm is not swung, but only the right wrist circles, like a "wrist flower" (wànhuā 腕花) in which the wrist circles.

25.2 Raise the Knee and the Sword

With the feet on the axis, turn the body to the right to face due West, and then raise the left knee to form a right one-leg stance, facing West. At the same time, hold the sword in the right hand, circle in front of the body, and lift and block upward, with the sword a little higher than the

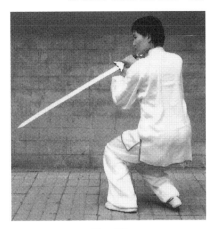

Fig. 84

head. Place the left sword-fingers on the inside of the right arm. Look straight ahead. (Figs. 84, 85)

Important Points

To lift (tuō 托) means to lift the sword and block from a lower to a higher position with the power in the bottom edge of the sword blade. In this movement, hold the sword loosely in the right hand, palm out, and hold the sword high above the side of the head. Keep the sword horizontal to the ground and the tip pointing forward.

Common Mistakes

● In back-cross step and circling the sword, the movements are not continuous and the arms and legs are not coordinated. In lifting the knee and raising the sword, one comes first, and one comes later; that is, the movements are disjointed.

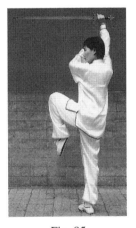

Fig. 85

● The sword tip drops so that the sword is not parallel with the ground.

● When pivoting on the ball of the foot and turning the body, the sword tip touches the ground.

26. Gōngbù Guàpī 弓步挂劈 (Bow Stance, Hook and Chop)

Also known as Zuǒ Chēlúnjiàn 左车轮剑 (Wheel the Sword to the Left)

26.1 Turn the Body and Hook the Sword

Land the left foot to the front crosswise, turn the body to the left, and cross the legs, with the right heel coming off the ground. At the same time, holding the sword in the right hand, hook it back passing the left side of the body, with the sword tip pointing behind the body. Place the left sword-fingers on the right wrist. Look at the sword tip. (Fig. 86)

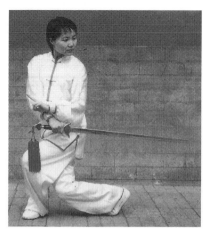

Fig. 86

Important Points

● To hook (guà 挂) is to hook and hang the sword back with the sword tip passing beside the body from the front to block an opponent's attack. In this movement, first bend the wrist to make the sword tip point down; swing the right arm downward and back as the body turns, with the web between the thumb and the index finger facing the rear; and then let the sword tip go first, hang the sword back close to the left side of the body, the route of the sword being a vertical circle.

● When hooking, turn the body fully, keep the torso upright and natural.

Common Mistakes

● The landing of the foot is too heavy and the distance is too far.

● When hooking, the sword is too far away from the body, or the sword tip touches the ground.

26.2 Bow Stance and Chop

Turn the body to the right. Move the right foot one step forward, and shift the body center forward to form a right bow stance. At the same time, hold the sword in the right hand, turn the wrist and hold it high to chop down to the front, with the sword horizontal to the ground at shoulder height. Reverse the left sword-fingers and circle from the left rear to the upper left of the head. Look straight ahead. (Figs. 87, 88)

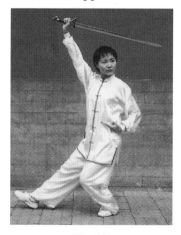

Fig. 87

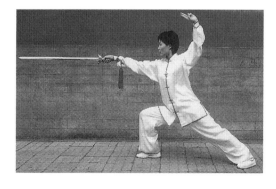

Fig. 88

Important Point

Make the direction of both the bow stance and chopping due West.

Common Mistakes

- When lifting the sword, the sword tip is raised.

- The right arm and the right leg are not in alignment.

- The turning of the body, the chopping, and circling the left sword-fingers are not completed at the same time.

27. Xūbù Lūnpī 虚步抡劈 (Empty Stance, Circle Sword and Chop)

Also known as Yòu Chēlenjiàn 右车轮剑 (Wheel the Sword to the Right)

27.1 Turn the Body and Make a Circle with the Sword

Turn the body to the right. Turn the right toes out, and bend the right leg, with the left heel off the ground, forming a back-cross stance. At the same time, holding the sword in the right hand, make a circle with the sword and swing backhand from the right downward to the back. Lower the left sword-fingers in front of the right shoulder, palm down. Look at the sword tip. (Fig. 89 front and rear views)

Important Points

- When turning the body, first shift the body center back, turn the right toes out, and then shift the body center forward into a back-cross stance.

- When making a circle with the sword to the rear, hold the handle loosely, swing the sword straight backhand behind the body, keep the sword tip pointing toward the rear, and bring the sword back in an arc close to the body; make sure not to touch the ground with the tip of the sword.

Common Mistakes

- The right arm is turned outward, and the sword tip is hooked and stabbed to the rear.

- The head and the waist are bent, and the back is hunched.

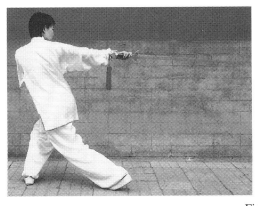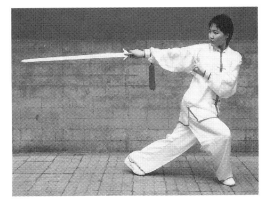

Fig. 89

27.2 Forward Step and Hold the Sword High

Turn the body to the left. Move the left foot forward with the toes out. At the same time, hold the sword in the right hand, turn the arm, circle and hold the sword high above the head. Lower the left sword-fingers in front of the abdomen, turning them in an arc and then lifting them to the side of the body. Look straight ahead. (Fig. 90)

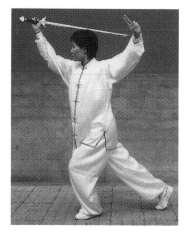

Fig. 90

Important Points

When making a circle with the sword and lifting the sword, do not straighten the right arm, and make sure that the sword handle is a little higher than the head, the sword tip a bit lowered and pointing to the rear, without touching the body.

Common Mistakes

The sword is held too tightly, the sword is lifted with the arm straight, and the sword tip is raised.

27.3 Empty Stance and Chop

Step forward with the right foot, land the toes to form a right empty stance. At the same time, hold the sword in the right hand, make a circle and chop to the lower front, with the sword tip at the knee level and the sword and the arm aligned on the same slant. Draw a circle with the left sword-fingers upward and then lower them to the inside of the right forearm. Look to the lower front. (Fig. 91)

Important Points

• When making a circle and chopping while holding the sword in the right hand, first draw a vertical circle to the right side of the body, and then chop with the momentum to the lower front, with the power in the middle of the sword edge.

• The whole movement should be integrated and consistent; do not break it into parts or pause halfway. Do not do the first movement as a slicing up and back, but rather as a part of the vertical circular motion.

Common Mistakes

• When holding the sword in the right hand and swinging backhand downward and backward, it is easy for the sword tip to touch the ground, or slant outwards.

• When swinging the sword, a lack

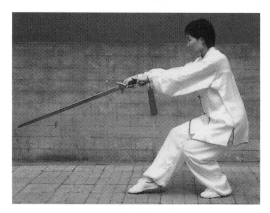

Fig. 91

of strength causes a pause halfway through the movement.

● When chopping downward, the power is not focused on the edge of the sword, and the torso leans. The sword is not in a straight line with the right arm.

28. Chèbù Fǎnjī 撤步反击 (Back Step and Strike Backhand)

Also known as Dàpéng Zhǎnchì 大鹏展翅 (Great Eagle Spreads Its Wings)

28.1 Lift the Foot and Draw Back the Sword

Turn the torso slightly to the right. Lift the right foot and pull it in to the inside of the left calf. At the same time, turn the right arm out, palm slanted up, and pull it back a little with the left sword-fingers. Look at the sword tip. (Fig. 92)

Important Point

Keep this movement closely connected with the next movement — withdraw the foot, without pause.

Common Mistake

The foot is lifted too high, forming a one-leg stance.

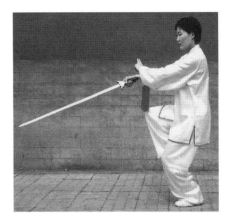

Fig. 92

28.2 Withdraw the Foot and Strike

Withdraw the right foot one full step to the right rear (Northeast), then shift the body center to the right, turn the torso to the right, push the left heel down and outward, and naturally straighten the left leg into a right side-bow stance (hip sideways stance). At the same time, hold the sword in the right hand, strike backhand to the upper right in the rear, with the power in the far end of the sword blade, the sword tip slanted up to head level. Bring the left sword-fingers to the lower left at waist level, with the palm turned downward. Look at the sword tip. (Figs. 93, 94)

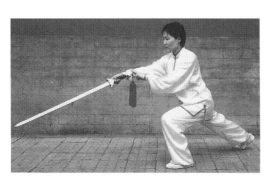

Fig. 93

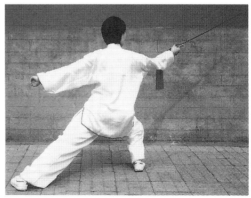

Fig. 94

Important Points

• The direction in which to withdraw the foot and strike is the Northeast. When withdrawing the right foot, land the ball of the right foot first, and while shifting the body center to the right, bend the right leg, then set the right foot firmly, push the left heel down and outward, and straighten the left leg to form a side-bow stance.

• To strike (jī 击) is a quick, light hit with the far end of the sword to the left (or right), with the power sent to the blade tip. To strike to the left is an obverse strike, while to strike to the right is a backhand strike. In the backhand strike, strike to the upper right with the drive of the turning the body to the right, bend the right arm first and then extend it, the power reaching the far end of the sword blade. Move the left sword-fingers to the lower left in symmetry with the sword.

Common Mistakes

• When withdrawing the right foot, the toes are not turned outward, the ball of the foot is landed too heavily; and the shift of the body center to the right is too sudden.

• In the side-bow stance, the toes of both feet are turned out too much, the direction of the right knee in is not the same as the right foot, which leads to a twisting of the hip.

• The power of the strike is not focused on the far end of the blade edge, the strength of the strike is not driven by the turn of the waist, and the right arm, elbow and wrist are not bent first and then extended, so that the strength cannot reach the front part of the sword edge. Striking is done as slicing (xuējiàn 削剑).

29. Jìnbù Píngcì 进步平刺 (Step In and Stab with a Flat Sword)

Also known as Huángfēng Rùdòng 黄蜂入洞 (Yellow Bee Enters the Cave)

29.1 Raise the Foot and Hold the Sword Horizontally

Turn the body first slightly to the left, then to the right. Lift the left foot and pull it to the inside of the right calf. At the same time, holding the sword in the right hand, first swing the sword to the left, then turn the palm and move to the right, and place the sword horizontally in front of the right chest, the sword tip pointing to the left. Circle the left sword-fingers up passing the face and lower them in front of the right shoulder, palm down. Look to the right front. (Fig. 95 front and rear views)

Important Points

• Drive the arm with the waist, move the sword by the arm in horizontal arcs.

• Complete at the same time lifting the foot, placing the sword horizontally and making a circle with the sword-fingers.

Common Mistakes

• The foot is pulled back too high, done as a one-leg stance.

• When swinging the sword to the left, the hand is turned so the sword tucks in.

● The movements of the hand, the sword, the feet and the waist are not coordinated or synchronized.

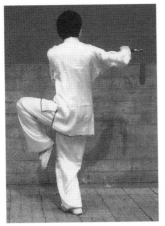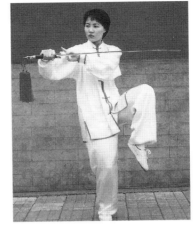

Fig. 95

29.2 Step Forward and Draw Back the Sword

Turn the body to the left. Step with the left foot to the front, the left toes out. At the same time, hold the sword in the right hand, roll and wrap it downward, and then draw it back to the waist. Meanwhile, turn the left sword-fingers and lower them in front of the abdomen. Look straight ahead. (Fig. 96)

Important Points

When rolling the sword and lowering it, turn the right arm out, turn the palm up, and point the sword tip directly in front.

Common Mistakes

The foot is landed heavily, and the direction is not correct.

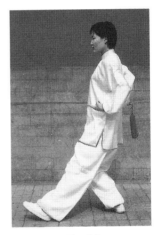

Fig. 96

29.3 Bow Stance, Stab with Flat Sword

Step forward with the right foot, and shift the body center forward into a right bow stance. At the same time, holding the sword in the right hand, stab to the front at chest level, palm up. Make a circle with the left sword-fingers to the left and up to the upper side of the head. Look at the sword tip. (Fig. 97)

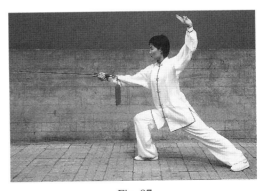

Fig. 97

Important Points

- When moving forward, do not rush the step.

- When stabbing, turn the waist in the same direction as the shoulder, keep the torso upright and the sword and the arm in the same line.

- Coordinate stabbing, bending the leg and the movement of the left sword-fingers in a synchronized way.

Common Mistakes

- The stabbing is not done at the same speed as the bow stance, and so the sword and foot do not come into position at the same time.

- The left arm is held up, but not bent into an arc; it is bent too much.

- When turning the body to the side, the hip is twisted and the head is tilted, the posture is not upright.

30. Dīngbù Huíchōu 丁步回抽 (**T-Stance and Pull Back**)

Also known as Huáizhōng Bàoyuè 怀中抱月 (Embrace the Moon)

Shift the body center back, pull back the right foot to the inside of the left foot, and touch the ground with the toes, forming a right T-stance. At the same time, holding the sword in the right hand, move the sword in an arc upward and backward, bend the elbow and pull back, the palm inward, and place the hand next to the left abdomen, with the sword slanted up and the sword tip pointing upward on a slant. Drop the left sword-fingers on the handle. Look at the sword tip. (Fig. 98)

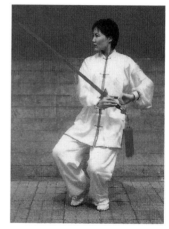

Fig. 98

Important Points

When drawing back the sword, first turn the right hand out, lift the sword handle a little bit, and then draw the sword in an arc back and down to the side of the abdomen.

Common Mistakes

- The T-stance is done as an empty stance.
- Refer to Step 7: Step Back and Pull the Sword Back.

31. Xuánzhuǎn Píngmǒ 旋转平抹 (**Turn Around and Smear Horizontally**)

Also known as Fēngsǎo Méihua 风扫梅花 (Wind Sweeps the Plum Blossoms)

31.1 Step with the Foot Pointing Outward and Hold the Sword Horizontally

Land the right foot to the front, with the toes turned out, and turn the torso slightly to the right. At the same time, turn the right palm down, and hold the sword horizontally before the chest. Place the left sword-fingers on the right wrist. Look at the sword tip. (Fig. 99)

Important Points

● Turn the torso due West.

● When holding the sword horizontally, put the right hand in front of the right chest, with the sword tip a bit higher. Bend the arms so that they form an arc.

● The movements of stepping with the foot pointing outward and holding the sword horizontally should be completed at the same time.

31.2 Step with the Foot Pointing Inward and Smear

Continue to turn the torso to the right. Step hooking in the left foot to the inside of the right foot, with the toes of the left foot and the toes of the right foot opposite to each other forming the shape of the Chinese character for eight (八). At the same time, hold the sword in the right hand, and smear horizontally from the left to the right as the body turns. Keep the left sword-fingers on the right wrist. Look at the sword. (Fig. 100)

Important Points

● Turn the body to face the same direction (South) as the beginning position.

● To smear (mǒ 抹) means to lead the sword with the hand and wipe horizontally from one side to the other, the focus of the power slipping along the edge of the blade. In this movement, place the sword horizontal to the ground in front of the chest, and smear on the horizontal to the right as the body turns to the right.

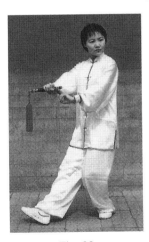
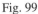
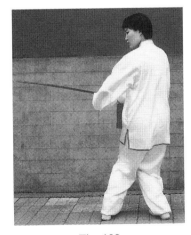

Fig. 99   Fig. 100

31.3 Empty Stance and Smear

With the left ball of the foot as the axis, turn the body to the right rear, move the right foot one step back and shift the body center back, and touch the ground with the left toes, forming a left empty stance. Hold the sword in the right hand, continue to smear horizontally when turning the body and withdrawing the foot, with the left sword-fingers still on the right wrist. When changing to empty stance, separate the hands to the left and the right and place them beside the hips, both palms down, and place the sword slanted at the right of the body with the sword tip in front of the body. Turn the body to the direction taken in the beginning movement. Look straight ahead. (Figs. 101, 102)

Important Points

● In this movement, turn the body to the right in nearly one complete circle, and be steady, continuous, and uniform in tempo when turning the body. Keep the torso upright, and do not bend the head or the waist.

● In executing the step of turning the foot out and the step of turning the foot in, land the feet near the middle line, at a distance that is less than shoulder-width apart. In particular, when stepping with the foot turned in, do not sweep the leg out or land the foot too far away from the body and do not step across the middle line too far to return to the original position.

● Pull back the foot as the body turns to the right, pivoting on the left ball of the foot, and turn the body to face South.

● In stepping with the foot turned out, land the heel first. In stepping with the foot turned in, land the ball of the foot first. And when pulling the foot back, also land the right ball of the foot first.

Common Mistakes

● The movements are not steady, the body center shifts up and down, and the body is not turned in an agile and flowing way.

● When hooking in the step, the leg is swept, the landing point is too far away from the body and the middle line, so that the closing step does not return to the original place.

● The torso is not upright, the head and the waist are bent.

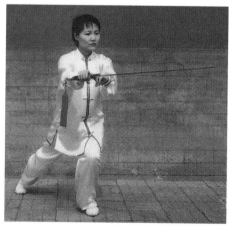

Fig. 101

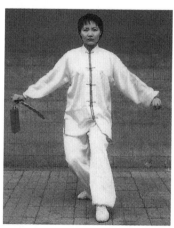

Fig. 102

32. Gōngbù Zhícì 弓步直刺 (Bow Stance and Stab Straight)

Also known as Zhǐnánzhēn 指南针 (Compass Points South)

Lift the left foot and land it in front, and shift the body center forward, forming a left bow stance. At the same time, holding the sword in the right hand, pull the sword back passing the waist, and stab forward with the edges of the blade vertical at chest level. Place the left sword-fingers on the right wrist. Look straight ahead. (Figs. 103, 104)

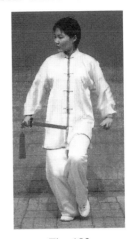

Fig. 103

Important Points

• Lift the left foot and pull it back to the inside to the right foot, and then make the left step forward.

• First draw back the left sword-fingers to the side of the waist, and then place them on the right wrist and stab with the sword.

Common Mistakes

• The bow stance is not coordinated or in sync with the stabbing.

• The sword is not stabbed forward after the hands have been drawn to the waist, but rather is sent forward when the hands are still to the sides of the body.

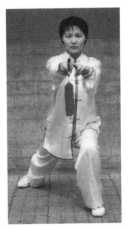

Fig. 104

Shōushì 收势 (Closing Position)

1. Sit Back and Take Hold of the Sword

Shift the body center backward, and turn the torso to the right. At the same time, hold the sword in the right hand, bend the arm and pull it back to the right side, palm facing in. Also pull back the left sword-fingers as the right arm is bent, and open the hand and place the left palm on the sword handle, ready to take hold of the sword. Look at the sword handle. (Fig. 105)

Important Points

When taking hold of the sword, turn the left palm out, thumb down facing the right hand. Both elbows are on the same level as the shoulders. Make sure to relax and lower the shoulders.

Common Mistakes

• The elbows are bent and the armpits are closed, causing tension in the arms.

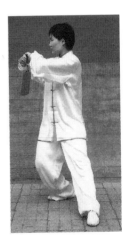

Fig. 105

● The torso is not turned to the right, and the sword held in the right hand is drawn in front of the chest instead of the right side.

2. Half-Step Forward and Close the Form

Turn the body to the left, shift the body center forward, move the right foot half a step forward to be parallel with the left foot, forming the stance with the feet apart. At the same time, take hold of the sword with the left hand, lowering it and passing the front of the body to the left side of the body. Change the right hand to sword-fingers, move them in an arc downward and backward and then lift them upward and then forward and then downward to the right side of the body. (Figs. 106, 107)

Important Points

After changing the hand to hold the sword, coordinate and synchronize lowering the sword in left hand in an arc and shifting the body center forward. And coordinate as one the lowering of the right sword-fingers in an arc and the stepping of the right foot half a step forward.

Common Mistake

The movement of the hands and feet is not coordinated or natural.

3. Bring the Feet Together and Return to the Beginning Position

Bring the left foot to the right one, and return to the Ready Position. (Fig. 108)

Important Points

● The posture is the same as that of the Ready Position.

● Pause a moment before moving on to relax.

Common Mistakes

The movements are slack, and the mind is not concentrated.

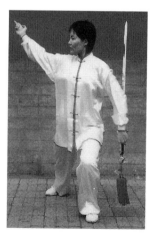
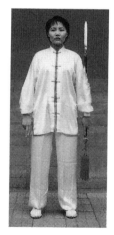
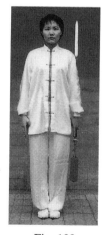

Fig. 106   Fig. 107   Fig. 108

CHAPTER X
WHY STUDY TAIJIQUAN?
A GLOBAL PERSPECTIVE

Beyond the popularity today of Taijiquan in China as described in Chapter I, all over the world people are taking up this traditional Chinese martial art. Why? After a brief introduction by the author, three of his students from Japan, Great Britain and the United States give their views on the benefits of Taijiquan.

Japan

Koike Rie, an architect born in 1950, is director of the Administrative Department of the Sino-Japanese Friendship Association of Taijiquan. She also instructs Taijiquan, having started Taiji practice in 1976. I first met Koike Rie when she came with a group from Japan to Beijing in 1980 at the invitation of my uncle, Li Tianji.

"My involvement with Taijiquan began after I graduated from college and had begun my career as an architect in 1972, around the time China and Japan had just re-established normal diplomatic relations that had been broken since World War II. In my study of the architecture of Shinto shrines and temples, I discovered in ancient Japanese architecture a strong Chinese influence in terms of style and art. This interested me very much, and I wanted to visit China to see the environment and life style of the Chinese people to trace the origins of Japanese culture.

"However, at that time China was not fully open to the outside world. With the exception of a few organizations related to China, no one could visit China without an invitation from the Chinese government. So that was my problem: How to contact the Chinese? Then I remembered that I had learned karate in college, and I knew there was a relationship between karate and the Chinese martial arts. Could I approach China through the martial arts? As I was researching this question, I got to know something about Chinese Taijiquan.

"The practice of Taijiquan in Japan really began with the Simplified 24-step form designed by the modern Chinese Taijiquan master Li Tianji who taught it to the Japanese Minister of Justice Fului Yosimi, in Beijing in 1959. Mr. Fului Yosimi subsequently established in 1967 the Japanese Taijiquan Association, thus formally beginning the popularization of Taijiquan in Japan.

"In 1976, some friends and I set up a classroom and invited an instructor from Mr. Fului Yosimi's Taijiquan Association as our teacher. From then on I began to realize my dream with Taijiquan. In 1980, the Chinese Delegation of Martial Art visited and performed in Japan, with Master Li Tianji as the secretary-general of the delegation. We were fortunate to meet with Master Li Tianji who agreed to support the cause of Taijiquan in Japan by welcoming us to study Taijiquan with him in Beijing. This led to our establishing a Taijiquan Committee with the help from the Sino-Japanese Friendship Association in Tokyo and the beginning of the widespread practice of Taijiquan in Japan.

"At the end of 1980, our group from Japan of 24 people arrived in Beijing in the cold winter and began our formal Taijiquan training there. As we were all beginners, Professor Li Tianji arranged a teacher for us in groups of three, personally demonstrating each movement and correcting our gestures one by one. The teachers were all top-level Chinese masters of Taijiquan, including Professor Li Deyin. We received training from many famous Taijiquan masters in a week and made marked progress in our skills, especially in our understanding of the basic concepts and the correct way of practice. The 24 members of the group that trained in Beijing in 1980 became backbone of the spread of Taijiquan in Japan, and our Taijiquan Committee developed rapidly.

"The following year, we succeeded in bringing Professors Li Deyin and Ye Shuxun to teach in Japan. From then on, we invited top-class Taijiquan masters from Beijing to Japan every year. Professor Li Tianji's daughter, Li Defang, began teaching Taijiquan in Japan following her father's instructions. All this enabled Taijiquan to become popular and to be practiced correctly by more and more people. Up until the present time, there are almost a million people practicing Taijiquan in Japan. Every year we have local and nationwide Taijiquan competitions and various kinds of activities for learning Taijiquan, making it one of the favorite sports in Japan. The Sino-Japanese Friendship Association of Taijiquan in Tokyo alone has 1,500 members, 75 classrooms and 20 instructors in the Tokyo area teaching students who range in age from 7 to 90 years old. The instructors of our association have all practiced Taijiquan for more than 20 years, and every one of them national Taijiquan championships in

Japan. Most now are over 50 and to assure future instructors, we started an instructors' training class two years ago with some 40 younger members of our association. They will be the backbone of the Sino-Japanese Friendship Association of Taijiquan in the coming years.

"For us who practice Taijiquan in Japan, we feel lucky that Taijiquan in Japan — in terms of either governmental exchanges or other Sino-Japanese friendship activities — developed under the support and care of Professors Li Tianji and Li Deyin and other masters with their superb skills. With their guidance and help, the correct standardized way of practice became the major Taijiquan trend in Japan. Having been spared any wrong turns in our initial practice, we were saved the trouble of later having to make corrections — something that is always even harder than learning something new.

"I have been practicing Taijiquan for over 28 years. Another reason I took it up in my youth was that I was rather weak, often laid up with a cold for days during the change of seasons. But in the last 20 years, I have become quite fit and never get sick. Further, I have made many friends through practicing Taijiquan. This has enriched my life without any feeling of pressure or fatigue. I am grateful that Taijiquan has brought me health, happiness and a full and colorful life. I am also very grateful for Professors Li Tianji and Li Deyin as well as many other warm-hearted Chinese teachers and friends who spread Taijiquan to Japan and taught and helped us personally."

Great Britain

Born in 1929, Richard V. Watson retired in 1996 from the reprographics industry and today is director of the Longfei Taijiquan Association of Great Britain. After studying judo and karate for over 20 years in his youth, he discontinued both activities to concentrate on his business career. He later discovered Taijiquan and studied it for many years in London. I first met Richard Watson in Beijing in 1989 when he came from England with a group to study at Renmin University.

"My early career as an apprentice in the reprographic industry was interrupted when I was conscripted for the army, serving from 1947 to 1949 in the Royal Army Medical Corps as a nurse and operating room assistant. The training I received in the body, its systems and functions for this work led to a life-long fascination with the body and its maintenance.

"I discovered Taijiquan in 1973 by coincidence when a friend asked me to accompany him to an introductory class in Taiji at the Renshuden Judo School in North London. The next year I began an 18-year association with Master Chu King Hung, one of three disciples of Yang Shouchung, the eldest son of Yang Chengfu. During our association I learned various Yang-style forms as well as various forms of Qigong. The international Tai Chi Chuan Association established by Master Chu enjoyed wide support and popularity throughout the 1970s and 1980s. His students came from many other martial arts disciplines and like me were intrigued by his skills.

"On my retirement in 1989, I decided to widen my Taiji horizons and joined a group of 40 people to Renmin University in Beijing. During my working years, I had managed to visit Hong Kong and Singapore several times and to study the Cheng Man Ching form in Penang, Malasia. But this journey to Beijing — the first of many — would change the direction of my Taiji studies irrevocably. At the welcoming ceremony, we were introduced to the head of the university's Physical Education Department, Professor Li Deyin, who would supervise the group's daily training program. During the trip, we also met Master Li Tianji, the creator of the 24-step Taijiquan we were to study. One afternoon we were treated to a demonstration of the newly created 42-Step competition routine by Chen Sitan (who later took the gold medal in the form at the 11th Asian Games). From that moment, I was hooked. I asked Professor Li whether I could return to learn this new routine on a one-to-one basis. He was kind enough to agree, and I returned in the autumn. Due to his busy schedule, our meetings took place before his university duties began. He cycled to the park near my hotel to coach me in the new routine from 7.30 to 9.30 a.m. I then had the day to myself to practice. This was a great situation to make good progress.

"When I returned home in 1989, my son, Simon, was keen to learn the new routine. He traveled to China with me to watch the Asian Games and with some encouragement from Professor Li, he became a dedicated competitor for the next eight years, representing Britain in four world championships.

"When I first encountered Professor Li, I was not aware of his status in the Taiji world or of these important contributions of the Li family to Taijiquan: His grandfather, Li Yulin was a contemporary of Yang Chengfu, his uncle Li Tianji is known as the father of modern wushu, and Professor Li is recognized as one of the top 100 martial arts teachers in China. This is a Dynasty that spans the 19th, 20th and 21st centuries!

"In 1991, with the help of the late Jifu Huang, I met with Master Li Tianji and Professor Li to discuss bringing the family's Longfei ("Flying Dragon," the martial arts name of Li Tianji) tradition to Britain. Over 12 years later, that connection has become well established. We have branches throughout England and in Scotland. During his annual tours, Professor Li has taught in Aberdeen, Glasgow, Manchester, Wolverhampton, Milton, Keynes and Herfordshire, the West Country and Jersey. All the students that train with Professor Li are touched by his brilliant coaching skills and his open friendship. I feel that one of the features of Longfei's influence on the international scenes is the openness and friendship. Long may it last."

The United States

Tim McGuire, 49, an electrical engineer, started studying Taijiquan some 12 years ago to help with a back ailment. He was able to continue to study under several teachers even as he moved to several different cities in the United States. I first met Tim McGuire when he came to Beijing as part of his engineering work for Motorola in 2001.

"Why do Taijiquan? In 1991, I took up Taijiquan to try to develop enough flexibility and strength in my waist and lower back that a constant sciatic nerve pain might be relieved. Two years earlier, I had limped into the finish of the New York City Marathon with a pain shooting down my leg, caused by damaged lumbar discs. I thought it most likely the end of my running career, but I hoped to continue the running addiction and so looked to other training regimens to cure my back. Physical therapy, swimming, and special stretching exercises all helped, but too little. Running was no longer a realistic possibility.

"I wish I could say that Taijiquan cured my back, but for me — as for most people — bad lumbar disks are something one just has to manage. And I found Taijiquan is wonderful for managing this kind of ailment as well as many of the other aches and pains brought about by the act of living. But more than that, the reason I have continued to practice for the last 12 years is for the many other benefits of Taijiquan I also found.

"At first, I bought a Taiji video and tried to learn the deceptively simple movements on my own. I was able to imitate a little, but I definitely felt something was missing. So I enrolled in a more formal learning environment at a local martial arts school in Andover, Massachusetts, run by a senior student of Yang Jwing-Ming, chief instructor of Yang's Martial Arts Association headquartered in Boston, who taught a traditional Yang-style Taijiquan form with 108 movements. The beginning class started with 25 students, and we were to learn the first 21 movements of the form in three months. By the end of this period, I was the only student left. There was nothing wrong with the instruction nor was there anything special about me, but Taiji needs patience and faith, faith that the slow movements are actually going to do you some good. Over the course of a year, I finally finished the 108-movement form.

"Regular and consistent training is important but occasional seminars with good teachers really get one more excited about Taiji. At the Massachusetts school, workshops were a regular occurrence, and I was able to learn the Simplified 24-Step Taijiquan along with a little Baguazhang and Xingyiquan from a visiting master, Liang Shouyu. Yang Jwing-Ming also held regular seminars on Qin Na, techniques of seizing and control.

"In 1996, I moved to Phoenix, Arizona. Eventually, I was able to find Zhu Ruhu, a White Crane master who was also a traditional Chinese medicine doctor and qigong healer. He taught me a Taiji style he called White Crane Taiji consisting of over 200 movements. I wish I could say I remember and practice it now, but I can't.

"In 1998, I had the unique opportunity to work in Beijing for Motorola in my work as an engineer. It was great watching the groups in the Purple Bamboo Park doing their Taiji and Qigong, but of course, I wanted to join in. A co-worker, back in Phoenix, e-mailed me the name of a Taiji master in Beijing I should try to meet. With the translation help of a co-worker in Beijing, I went to Renmin University and met with Professor Li Deyin. He very kindly talked with me and watched my meager efforts at doing Yang-style Taijiquan and Taiji sword for several hours. Professor Li graciously agreed to meet me on Sundays at Renmin University when he was not traveling. He taught me some of the more modern Taiji forms starting with the 32-Step Sword form and then with the help of his wife, Fang Laoshi, also an accomplished Taiji performer, the combined 42-Step Taijiquan form. The 42-step Taiji is Professor Li's creation.

"It wasn't until I accompanied Li Deyin to Chengde for a Taiji workshop that I realized how famous in China he is. Professor Li told me to meet him at 6 a.m. to do a little Taiji with few friends in a local park. As we walked through the gate of the park there were over 300 people waiting, in T-shirts specially made for the occasion to welcome Professor Li. We did Taiji all morning and had a great meal, with lots of beer, afterwards. This is what I call Taiji heaven.

"A great part of Taijiquan practice is the Taijiquan people one meets. In China, Taiji tends to be more of a social experience than in the U.S. I believe that is mostly because in the U.S. one needs to attend a school to learn it while in China you can just join a group in the local park.

"Before Professor Li went to England for the summer in 1999, he introduced me to Li Jianwei and Gao Shufen, a couple who lead a large Taiji practice group in the Temple of Heaven Park in Beijing. They treated me like family, and the entire group accepted me without question. Someone was always helping, despite my poor Chinese language skills. But Taiji practice can be a language unto itself, so communication on this level was easy. I really loved coming to the park on weekend mornings to study with the group, so it was upsetting when I had to return to the U.S. in the summer of 2000.

"The next year and a half, back in Phoenix, was a time of consolidation in my Taiji practice, practicing what I'd learned in Beijing on my own or occasionally with a friend. In the summer of 2001, Professor Li gave a workshop in San Diego on competition Chen-style Taijiquan. I attended the workshop, and it really solidified what I had learned in a group course on Chen Style in Beijing taught by Professor Li as well. I was also studying an instructional VCD on the same form. After enough years doing Taiji, I find I can now learn from a video, something I could not do back when I started in 1991.

"Taiji is something I do for myself, practicing daily at home, but it is still good to do it with a group, so when I took a new job in Portland, Oregon at the end of 2001, I immediately searched for a local school. I was lucky to find one run by Yu Shaowen, a top wushu performer, and his wife Gao Jiamin, on of China's best Taiji performers. As one learns more styles, one can see the common threads that weave through all of them, making it easier to learn the next one. I still find beauty and stillness in the Simplified 24-Step Taijiquan, always surprised by the levels of understanding I can still uncover, always surprised about how much I still have to learn.

"Why do Taijiquan? After 12 years this question no longer has much meaning. It is a part of what I am. It is a part of what makes me whole. So, I'll keep exploring this Taijiquan, still trying to peel back the layers of this deep art, hopefully making myself a little better person along the way."

APPENDICES

I. Note on Language

Chinese is a tonal language with four tones called the first tone, second tone, third tone and fourth tone. The first tone is high and steady, the second tone starts low and rises, the third tone starts high, drops, and rises; the fourth tone starts high and drops. In pinyin, the romanization system used in China to express Chinese characters, the tone can be indicated by a mark over the vowel. For example, the Chinese word "ma" can be pronounced four different ways, all with different meanings: First tone, mɑ; second tone, má; third tone, mǎ; and fourth tone, mà. Mɑ is the Chinese word for "mom," má is a kind of linen, mǎ is the Chinese word for "horse" and mà means to swear. The capital of China, Beijing, in pinyin is Bǒijīng. Taijiquan in pinyin is Tàijíquán. The other symbols in pinyin are close to English except for "c," pronounced "ts;" and "q," pronounced "tch;" and "x" pronounced "sh."

In part because Taijiquan is rooted in oral tradition in a tonal language, the names of some Taijiquan movements have come to take on different meanings simply because the tones have been pronounced in different ways. For example, a relatively quick striking movement in Taijiquan described as "shan" (See Step 20 in 24-Step Taijiquan or Step 22 in 81-Step Taijiquan) has been interpreted in Chinese as meaning either "fan" or "lightning." It depends on how one hears the tone of the word "shan." In 24-Step Taijiquan the movement is called Shǎntōngbì (third tone of shan with "bi" meaning "arms") in pinyin or 闪通臂 in Chinese or Send a Flash Through the Arms in one possible English translation. In 81-Step Taijiquan it is called Shàntōngbèi (fourth tone with "bei" meaning "back") or 扇通背 or Fan through the Back: An image meant to evoke the quick opening of the fan with the opening of the arms generated through the power of the back.

Another example of the variations in names is 揽雀尾, sometimes translated as "Grasp the Peacock's Tail" and sometimes as "Grasp the Sparrow's Tail." According

400

to Professor Li, the "bird" could be a sparrow and represent the famous story of the Taiji master who had such control that if a sparrow stood on his hand, the sparrow could not fly away because every time the sparrow started to kick off for flight, the master withdrew his "qi" or energy leaving the bird no platform from which to kick off. As for peacock, this gives the idea of gathering in the long tail of that bird and is the definition that Professor Li prefers as better related to the meaning of the movement.

Taiji students the world over use the Chinese names for Taiji movements, a practice that acknowledges the Chinese cultural roots of Taijiquan while providing a linguistic standard for modern international Taijiquan gatherings and sports competitions whatever the language of the host country. In that regard, we have provided the Chinese names in pinyin as well as the Chinese characters themselves and English translations for every movement as well as for basic terms and principles. In general, we have sought in the English translation of the names of Taijiquan movements to come as close as possible to something that represents the meaning of the movements as illustrated in the photographs and explained in the text.

II. Contact for Information on the Author's Teaching Schedule and Other Teaching Materials by Li Deyin

Deyin Taijiquan Institute (GB)
8 Flamborough Way
Coseley, West Midlands
WV14 9UD
UK
Email: deyintji@msn.com
Tel: +44 1902 883565
Fax: +44 1902 564782

III. Books in English by Li Deyin's Uncle, Li Tianji:

A Guide to Chinese Martial Arts
By Li Tianji and Du Xilian
Foreign Languages Press, 1991
24 Baiwanzhuang Road
Beijing 100037, China

Li Tianji's *The Skill of Xingyiquan*
A translation from the Chinese by Andrea Falk, 2000
tgl books
P.O. Box 6550
Victoria, B.C.
Canada V8P 5n7
tgl@thewushucentre.ca
www.thewushucntre.ca